D1526111

PARACELSUS

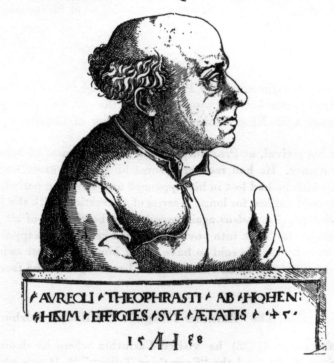

ALTERIVS NON SIT ✦ QVI SVVS ESSE POTEST

✦AVREOLI ✦THEOPHRASTI ✦AB ✦HOHEN:
✦HEIM ✦EFFIGIES ✦SVE ✦ÆTATIS ✦ 4 5
1 AH 83

PARACELSUS
MEDICINE, MAGIC AND MISSION AT THE END OF TIME

CHARLES WEBSTER

YALE UNIVERSITY PRESS
NEW HAVEN AND LONDON

For information about this and other Yale University Press publications, please contact:
U.S. Office: sales.press@yale.edu www.yalebooks.com
Europe Office: slaes@yaleup.co.uk www.yaleup.co.uk

Set in Adobe Caslon by Carnegie Book Production, Lancaster
Printed in Great Britain by T J International Ltd, Padstow, Cornwall

Library of Congress Cataloging-in-Publication Data

Webster, Charles, 1936–
     Paracelsus: medicine, magic and mission at the end of time/Charles Webster.
        p.; cm.
     Includes bibliographical references and index.
     ISBN 978–0–300–13911–2 (alk. paper)
   1. Paracelsus, 1493–1541. 2.   Physicians—Biography. 3.   Science and magic—
History—16th century. I. Title.
     [DNLM: 1.   Paracelsus, 1493–1541. 2.   History of Medicine—Biography.
3.   Physicians—Biography. 4.   History, Early Modern 1451–1600—Biography.
5.   Philosophy, Medical—Biography. WZ 100 P221Wa 2008]
     R147.P2W33 2008
     610.92—dc22
     [B]

                                                                    2008027973

A catalogue record for this book is available from the British Library.

10 9 8 7 6 5 4 3 2 1

to Helena and Charles

CONTENTS

ILLUSTRATIONS

Preface and Acknowledgements

Paracelsus has always provoked curiosity extending well beyond the academic audience. Overall he may possess the distinction of having attracted more comment than any other medical doctor in history. Amid this profusion, serious contributions are greatly outnumbered by popular biographies, which continue to dominate the market. Walter Pagel's pioneering book on Paracelsus, dating from 1958, remains the one outstanding general study available to the English-language audience. Among the limitations of Pagel's work was his lack of access to the theological, social and ethical writings of Paracelsus, which are voluminous and self-evidently a central preoccupation, perhaps even our reformer's paramount concern. The irregular advance of the critical edition of these non-scientific writings in the course of the last fifty years has at last provided access to some important sources, and therefore a basis for a much better understanding of the whole outlook of Paracelsus. Scholarship has been slow to catch up with these materials, but the best of the recent specialized literature has at least demonstrated the intrinsic interest of the theological writings.

Given the fifty years that have elapsed since the appearance of the book by Pagel, there is urgent need for a new perspective, taking into account the fuller body of primary resources, recent research and also injecting a new level of historical awareness. Without diminishing regard for his involvements in science and medicine, I also draw attention to the role of Paracelsus as a religious and social controversialist. Unquestionably Paracelsus was committed to the transformation of medicine and related sciences, but it is important to appreciate that this mission was inseparably associated with his broader philosophical and religious aspirations. Accordingly, this study avoids treating his diverse activities in isolation, but attempts to establish their interrelations and correct place within the order of priorities to which, I argue, Paracelsus himself would have subscribed.

The adoption of a broader framework inevitably requires engagement with the social and intellectual environment in Germany during the early Reformation and the German Peasants' War. It is unrealistic to consider the career and aspirations of Paracelsus without reference to the crisis that gripped the German region at this date. Depending on the point of view of the observer, it was either the good fortune or the misfortune of Paracelsus to be located in the eye of this storm. The course of his career consistently exposed him to the full effects of the turbulence of his times. There is little chance of understanding the revolutionary programme of Paracelsus without reference to the revolutionary situation in which he lived. Not only do such factors contribute to a more balanced understanding, but these seemingly remote and alien circumstances help to explain some of the difficulties experienced by later generations in engaging with our turbulent reformer.

My fresh look at Paracelsus from the contextual perspective has inevitably generated a study containing many innovative features. However, greater concentration on his religious and social commitments, attention to like-minded radicals among his contemporaries, and reference to the broader historical context by no means reduce the interest or standing of Paracelsus, who continues to justify his reputation as a creative thinker and dominant presence within the scientific movement and among the alienated intellectuals of his age. The massive body of his writings testifies to the scale and audacity of his programme. Given the profound limitations of the situation, the new science and New Jerusalem to which he aspired represented unrealizable goals, but the ambition of his mission stimulated an outburst of creative energy and constructive effort which still have the capacity to surprise and impress.

The speculations of Paracelsus will surely seem relevant, and even in some respects particularly resonate with a modern readership. Given the anxieties that have accompanied the onset of the present millennium, the current observer will be impressed by some analogies between past and present. Turning the clock back exactly five hundred years, the early sixteenth century emerges as a comparable notable crisis point. Paracelsus emerged as one of the leading analysts of the mounting catastrophe, trying to make sense of the collapse of confidence in the old church and the professions, the perceived menace to the west from the Ottoman

Empire, and a regime of ruthless exploitation that seemed to characterize the incipient capitalist system. The writings of Paracelsus impart a real sense of a civilization living on borrowed time and facing the threat of extinction. As arguably the leading scientific intellectual of the day, he applied his aptitudes to achieving a better understanding of the apparent end of time crisis. While not minimizing the seriousness of the predicament, he held out the prospects of true consolation through the exercise of sacrifice and reformist altruism. The apocalyptic constructs of Paracelsus were therefore very different from the deranged and fatalistic speculations of some other leading radical activists and commentators. Paracelsus provides a particularly sensitive and significant insight into the crisis affecting Germany and the Christian west, which constituted one of the striking features of the early modern period and which deserves to be more widely known.

In most respects the pattern of this book and its various conventions are self-explanatory. Just a few points call for special mention. In the first two chapters I discuss why 'Theophrastus von Hohenheim' adopted the name Paracelsus for literary purposes. Quite quickly the name Paracelsus passed into general usage. However, throughout his lifetime, Theophrastus von Hohenheim remained in use in many contexts. Accordingly, at various points in this study it seems appropriate to retain this baptismal name, particularly with respect to events before 1530.

Sometimes I need to refer to one of the many writings by Paracelsus that have not yet been published. For the purposes of this general study it has been sufficient to rely on summaries and excerpts in standard reference works, such as the second part of Karl Sudhoff's *Versuch einer Kritik der Echtheit der Paracelsischen Schriften*, the full details of which are provided in Part I of the bibliography.

All writers on this period face some awkward problems in their use of terminology for conceptual categories. I appreciate that many problems surround the terminology for the confessional groupings of the 1520s. Particularly relevant to this study is the extensive discussion about the use of the magisterial/radical distinction with respect to the early Reformation. Along with many other specialists in this field, I am satisfied that this division retains its value and that no better alternative has emerged. Accordingly, it is retained in this study, with due care being taken not to suggest any kind of artificial homogeneity in the radical movement. I also know that terms like science or its specialized divisions were either not in use at the time, or were applied differently from their modern sense. However, they are sometimes the best words to adopt for specific circumstances. Similarly, I have used terms like chemistry sparingly, and only when such usage seems more appropriate than the older terms such as alchemy. The latter suggests engagement with problems such as transmutation that was not interpreted in the traditional manner where Paracelsus was concerned.

Over the years I have benefited from contact with many Paracelsus scholars, the earliest being Walter Pagel, who was kind enough to encourage my first studies in this area. Despite some notable differences of outlook between us, Pagel's prolific output has been a continuing source of reference and gain. More recently this aspect of my work has been generously assisted and encouraged from time to time by many others, including Udo Benzenhöfer, Stefano Carotti, Pietro Corsi, Andrew Cunningham, Antonio Clericuzio, Dane Thor Daniel, Thomas Earle, Ute Gause, Ole Peter Grell, Carlos Gilly, Yosef Kaplan, Peter Mario Kreuter, Michela Pereira, Hartmut Rudolph, the late Robert Scribner, Joachim Telle and Siegfried Wollgast. Disappointingly, owing to the special points of concentration of this study, I have not been able to do justice to the work of many colleagues, including Erik Midelfort, William Newman, Owsei Temkin and Gerhild Scholz Williams, who have in recent years written with great insight about some important and specific interventions of Paracelsus. I must also thank many librarians in various parts of Europe, and especially the staff of the Bodleian Upper Reading Room and the Taylorian Institution, for their patience and general helpfulness during the periodically interrupted work on this project.

As already indicated, my interest in Paracelsus is of long duration. My main regret is that, until recently, the weight of other obligations has prevented more than sporadic attention to this aspect of my work. I must thank my many immediate colleagues, especially in Oxford, for having periodically provided platforms allowing me to discuss my ideas and sometimes to contribute short written presentations. My final thanks are directed to my family for their cheerful encouragement, but especially to Carol for her continuing support, patience and forbearance, without which this book would never have been completed.

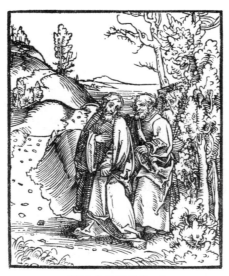

CHAPTER I

LIFE AND LABOUR

Worumb seind sie mir so gehaß? darumb muß ich ein Luther heißen und ich bin Theophrastus, nit Lutherus: Lutherus verantwort das sein; ich wird das mein auch beston.[1]

In light of the relentless experience of humiliation and disappointment that he endured during his lifetime, Paracelsus would have taken comfort from the subsequent course of events. In the short term, owing to the commitment of his earliest followers, his unpublished manuscripts were retrieved and an ambitious publishing programme was initiated. The immediate and profound impact of his writings, as well as enduring curiosity about his ideas, demonstrated beyond doubt that his hardships and self-sacrifice had not been in vain.

As later generations became acquainted with the massive corpus of his writings, he emerged as a more substantial, original, multifaceted and inspirational figure than could have been anticipated from the evidence available during his lifetime. Certainly, his audacious confrontation with the entrenched establishment of his profession, his demand for root and branch reform, the wide range and originality of his thinking and the fertility of his influence are sufficient to establish his credentials as a pioneer, indeed one of the main instigators of the great scientific movement that is a defining characteristic of the early modern age. In particular his contribution to the understanding of health and disease, as well as his broader humanitarian concern, led to his inclusion in the ranks of the 'Great Doctors' and there he has obstinately remained, notwithstanding the cavils of generations of detractors.[2]

This sense of the grandeur of his enterprise is not the invention of modern analysts. Within a few decades of his death Paracelsus was being ranked alongside Dürer and Luther in estimates of his importance. Even his earliest editors confidently branded him as 'Paracelsus the Great'. During his lifetime, our reformer was well aware that he was being called the Luther of medicine, an epithet originally intended to parody, but also indicative of intuitive fear of his capacities as a rival and innovator. He scornfully rejected the Luther analogy. Recognizing that he was being lured towards a poisoned chalice, he denied that he was any kind of heretic ringleader, appreciating that identification with heterodoxy was likely to expose him to the charge of sedition and thereby the risk of the severest penalties.[3]

Paracelsus proved well able to exercise prudence when this was required for his survival, but he made no attempt to disguise the radical nature of his mission. Self-evidently, the programme that he laid down for his *secta theophrasta* not only was designed to change the culture of medicine but also possessed implications for the entirety of spiritual and social existence. Fuller exploration of the medicine of Paracelsus within this wider context is one of the main purposes of this study.

Modern Times

The life and work of Theophrastus von Hohenheim (from late 1529 also known as Paracelsus) might well have been pervaded by good fortune.[4] After all, he was born into an age and land of opportunity. His medical contemporaries, as well as others among the learned classes, were conspicuous for their prestige, prosperity and even opulence. The lifetime of Theophrastus, between 1493 and 1541, coincided with dynamic developments in the economy and culture of the German-speaking regions of Europe. For the beneficiaries of this expansion, modern times generated a greater level of affluence than had ever before been witnessed in this part of Europe. The incessant travels of Paracelsus gave him a broad familiarity with the Upper Rhine, south-western Germany, Austria and parts of the Swiss Confederation. Thereby he achieved sound first-hand experience in the heartland of economic growth and he witnessed its full social effects. As a chemist he drew on the latest knowledge of old industries like mining and metal-working that were currently undergoing revolutionary expansion and experiencing the full benefits of technical innovation. Among the offshoots of the metallurgical trades was the new printing and publishing industry which, for any active writer and propagandist like Paracelsus, represented an indispensable point of focus. As a medical practitioner by vocation, he was assessed on his ability to exploit the growing range of drugs, now drawn from the New World and Asia as much as from Europe, and he was dependent for his livelihood on the patronage of families who drew their wealth from the new economic order.

Cities associated with the career of Paracelsus, like Augsburg, Basel, Nuremberg and Strasbourg, exploited traditional manufactures and developed regional and international industry and trade. These cities employed the skills of the learned professions, fostered the arts, crafts and new trades, and thereby emerged as cosmopolitan cultural centres and homes to a characteristic northern Renaissance. Such towns were proudly independent, competitive and affluent. Their prosperous classes supervised the embellishment of churches, instigated other ambitious building projects, commissioned important works of art, even arranged for the paving of streets. Indeed, they exhibited all the miscellaneous signs of consciousness of belonging to cities of European importance. Patricians and their newly enriched neighbours cultivated an affluent lifestyle, but also gave high priority to the display of traditional piety. In both their lay and religious capacities, their surplus wealth was directed to the patronage of the arts and architecture on an impressive scale. This philanthropic effort was reinforced by the patronage exercised by collective groups such as fraternities and guilds.

The projects of this age were ambitious and expensive, often taking decades to complete, which resulted in the strange paradox that the acceleration in the embellishment of churches and monasteries, and the multiplication of religious charities, continued without interruption right up to the moment of the Reformation, when in areas affected by regime change most of these investments were brought to a sudden end. Splendour was by no means limited to the big cities. As indicated by the magnificent altarpieces at Issenheim, Sankt Wolfgang and Kalkar, the period before the Reformation was a time for ostentatious refurbishment of all manner of parish churches and old-established rural shrines.[5] Such remarkable productions enhanced the attractions of such sites as places of pilgrimage and healing. Thereby the Church reinforced its profile in the medical market-place and reminded secular healers of the limitations of their role.[6]

The early sixteenth century was a busy time for the workshops of craftsmen throughout the Empire. In Nuremberg there was by this date a veritable army of goldsmiths, silversmiths, bronze and medal casters, armourers, glass workers, jewellers, instrument makers, painters, sculptors and printmakers.[7] Many of the craft families embraced a good number of these arts. Artisans emerged as a numerous and assertive class. Among medical practitioners Paracelsus was unusual in the extent of his involvement with these groups and in his high estimation of their intellectual gifts and technical capacities. It seemed to him that physicians had much to learn from artists and even humble artisans. Without a more equal partnership, he warned that the elite of his own profession was likely to be left behind in a sterile cul-de-sac.

In practice, such mutual respect and equal partnership was already beginning to yield a substantial dividend, as indicated for instance by the relationship of Conrad Celtis and Albrecht Dürer.[8] The latter not only epitomized the creative genius, inventiveness and diverse skills of the artist and craftsman, but also provided an avenue of contact with the academic humanist. Besides their artistic merit, Dürer's own works were demonstrations of great technical virtuosity, as was the case with other artistic undertakings, which were often the inspired result of partnerships requiring the input of various skills as well as involving complex arrangements for financial backing.[9]

From the outset, the new printed book industry enhanced the value of its products by utilizing the most advanced skills of artists. Apart from the Gutenberg Bible, the most ambitious publication before 1500 was the *Nuremberg Chronicle*, a massive compendium of world history compiled by Hartmann Schedel, a Nuremberg physician and humanist.[10] Schedel's input is not without its interest, but the overwhelming significance of this project relates to its place in the history of graphic design and the art of the woodcut. Further valuable collaboration between humanist physicians and artists emerged in the scientific field, as witnessed in the period 1530–58 by the magnificent herbals associated with Otto Brunfels and Leonhart Fuchs, or illustrated anatomies, the most important deriving from Andreas Vesalius; slightly later examples included the first three volumes of the natural histories complied by Konrad Gessner, and the encyclopaedic survey of mining and mineralogy undertaken by Georgius Agricola. In their different ways, all of the aforementioned publishing ventures illustrated the fruitfulness of the partnership between the scholar and the artisan.

The above projects indicated the vitality of the work of medical humanists and their associates, and they constituted proof of their capacity to contribute to the prestige of their local communities and trades. On account of this broad cultural contribution, as well as their professional work, these doctors were recognized as assets and they became valued as citizens of importance. The success of physicians in achieving upward mobility is indicated by the ability of total outsiders, in a short time, to establish a strong foothold, secure entry into the best circles, marry into rich and influential families and establish dynasties that often supplied doctors for many generations in unbroken succession. Augsburg provides plenty of examples to illustrate this phenomenon, one of the best known being the Occo family, where Adolph Occo I, II and III were the dominant humanistic medical presence in the city for the best part of a century.[11] In their locality, humanist physicians were likely to be an integral part of the civic bureaucracy and members of the social elite. Fiercely protective of their image, they accepted newcomers only on condition of strict respectability and an impeccable regard for propriety.

By the time of Paracelsus, both medicine and the professions in general constituted an attractive career opportunity in Germany, meriting investment in a prolonged period of study and training, usually including time spent in various universities, some of them abroad, especially in Italy. Apart from private patronage, upon which they relied, there were also plenty of other professional niches such as association with the courts of secular or ecclesiastical rulers, appointments as municipal physicians, or posts made available through the endowment of university medical faculties or attached to various municipal or charitable institutions for the sick.

Notwithstanding the auspicious circumstances, the path to security and prestige was not without pitfalls. Of the above-mentioned physician humanists, Brunfels had the hardest career. As a former priest and latecomer to medicine, he did not obtain his doctorate until 1530 at the advanced age of forty, shortly after which he was appointed as town physician to Bern, but he died within a couple of years of taking up office. Others experienced a much more secure career progression. After a shaky start at Ingolstadt University, under the patronage of the newly restored Duke Ulrich of Württemberg, Fuchs was appointed to a chair of medicine at Tübingen, where he remained for the rest of his career. Vesalius first taught at the University of Padua and then became physician to Charles V and Philip II. After various teaching posts at Lausanne University, Gessner became the town physician of Zürich. Agricola was town physician in St Joachimsthal; then he was promoted to Chemnitz, where under the patronage of Moritz of Saxony he served three times as Bürgermeister. Joachim von Watt (Vadian) at St Gallen, or Heinrich Stromer in Leipzig, provide other examples of the rise of doctors into positions of influence, office holding and, in their cases, a key role in the politics of religious reformation in their areas.

The preceding profiles give some indication of typical career prospects available to the contemporaries of Paracelsus. For many doctors the expectations were much less. Even those appointed as municipal doctors might receive a miserable salary and only be ranked for tax purposes among middling handworkers. Nevertheless, even humbly qualified medical practitioners could aspire to a viable and stable subsistence. For instance Wilhelm Bombast von Hohenheim, the father of Theophrastus, was a mere licentiate in medicine, but he settled into a minor medical appointment at Villach in Carinthia, where he remained until his death, thirty-two years later. An alternative route was taken by Lorenz Fries, erstwhile friend to Theophrastus, who made his reputation in publishing, but was also a medical practitioner in the various places where he settled; however, he was equally well-known as an exponent of the mathematical arts.[12] As indicated by the example of Erhard Etzlaub, the illustrious mathematical practitioner, career diversification often operated in the direction of medicine.[13] At this date medicine was by no means a watertight profession.

There was in fact ample work for every class of entrant into medical work. Academically qualified medical practitioners spent a great deal of their time counselling the affluent about symptoms associated with their way of life. At the same time they had ample opportunity to demonstrate their professional competence and ethical standing by meeting the manifold challenges posed by diseases associated with poverty or by public health vagaries such as industrial diseases, periodic and severe outbreaks of epidemic diseases such as plague or sweating sickness, or the menace of syphilis, the major new disease of the day, which was exercising a terrifying effect during the lifetime of Paracelsus. With tolerable luck the doctors might satisfy their clients, enhance the status of their profession and grow rich in the process.

During the Renaissance, academically qualified physicians asserted themselves as top dogs, and they were determined to stay in this position. But the downside of their existence was difficult relations with other occupations involved in health care, many of which were in direct competition with the physicians. In practice, physicians experienced the greatest difficulty in imposing their hegemony, either over their long-standing professional partners, the apothecaries and surgeons, or over a host of inferior categories such as itinerant general medical practitioners and specialists, barbers, bathhouse keepers, veterinary experts and purveyors of local medical wisdom. All of these types appreciated that medicine was the means to a good living and upward social mobility. They knew that there was plenty of work to go round and were determined that physicians should not enjoy an unchallenged monopoly of this opportunity.[14]

The Bleak Age

The previous section gives some insight into the positive aspect of the socio-economic picture in the first part of the sixteenth century. The successful physician and his family were well placed to enjoy the full benefits of the system and insulate themselves from the disabilities affecting their less fortunate neighbours. Guided by their humanistic ideology, physicians had good reason to believe that they were witnessing the realization of a utopian social order, and they were not short of practical ideas for the further enhancement of their status. Of course, in the prevalent market situation, their aspirations to harmony and order in the practice of medicine were never more than imperfectly fulfilled, even with the help of collegiate organizations set up for the purpose of consolidating their political influence. Physicians were nevertheless able to maintain a reasonable degree of solidarity and keep their humanistic ideology alive from one generation to the next. Humanists in general were successful in furthering their aims, but in the field of medicine the figure of Paracelsus emerged as a powerful obstacle to their progress.

In the short term, our reformer was just another irritant rather than the catastrophic threat he was to pose in the course of time. As Paracelsus himself often bitterly reflected, modern times were hard times for those who experienced the downside of the system. Despite all of his earnest efforts as a medical practitioner, at every stage of his mature career patronage proved elusive; expectations of security failed to materialize. Frequently victim of the machinations of envious competitors, he was subjected to humiliation and was ultimately virtually turned into a vagrant among his peers, drifting from place to place in the vain hope that better prospects, or at least an adequate subsistence, might materialize in some other, usually distant, location. As a writer he fared only marginally better. He generated a mountainous body of writings, in draft form, surveying the whole field of medicine and many aspects of the natural sciences. Similar in amount, and of equal importance to him personally, were the dozens of drafts of theological and ethical writings which confirmed his engagement with many of the most topical secular and spiritual issues of the day. Paracelsus possessed abiding confidence that he was making a decisive contribution to the reform of the medical sciences, social amelioration and spiritual regeneration. From his immense body of writings he succeeded in securing the publication of very little, apart from a series of popular astrological pamphlets. Lack of a publishing outlet naturally prevented him from reaching the wide audience for which his writings were designed, which was a source of deep frustration and added to his sense of injustice and anger. His own bleak experiences served to reinforce his conviction that, despite all of the cultural pretensions of the modern age, both church and state were fundamentally flawed, as a consequence of which they were heading for a catastrophe.

Such a pessimistic conclusion seemed to Theophrastus the only legitimate reading of the recent course of events. Professional experience brought first-hand knowledge of the accumulating litany of uncontrolled and seemingly uncontrollable diseases that were afflicting western Europe. To this crisis was added the impact of periodic famines. Often exceeding natural disasters in their effects were political and religious discord and social unrest, all of which undermined internal stability and weakened the capacity to respond to destructive external threats, not the least of which was the Ottoman Empire. In Germany, many of these problems came to a head in the 1520s, thus heightening the atmosphere of crisis and instability during the early maturity of Theophrastus. As outlined at various points in this study, the year 1525, which marks the first known point in the career of Paracelsus, was a notoriously bad year for civil unrest. Salzburg, the place of his first known domicile, discovered that its renaissance opulence melted away, and for a time the city was on the brink of anarchy. The siege mentality prevalent among old and new regimes was likely to spark off suppression of basic liberties and even campaigns of merciless persecution. At the worst, civil society almost anywhere showed itself capable of relapsing into a bloodbath.

In the aftermath of the German Peasants' War of 1525, the atmosphere was particularly hostile to nonconformists. Catholic regimes reasserted their authority with as much severity as was allowed by the political realities of the situation. Where the Reformation held sway, hostility was shown to those failing to conform to the dictates of the religious party that assumed control. The atmosphere of crisis and intolerance was not universal, but few places completely escaped the adverse consequences. Collectively, the adversity and ill omens invited representation as a pattern demanding the most pessimistic conclusion. As a consequence, premonitions about the end of time and imminence of the ordeal of divine judgement were taken as well-founded hypotheses. Pessimistic views of this kind seemed to have intellectual credibility and they were as rife within the mainstream, both Catholic and Protestant, as among the radicals. Apocalyptic deliberations by Paracelsus were accordingly not indications that he was subject to the delusions of an isolated crank. Although not identifying with any kind of mainstream, he was certainly not a lone visionary. Rather, he belonged to a substantial and responsible segment of opinion that was sceptical about the chances of reform within the old order, but had no grounds for optimism about the reformation that was taking effect under its feet.

The thinking of Paracelsus must be set against the bleak and oppressive age about which he lamented in all classes of his writings. The sense of living at the end of time was one of his responses. In some circles the doom-laden scenario generated pessimism, fatalism and an obsession with martyrdom. In the case of Paracelsus, the response was altogether more constructive. Displaying total self-confidence, demonic energy and a strong sense of purpose, he mounted his own audacious campaign of reform, determined, in the short time allocated at the dawn of the apocalyptic age, to produce a blueprint for scientific and medical reform as well as social transformation.

Against the Tide

At this stage it is helpful to provide a summary of the career of Paracelsus, with a view to arriving at a better understanding of the seemingly relentless succession of his adverse experiences as he habitually found himself swimming against the prevailing tide.[15] It is also necessary to counteract parts of the elaborate mythology that surrounds Paracelsus and constitutes the staple of popular biographies, even infiltrating more serious studies. Why Theophrastus von Hohenheim elected to call himself Paracelsus also deserves fuller consideration, which is provided in later chapters. Since his father, Wilhelm, was an illegitimate child and also because his mother seems to have belonged to a family in the service of the Benedictine order at Einsiedeln, Theophrastus was himself in a position of minor but distinct social disadvantage. Although Einsiedeln, in the Canton of Schwyz, the location of Theophrastus's birth and early childhood, was a thriving community, Wilhelm may well have found it difficult to practise medicine in competition with the miraculous works associated with the local cult of the Virgin Mary. This may account for the distaste for the pilgrimage practices at Einsiedeln that Paracelsus recorded in later life.[16]

Perhaps it made good professional sense, after the premature death of his wife, for Wilhelm to abandon Einsiedeln to take up the modest medical post in Villach. Thereafter he made no attempt to follow the example of figures like Georg Agricola and compete for more prestigious posts in more prosperous mining towns. Such humdrum existence may have been unglamorous, but it conferred some big advantages on the young Theophrastus, who gained from the professional experiences of

Wilhelm and derived invaluable insight into the mining and metallurgical industries in one of the main hubs of their operations.

Virtually no reliable evidence is preserved concerning the formal education and early career of Theophrastus. Understanding of events in his formative years is not helped by some loose comments in his own writings. In particular, the popular notion that he received direct tuition from high-ranking clerics, including the famous Johannes Trithemius, abbot of Sponheim, must be treated with scepticism.[17] On the face of it, Theophrastus pursued a normal course of professional studies, ending with a medical doctorate at an Italian university, which was a common pattern for German physicians of his generation. On taking up his citizenship in Strasbourg in 1526, it was recorded that he was an *Artzney Doctor*;[18] in the following year in Basel in a legal document he testified that this doctorate was derived from the *hohen schul zu Ferraria*,[19] while on many other occasions he was identified as 'doctor' in a variety of styles.[20] There is in fact no decisive evidence to support his presence at any university and nothing to confirm the Ferrara doctorate. It is also striking that almost every reference in his writings to universities, medical faculties and to those possessing doctorates is negative or often abusive. It is quite possible that he possessed no university degree of any kind. As with many others lacking formal qualifications, it is likely that he was honoured by the title of doctor in both internal medicine and surgery for the understandable reason that his clientele recognized his competence in both directions.

The activities of the young Theophrastus in the period before his arrival in Salzburg in 1525 are a matter of speculation. His own testimony speaks of widespread travels, perhaps extending to the fringes of Europe in all directions.[21] Such journeys in search of relevant professional experience were by no means uncommon. The sources of his subsistence during these travels are uncertain, but it is likely that he worked as a military surgeon and also at some stage in a medical capacity in the metallurgical industries.[22] His detailed knowledge and ability to draw upon unusual terms of art in these areas suggests more than a casual acquaintanceship. In the course of these activities he picked up a wide competence, including knowledge of the healing powers of mineral waters and springs.

There is some evidence that his difficulty with professional competitors began at this early stage. Writing in about 1528, he pointed out that he had been driven out of Lithuania, Prussia, Poland and the Netherlands. He ascribed his troubles to the jealousy of local physicians, whom he seems to have treated as incompetent cheats. In return they were unappreciative of his abilities. He took consolation from the effectiveness of his treatments and the support of his patients.[23]

Tiring of his wandering existence, understandably he opted to try again on home soil. Salzburg made sense, since it was a major administrative centre for the wealthy archdiocese and was close to the thriving salt and mining industries. There was potentially ample work for the incomer, although in this conservative stronghold he was likely to suffer from legal disadvantages. Nor was he helped by the poor development of autonomous civic structures, which had been inhibited by the ecclesiastic powers. On this account Salzburg had no chance of becoming a pluralistic centre for publishing or commercial development. Given such constraints, it seems that Theophrastus found a niche for himself living and working in the best-known bathhouse community in the town. Nothing is known about his medical work, but there is firm evidence that at this stage he was actively producing theological tracts, among them the inflammatory *De septem punctis idolatriae cristianae*, from which it is evident that he was known at this date as a lay preacher. In this capacity he entered into dispute with two theologians who accused him of picking up his ideas from peasants. In his indignant response, Theophrastus insisted that he knew all about the universities and listed a handful that he had visited, but he denied that they were any use to an aspiring theologian. He decided to follow the example of the apostles and rely on the teachings of Christ.[24]

At exactly this moment, when Theophrastus was establishing himself as a vitriolic critic of the Roman church, peasant unrest boiled over into a full-scale insurrection. Salzburg emerged as one of the principal targets of protest and it was among the few locations where the peasant movement was not subjected to military humiliation. No doubt on account of his vulnerable social and legal status, acting perhaps out of prudence more than any other instinct, at the start of hostilities he precipitously abandoned the career that he had just started and conspicuously distanced himself from Salzburg, its archdiocese, and the whole of Habsburg Austria. He must have realized that he had made himself vulnerable to the accusation of implication in the peasant movement. Given the prolonged regime of recrimination that followed the uprising, he can be judged to have acted wisely and no doubt knew that his precipitous departure was likely to turn into prolonged exile.

An unfortunate episode during his early exile indicated a vulnerability to exploitation that must have been a common experience among peripatetic medical practitioners. It seems that in the late summer of 1526, on account of the lack of success of Markgraf Philipp I of Baden's own physicians in treating a gastrointestinal disorder, Theophrastus was called to attend to the problem. He completed the treatment to the Markgraf's satisfaction, but was then cheated of the promised fee, trouble that he blamed on rival practitioners at the court.[25]

Perhaps influenced by this experience, Theophrastus decided to avoid dependence on the princely courts, no doubt a wise decision, although in the longer term such dependence on rich patrons was impossible to avoid. In the short term his fortunes showed signs of distinct improvement. Indeed, Strasbourg seemed like an ideal choice for a new start on an urban medical career. Strasbourg was a major imperial city in which the old church was on the wane and the conservative ecclesiastical hierarchy was being supplanted by a new and independent-minded clerical elite. In Strasbourg Theophrastus would have encountered such a tolerant and vibrant cosmopolitan culture that exile from Salzburg would have seemed like a blessing in disguise.

By the date of his arrival, probably in the autumn of 1526, Strasbourg had developed into a major publishing centre. The city was also attractive to religious nonconformists, many of them exiles from less tolerant places to the south, precisely the environment from which Theophrastus himself had emanated. In this vibrant community, incomers with talents to offer were welcome. Without impediment, Theophrastus was able to assume citizenship, join a relevant guild without delay and embark again on his medical career. By contrast to his experience in Salzburg, he seems to have avoided drawing attention to his lay theological activism, and there is no sign that he publicized any unorthodox medical ideas that had been developed by this stage. The diary of the influential Nicolaus Gerbel gives insight into the social and professional calendar of Theophrastus.[26] Neither this source nor others give an indication of anything except exemplary conduct and a conventional approach to his medical duties.

On account of such impeccable behaviour, it is likely that Gerbel recommended Theophrastus to the great humanist publisher, Johann Froben of Basel, who had been written off by his own doctors, supposedly on account of a gangrenous foot. A six-week visit from Theophrastus early in 1527 produced tangible relief, as a consequence of which the young doctor was generously rewarded and invited to become town physician of Basel, a post that provided a link with the university medical faculty. Naturally, the backing of Froben gave Theophrastus access to such great names as Erasmus, Oecolampadius and the bothers Bonifacius and Basilius Amerbach. With respect to his career, Theophrastus had in one stroke caught up any lost ground and landed a prestigious post in one of the great centres of commerce and the arts.

On this occasion the professional opportunity was less attractive than it seemed. Basel had emerged as a major publishing centre, and was almost as welcoming to outsiders as Strasbourg. But its distinctive contribution lay in the humanistic field, whereas Theophrastus had firmly moved in the opposite direction. Basel was in a state of turmoil over the direction to assume in reforming the church. The various interests were finely balanced and the radical forces less assertive than in Strasbourg. In addition, Theophrastus faced professional jealousy from local doctors and members of the medical faculty. The local medical establishment was uninviting. Despite his protests they effectively prevented him from gaining access to medical faculty premises to deliver the lectures for which he had a statutory responsibility. After Froben died in October 1527, their latent jealousy turned to open hostility.

Up to this point, notwithstanding the unfriendly climate, Theophrastus seems to have pressed on with his duties. There is ample evidence to show that he was active in both teaching and writing. In the context of this growing self-confidence, he decided to mount a trial of strength with the local medical establishment, which was a grave miscalculation on his part. He threw down the gauntlet in the form of a manifesto or *Intimatio*, declaring his intention to pursue an entirely independent approach to medicine.[27] He openly rejected reliance on the standard ancient authorities, instead calling for a fresh spirit of enquiry. From the lampoons of his critics it is evident that he had the audacity to suggest that his own speculative ideas were a superior option for the future of medicine. Furthermore, to give his heretical notions even more currency, he delivered his lectures in German.

The actions of Theophrastus inevitably inflamed the situation, with the result that he rapidly squandered his credit and became an embarrassment to his erstwhile supporters. Denunciation of the medicine of antiquity, and, by implication, the whole humanistic endeavour, was not likely to recommend him to the humanist publishers and their clientele Prominent among these was Hieronymus Froben, the son of Johann, who had no reason to extend the patronage offered by his late father. In these circles some notoriety was occasioned by the reformer's provocative act of burning a medical textbook on a bonfire marking the eve of the feast of St John the Baptist (23 June 1527).[28] News of this act of defiance travelled far afield. It was for instance one of the few things about the background of Theophrastus reported by Sebastian Franck.[29]

Two specific moves by his enemies made the situation of Theophrastus in Basel untenable. First, in the winter months of 1527–28 some scurrilous verses against him, supposedly emanating from the ghost of Galen, were nailed at the entrances to important public buildings, an important episode that is further considered in the next chapter. Secondly, at about this time, a prominent member of the cathedral chapter refused to pay the medical fee due to Theophrastus, who turned to the magistrates for support but, as on previous occasions, his complaints were rejected.

Publicly humiliated in Basel, Theophrastus promptly vacated his post and went in search of a means of retrieving his reputation. Especially important was finding avenues for disseminating his ideas about the reform of medicine to which he was now irrevocably committed. Even though he lacked stable employment, a career as writer was a viable secondary possibility, especially since medical publishing was a boom industry.

For this purpose he soon adopted the name Paracelsus. He immediately discovered that a freelance career was no easier than his disastrous assignment in Basel. His first instinct was to move back towards Strasbourg. For a short time he settled in Colmar, where he seems to have again been successful as a general medical practitioner and was regarded as a congenial social companion. For a time he accepted the hospitality of Lorenz Fries, who was already an established writer. It soon emerged that Fries and Theophrastus were at odds in their outlook. Given the established position of Fries in the Strasbourg book trade, it was natural that his ambitious younger rival should try to locate himself in an alternative publishing centre.

It was entirely sensible that Theophrastus should head for Nuremberg. Sebastian Franck, who lived in Nuremberg at this time, is a reliable and reasonably sympathetic witness to this next round of controversy. The new arrival struck Franck as being strange, indeed remarkable, indicating a striking tendency to forthright rejection of nearly all the practitioners and nearly everything written in medicine and astrology.[30]

Theophrastus decided to prove his worth with a series of writings on syphilis, an apparently sound decision on account of the high level of anxiety about this disease and the obvious room for some new thinking. One short pamphlet and one longer tract on syphilis were successfully launched; in parallel he interested the same publisher in his capacities as an astrological commentator. At this date he was actively drafting further works on both fronts. This was a good start, but his general iconoclasm and self-evident lack of respect for his medical rivals was calculated to stir up trouble.[31] His apprehensions were promptly realized. With the help of the rich and well-connected doctor, Heinrich Stromer von Auerbach of Leipzig, the Nuremberg medical establishment was able to prevent publication of a further and more ambitious work on syphilis.[32]

Although the author complained to the authorities, he was not received sympathetically. In fact this episode had wider ramifications since Stromer's network helped to inspire a more extensive embargo on the publication of medical writings by our reformer, which remained largely in force until after his death.

Even before he had come to terms with his humiliation in Basel, Theophrastus was again wounded by his treatment in Nuremberg. His frustrations were expressed in emotional terms in draft introductions to his *Paragranum*. He knew that he was accused of knowing nothing about syphilis and of being unworthy of the title of doctor. Undaunted by these taunts, he promised that he would write authoritatively, not only on syphilis, but about all the diseases known to his profession. He now attacked his rivals mercilessly, making even clearer his lack of confidence in their treatment of syphilis. He called them *holz-* or *schmier-doktoren*, the epithets usually used for mountebanks peddling guaiacum or mercury cures. Despite their pretensions, doctors emanating from the medical faculties were no more competent than the mountebanks. He warned them to be prepared for further humiliations when the wider range of his writings reached publication.[33]

At this point of reassertion, for literary purposes, Theophrastus von Hohenheim evidently decided to style himself 'Theophrastus Paracelsus', a rebranding that was tried out in late 1529 on the title-page of a short astrological pamphlet.[34] Indicative of the growing familiarity of this name, in a further short tract on the Comet of 1531, his name was for the first time given simply as 'Paracelsus'.[35]

Notwithstanding his audacity, Paracelsus faced frustration on all fronts. He was effectively blocked from further work as a town and court physician, or as a freelance writer. Consequently, he risked a future starved of patronage, patients and publishers. There was no choice but to revert to the market-place of private patronage. This search for work took him at the beginning of 1531 to St Gallen, where the rich, retiring Bürgermeister, Christian Studer, became his patient. Studer was seventy-three years old and fatally sick. The St Gallen assignment lasted for the best part of a year, in fact until the death of the patient, but Paracelsus seems to have remained in the area at least until 1533, which represented one of his longest stays in any locality. However, there is no evidence for any real upturn in his fortunes. In 1533 he complained that he was being oppressed by his critics among the old and new churches. He managed to maintain something of a subterranean dialogue with a few independent-minded local clerics. Deterioration in his health was given as the reason for setting off again on his travels.[36] As always, he remained active as a writer, but his mood hardened and he became more resentful. His grumbles also indicated that he was leading a hand-to-mouth existence, which again placed him at the mercy of exploitative patrons.

St Gallen was unusual in that its dominant citizen was a physician, Joachim Vadian, who was firmly entrenched as town physician; also he served periodically as Bürgermeister. Paracelsus had every reason to fear the disapproval of Vadian. The latter was a famous humanist scholar; he was a robust champion of religious reform, but also conservative in his values. Our reformer knew that Vadian's medical outlook was humanistic and that he was no friend of Studer. The presence of Vadian and the upstart Paracelsus in the same small town had the makings of an explosive situation.

In this case Paracelsus reverted to his Strasbourg mode of behaviour. He seems to have shown every restraint, and thereby attracted little attention. Various pieces of direct evidence about his activities show that he expressed some firm and unconventional views, but there was nothing to suggest that he made any public display of his instincts as a medical innovator or religious radical. In a significant conciliatory gesture, he dedicated his important and actively reworked *Opus Paramirum* to Vadian, who was made the subject of a graceful prefatory tribute. On his side, Vadian showed little awareness of the presence of the reformer. Vadian's only known response was a query addressed to Christoph Klauser, the town physician of Zürich, seeking an opinion about a tract on a recent comet published by Paracelsus. Vadian and his friends had observed the same comet. Klauser's reply is not recorded, but he is known to have adopted an unfriendly attitude towards Paracelsus and possibly he prevented publication of the latter's medical works in Zürich.

Given the absence of security, Paracelsus embarked on some further abortive career moves, which took him back into the Habsburg lands of Austria and the Tyrol, the province of influence of the fatal partnership of Prince Ferdinand and Archbishop Lang. Even with the passage of a decade, the spirit of unrest had not finally been extinguished; on their side, the authorities were vigilant in rooting out the agents of discontent. Predictably, the short visit of Paracelsus to Innsbruck, the Habsburg administrative centre, produced a negative reception. He then headed for Sterzing, the chief town of the south Tyrol and the seat of a bishop, but also remembered as a former peasant stronghold. To help with an ongoing plague problem, Paracelsus drafted a short tract, quite conventional and strictly utilitarian in its design, but to no avail, since here also his services were spurned. He retreated to nearby Meran, another former peasant stronghold, where at least he was well received; this allowed him the opportunity to spend the winter months of 1534–35 in companionship and safety.

Paracelsus now headed north, partly in search of further patients, partly to find a publishing outlet. Some details of his prescribing habits at this date are known from treatment given to the reform-minded Bendectine, Fürstabt Johann Jakob Russinger, at Bad Pfäfers and Adam Reißner at Mindelheim.[37] Both furnish confirmation of the relatively simple and conservative character of his prescribing. Paracelsus also dedicated to Russinger his little tract on the local mineral waters, suggesting that the two enjoyed friendly relations. A short stay in Augsburg contributes further evidence concerning his prescribing habits, but this visit was mainly important for the triumph of achieving publication of his *Grosse Wundarznei*. This was the only substantial medical work by Paracelsus published during his lifetime. The publisher, the experienced Heinrich Steiner, evidently identified the commercial opportunity presented by this book and without delay published a fine edition, which was immediately successful and continued to be in vogue for the next century.[38] The *Grosse Wundarznei* is recognized as a successful addition to the already formidable tradition of vernacular surgeries produced by German authors. The *Grosse Wundarznei* episode was a much-needed boost to the morale of Paracelsus; furthermore, it was recorded in one of the main homes of the humanistic medical establishment. Even on this occasion, success was not achieved without controversy. The author had to contend with a rival and incompetent edition produced by Hans Varnier in Ulm. The Augsburg edition opened with the author's denunciation of the Ulm edition, followed by an exchange of letters with Wolfgang Thalhauser, an Augsburg town physician and a known patron of avant-garde thinkers. His congratulatory letter was an embellishment to the edition but it infuriated Thalhauser's colleagues, who issued a censure and successfully petitioned for the offending letter to be removed from the 1537 Steiner edition.[39]

A further *coup* was achieved in Augsburg when Steiner also took on the publication of the most ambitious of the prognostications that Paracelsus had yet produced. This expensive, illustrated work counted as another rare publishing success for our author. At last, in Steiner, Paracelsus seemed to have located an ideal business partner and apparently a successful publisher. Steiner had a long track record of liberal publishing, including associations with Haug Marschalck, Utz Rychsner and Sebastian Franck; among his productions was the latter's pacifist-inclined *Kriegbüchlein* (1539), which was partly derived from the *De incertitudine et vanitate scientiarum* of Cornelius Agrippa von Nettesheim. Steiner's tendency to brush with the Augsburg authorities and his habit of overreaching himself at a time of economic recession soon led to a spectacular bankruptcy, the complete end of his business career in 1545 and death in 1548.[40] Accordingly, the seemingly auspicious partnership with Paracelsus may well in practice have contributed to deepening the difficulties of both of them.

After the Augsburg interlude, Paracelsus fell back on his peripatetic way of life, in Austria and Moravia moving from one aristocratic patient to another, pressing on with his writing as the occasion permitted. He passed through Vienna, perhaps with the hope of bringing further publications to fruition, but continuing opposition of the medical establishment frustrated his efforts. Carinthia provided the next place of shelter, where he spent a couple of years, at one time living in Villach, the home of his father, who had died as recently as 1534. In Carinthia he made substantial progress on his ambitious *Astronomia magna* and drew together a collection of writings, the so-called *Kärntner Schriften*, which were prepared and accepted for publication by the local grandees. Perhaps in connection with this project, an obscure master, known only by his monogram AH, produced an engraved profile portrait. This sombre and minimalist study is thought to be the only authentic representation of Paracelsus among the many hideous and fictitious efforts that are regularly reproduced in the literature.[41]

At last, in Carinthia, Paracelsus seems to have been well received, but this reward came too late; he remained in a state of restlessness and his health was deteriorating. It seems that he felt no relief from the oppression that had been the dominant circumstance of his life. Just occasionally, his frustrations surfaced: he then tended to complain about being in bondage or about his lack of freedom, perhaps reflecting residual resentment about the inferiority of his social status that derived from the conditions of his birth in Einsiedeln. Whatever literary and professional fame he achieved, he remained a bondsman to his native Benedictine cloister. To this were added the indignities of a life of servitude to individual patrons and victimization by jealous competitors among the medical faculties and the local medical establishments in most places where he tried to settle. It comes as no surprise that periodically, even in the harmonious circumstances of Carinthia, he complained that he had never enjoyed freedom, was destined always to carry a cross, and was continually harassed by his critics.[42]

In view of this abiding sense of frustration, the inveterate reformer was constantly tempted to hazard his chances in new pastures, and when all of these had been exhausted, he reverted to his old haunts.

Particularly tempting was the chance to return to Salzburg, where his meagre possessions were still in storage after his precipitous retreat in 1525. The death of Matthäus Lang at last made it safe to return. On 15 April 1541, at Strobl near St Gilgen on the Wolfgangsee, he dispensed his last known medical advice to a local patient. Shortly afterwards he must have made the short journey back to Salzburg. Nothing is known of his last days, except for the details contained in his final testament, which is dated 21 September 1541. He died three days later, having reached the age of forty-eight. According to his wishes he was buried in the churchyard of St Sebastian, where his remains are still preserved. In his manuscript annotation to the terse biographical notice by Konrad Gessner, Basilius Amerbach provided a date for the death of Paracelsus and noted with satisfaction that his epitaph suitably immortalized the fame of deceased.[43]

Demonization

As indicated by the preceding biographical summary, apart from the brief period in Basel, Paracelsus led a shadowy existence. Given the absence of firm evidence, his subsequent reputation was determined mainly on the basis of rumour. After his death, fierce competition ensued to determine what characterization would be handed down to posterity. While his advocates concentrated on retrieving and editing his writings, his detractors applied themselves to the demonization of his personality. The latter campaign established a deeply rooted tradition that attributes the misfortunes of Paracelsus to fundamental flaws in his character.

The basis for a negative verdict was provided by the compelling and colourful testimony of Johannes Oporinus, the famous Basel humanist and printer, who for a short period during his youth had worked as an assistant to Paracelsus. Reflecting his experiences around the date of the notorious Basel episode, Oporinus produced a character sketch of Paracelsus written for the benefit of Johann Weyer (best known for his writings on witchcraft) and other humanist doctors in Cologne, who were in controversy with a troublesome early Paracelsian.[44] The Oporinus testimony was similar in spirit to a much shorter statement by Heinrich Bullinger, the Zürich reformer, stemming from the briefest of contacts with Paracelsus in 1527, which were reported in a letter to Thomas Erastus.[45] Both sources were based on first-hand experience, but they related to a short phase in the life of Paracelsus and they were not spontaneous expressions. Rather they were intended, more than thirty years after the events they describe, as contributions to the campaign against Paracelsus and his earliest disciples waged by his humanist opponents. The background involvement of Thomas Erastus and Johannes Weyer with these testimonies is suggestive of a link with this defensive initiative. Both were prominent critics of Paracelsus and defenders of Galenic medicine. Accordingly, the letters they instigated were not spontaneous and independent opinions but responses inspired by committed activists and tailored to the known expectations of a clique of embattled humanist doctors. It is necessary to consider whether any serious points are raised by these products of the humanist propaganda campaign. Certainly, Bullinger and Oporinus are weighty authorities, and the characterization they promote has been widely used over the centuries to trivialize, marginalize and generally evade treating Paracelsus with the seriousness merited by the content of his writings.

Oporinus's perspective concentrated on erratic behaviour, the blame for which was laid at the door of drink, to which, he stated with confidence, Paracelsus was only introduced at the age of twenty-five.[46] Bullinger too accused Paracelsus of drinking too much wine, while his convivial habits were also recorded in another source dating from the same period.[47] Both Oporinus and Bullinger hinted at impropriety in other spheres of his behaviour. At the same time Oporinus frankly admitted that, to his amazement, his master possessed remarkable accomplishments as a medical practitioner, displayed sound knowledge of the pharmacopoeia across a broad front, and he had no doubt that Paracelsus's bizarre antics in the laboratory reflected genuine competence in the chemical arts. Many specific points of detail were provided to back up these positive conclusions about the technical abilities of his former master.

The drink problem was so endemic in Germany that it aroused active social concern. Drink, especially the taste for expensive foreign wine, was highlighted by Hutten and it was the subject of the first original work published by Sebastian Franck.[48] The peripatetic existence of Paracelsus necessitated reliance on inns, and these places were likely to have been a main location for his activities as a hedge preacher and for general banter about issues of the moment. Such habits reflected attitudes prevalent in all social classes, where alcoholic drinks of one kind or another featured among the staple beverages. Theophrastus himself had responded with righteous indication when his clerical critics complained about his habit of mixing preaching and drink during his time in Salzburg.[49] Applying a standard weapon from the armoury of the anticlerical campaign, Theophrastus had attacked his critics for their over-indulgence in food and drink; thereafter the same accusations were regularly applied to discredit both the clergy and the prosperous classes in general.[50] He never tired of elaborating on the contrast between the debauchery of the rich and the chaste existence of the poor. His writings left no doubt where his own sympathies lay. It is evident that he regarded his own social behaviour as moderate and unexceptionable. Even if he failed completely to meet his own ascetic aspirations, there is no evidence that his social habits impeded his professional work or literary productivity. He was consistently prolific on both fronts.

Indicative of their difficulty in finding evidence of serious fault, in desperation, the critics highlighted the failure of Paracelsus to observe the expected code of dress for physicians. This criticism was offered by both Bullinger and Oporinus. The latter observed that his master was not in the habit of changing his clothes, so that his outer garments were quickly ruined by their all-purpose use, a problem which was addressed by the regular purchase of new overcoats. In his dress and manner, Paracelsus reminded Bullinger more of a drayman than a physician. Paracelsus reflected bitterly on his humiliation at the hands of medical colleagues in Innsbruck who would not accept his presence on account of his failure to dress according to the conventions of their profession. Urban statutes tended to lay down rigid rules for the costume of all classes. Physicians were protective of their image, which they believed reflected on the dignity of their profession and on their capacity, on which they depended, to exercise dominion over inferior practitioners. By ignoring these conventions Paracelsus broke rank with his professional counterparts, allied with inferior practitioners, and indeed with the artisan class. That he remained unrepentant on the issue of dress is indicated by the revealing copper-engraved portrait produced by Master AH in 1538.[51] This modest portrayal was probably intended to grace a major medical publication, but it showed Paracelsus in the dress of an artisan. Such a mode of representation was alien to the contemporary physician, for whom ostentatious portrait frontispieces or portrait medallions represented the rule and indicated a degree of competition over the complexities and costliness of dress.[52]

The threadbare nature of the adverse sides of the characterizations by Bullinger and Oporinus shows that they limited themselves to the commonplaces of conventional social criticism. All controversial figures were likely to attract such caricature, and often this was publicized in the form of defamatory illustrations included in broadsheets and pamphlets. As in the case of Paracelsus, the character of Luther was subjected to grotesque caricature, including of course the accusation of addiction to drink.[53]

Probably since his exile from Salzburg and certainly after his catastrophic experiences in Basel, Paracelsus knew that his critics were on the look-out for opportunities to undermine his credibility. Klauser's passing remark about Theophrastus's bias towards alchemy was no doubt intended to be disparaging. Fries urged that Theophrastus's astronomy was a cover for *teuffelische Necromantia*.[54] Such slurs reinforced the image established by his detractors in Basel. As he moved into his Paracelsus mode, the young innovator must have realized that his declared bias towards natural magic opened him to the accusation of involvement in the dark and insidious sides of demonic magic. In the 1560s the humanist doctors cultivated such adverse rumours to build up the impression that Paracelsus was implicated in heresy and black magic. Gessner was particularly committed to this construction and he claimed to have obtained supportive evidence from Oporinus, although the latter noticeably failed to include any references to consorting with demons in his 1565 character sketch. Attempts by Erastus to extend this argument in order to raise doubts about the religious orthodoxy of Paracelsus might have been more damaging, but in practice Erastus made incompetent use of the documentation, as a consequence of which his accusations of heresy, although protracted, must have seemed lacking in substance and therefore unconvincing to any informed readership.[55] As the objective evidence concerning the outlook of Paracelsus unfolded in the course of the 1560s, his audience would have discovered the truth for themselves. It then became apparent that Paracelsus's worldview embraced both natural and demonic magic, but he strongly denied participation in any of the magical arts possessing sinister associations and frequently condemned the more dubious types of practitioner. Although the published writings contained many hints of his religious radicalism, he disclaimed any susceptibility to anti-Trinitarianism or pantheism, two of the most commonly asserted heresies associated with Neoplatonism.[56] Since the much fuller body of evidence on this front was buried from sight in the private manuscript collections of the guardians of his non-scientific writings, it was impossible for his enemies to make headway with their criticisms. It was only later generations of Paracelsians who were able to absorb the full flavour of his religious unorthodoxy and promote these ideas in their conventicles.[57]

The historical Paracelsus comes as a disappointment to those expecting evidence of his involvement in occultist cells or other bizarre encounters. With the notable exception of the episode in Basel, the evidence of his mature years as a whole suggests that his personal behaviour attracted little comment in most of the places where he settled. Generally, he seems to have led a private existence and for the most part avoided involvement in the controversies that surrounded him. Given that he generally gravitated to tough professional assignments, relating to patients who were terminally ill, his professional services seem to have given satisfaction. The information concerning his prescribing habits, which is detailed and not inconsiderable in amount, suggests that he was remarkably cautious, mainly conventional, and certainly not prone to wild clinical experimentation. His abilities as a doctor were reluctantly conceded by his critics. Oporinus acknowledged that Theophrastus had affected some remarkable cures, while in Alsace his late master had been fêted by the nobility and peasantry alike as a second Aesculapius.[58] Marstaller even conceded that Konrad Gessner credited Paracelsus with the cure of many intractable diseases.[59]

Paracelsus was certainly a colourful personality but, had it not been for the Basel incident, there would be little grounds for considering his manner of expression to be unacceptable according to contemporary norms. There is no doubt that his inflammatory behaviour in Basel had a permanently damaging effect which was precisely what was intended by his critics who, from the moment of their first confrontations, drew every ounce of benefit to themselves from any scrap of information adverse to the reputation of the young reformer. In Basel Paracelsus undoubtedly over-reacted, but in retrospect it is possible to have some sympathy for his situation and an understanding of the frustrations that he must have experienced in attempting to perform his duties in an overwhelmingly hostile environment.

It is striking that early critics of Paracelsus passed little comment on his tendency to argumentativeness. His habit of robust expression was taken for granted. What was evidently the norm in the sixteenth century is more troubling to some recent commentators. Dietlinde Goltz complains that interpreters of Paracelsus are apt to gloss over his 'paranoid tendencies and an argumentative character', while Weeks scalds the mainstream of modern scholarship for failing to confront this dimension of Paracelsus, suggesting that scholars are in a state of denial about the 'outrageous boasts and bouts of rage' that Weeks regards as the hallmark of the writings of our reformer.[60]

When viewed in context, the vigorous style of expression of Paracelsus is not itself indicative of any lack of equanimity. Expressions of extreme tendentiousness are for the most part confined to particular and appropriate locations in his work. The long stretches of his writing devoted to technical exposition are relieved by only occasional deviations from the main subject-matter. Since he advocated an innovative programme, it was inevitable that he should criticize all the various opposing sides as effectively as possible and present his own alternatives in the most favourable light. This exercise was accomplished using the accepted rhetorical tools of the day. As something of a pioneer in the popular and vernacular exposition of medicine, he was exploring new ground, but his readership would have regarded his presentations as entirely appropriate for their purpose.

The main cause for concern of recent analysts seems to be the intemperate tone sometimes employed by Paracelsus in his expressions of disapproval. This again is understandable given the situation in which he found himself. His approach was very similar to that of other minority figures who confronted powerful vested interests. His writing may seem unconventional or even rebarbative from the modern standpoint, but it was not out of place among advocates of the Radical Reformation. Finally, by comparison with other relevant contemporary authors, Paracelsus was not exceptional in the robustness of his expression.[61] Before jumping to conclusions, it would be helpful to look more closely at the multiplicity of heated debates that enlivened the reformation landscape. Pamphilus Gengenbach devoted one of his celebrated satires to scorning 'Doktor' Lorenz Fries, whom he called, among other things, a pox-ridden horsefly (*ölschencklige hundßmuck*).[62] Fries was also the target of merciless attack from humanist physicians headed by the celebrated Leonhard Fuchs. In return Fries, erstwhile friend and something of a literary model for Paracelsus, defended his corner in the same vitriolic spirit. A glance at the scornful attacks by Luther and Zwingli on their competitors,[63] many of whom were their former allies and friends, also suggests that Paracelsus was not out of line with expectations among his contemporaries about the zealous defence of principle, which is precisely what our reformer believed was the object of his literary efforts.

In the event, the storm of disapprobation that Theophrastus von Hohenheim brought down on himself in Basel proved to be self-perpetuating, and has indeed echoed down to the present day. At no stage, notwithstanding all the disincentives, was there any indication of collapse in his determination to pursue his programme for comprehensive and radical change. This enormous and constructive task imposed a demanding regime and required the highest motivation, far beyond the usual expectations of even the most assiduous practising doctors or humanist scholars.[64] In their demonization of Paracelsus, his critics overlooked his capacity for productive labour and consistent resolve, intellectual attributes that are only intelligible in the light of his wider religious aspirations.

Jammertal

While the disrupted pattern of existence of Paracelsus was unusual when compared with the predominantly settled careers of his professional counterparts, his unsettled way of life was extremely common among the growing tide of religious nonconformists. The Harder pen portrait drawing attention to similarities between Conrad Grebel and Ulrich von Hutten is also to some extent relevant to Theophrastus von Hohenheim. Harder points out that Grebel and Hutten came from a noble background, experienced separation from their parents, were 'sojourners in foreign lands, living dissolute lives, suffering from similar symptoms of ill-health, attracted by the new liberating humanism, achieving self-identify as poets rather than scholars, debunkers of society, disillusioned by the fence-straddling of humanist-oriented Reformers, fugitives from arrest and persecution, yet sharp and witty in their writings, and finally experiencing premature deaths as fugitives'.[65] All three in their early maturity were converted to revolutionary objectives to which they became irrevocably committed, occasioning great personal inconvenience and sacrifice. At their deaths they seemed to be completely thwarted and humiliated, but all exercised immense longer-term influence, Grebel through his sectarian associations, Hutten through his writings, and Paracelsus both through his writings and his Paracelsian 'sect', in both its medical and spiritual guises.

Ulrich von Hutten was a literary prodigy, in many respects the natural leader of a class of knights with similar aspirations. In Strasbourg, Eckhart zum Drübel and Mathias Wurm von Geudertheim produced effective and vituperative pamphlets echoing Hutten's distaste for racketeers and the commercialization of religion.[66] Coming from a similar background to Theophrastus von Hohenheim, this group shared many of the same ideas about honour and the decline of values. As a working professional, Theophrastus was more in touch with commercial realities and in sympathy with the ethos and aspirations of the rising artisan classes than were the disenchanted knights, who often generated their social criticism from the isolation of their rural retreats, a luxury not available to Theophrastus.

Also reminiscent of the situation of Paracelsus was that of a broader segment of youthful religious reformers. By coincidence, this type was particularly strongly represented in the locations associated with Paracelsus. As already mentioned, Strasbourg at the date of his stay was a main haven for nonconformists. Basel was also a temporary home to many radicals, although those identified as Anabaptist leaders were periodically expelled. Conrad Grebel both studied in Basel and worked there as a proof-reader. Grebel mounted one of his most successful missions in the St Gallen area, which was home to Joachim Vadian, his powerful brother-in-law. Grebel then retreated to Graubünden, where he was imprisoned, escaped, but then died of plague in August 1526 at the age of twenty-eight. A few years later Paracelsus also sought refuge at St Gallen. Hans Denck found safety in Basel under the protection of Oecolampadius in 1522 and he died there from plague on 15 November 1527 at the age of thirty-two. Nuremberg, Augsburg and Strasbourg bore the marks of the influence of Denck. His main collaborator was Ludwig Hätzer, who became the victim of hostile authorities at Constance, where he was peremptorily imprisoned, tried on spurious charges and executed in 1528 at the age of twenty-nine. Felix Manz left Basel shortly before the arrival of Paracelsus and found his way to Zürich where he was imprisoned, tortured and then executed in January 1527, having not yet reached the age of thirty. In 1525 Michael Gaismair abandoned his career as an episcopal bureaucrat and discovered a vocation as peasant leader and architect of constitutional reform. For a short time after Paracelsus's flight from Salzburg, Gaismair dominated events in that vicinity. With the collapse of the peasant movement he retired to the safely of the Venetian Republic, where he was assassinated in April 1532, at about the age of forty-two.

The cruel fate and early deaths of these religious dissidents constituted an important object lesson for Theophrastus. He fearlessly pursued his confrontation with the medical humanists, in the course of which he was forced to reckon with their disparagement of the magical aspects of his beliefs and practice. This side of his reform endeavour incurred unpopularity, but it offered no threat to his safety. Operating to his advantage, influential figures everywhere favoured maintaining the open market in medical ideas, not least because they themselves were often philosophically curious about magic and alert to its potential benefits to them personally.[67] Granted, magic, kabbalah, astrology, prophecy and commentary on magical figures, all of which were promoted with gusto by Paracelsus, represented a grey area and a source of his vulnerability to criticism on various fronts. He also courted the charge of philo-Judaism, and even risked accusations of having participated in rites of sorcery or witchcraft. However, by artful presentation it was possible to avoid the impression of dangerous thinking. In these spheres, Paracelsus also had the advantage of a rising tide of sentiment in favour of Neoplatonism among the intellectual elite. Accordingly, such areas of speculation were proving to be more secure as a means of packaging radical thoughts.

Indeed, innovators like Paracelsus turned the tables on their traditionalist critics by claiming to occupy the moral high ground and insisting on their greater philosophical consistency with the new evangelical movement.

The situation was entirely different when it came to religion and social activism. No doubt guided by his experiences in Salzburg, appreciating that he was susceptible to the charges of heresy and sedition, Paracelsus observed a high degree of caution and a conspicuous capacity for sanguine judgement. In the prevailing atmosphere of intolerance and suspicion, of which he was only too aware, it was evident that straying outside the boundaries of his profession was likely to invite exactly the same fate as that of the figures listed above, many of whom were labelled as Anabaptists and thereby made specific targets for persecution. On this account Paracelsus concentrated his public energies on issues relating to medicine, reserving his social, ethical and religious programme for his more private deliberations.[68]

In public, Paracelsus balanced the demands of reforming zeal and necessary circumspection with reasonable success. Behind the scenes his writing regime continued on all fronts. There is no sign that fear of retribution caused any interruption in the flow of his social, ethical and religious writings. He remained cautious about drawing attention to this side of his work. As a consequence, his religious writings were so little known that they risked being completely lost from sight. Only in recent times have they received the attention they merit. Had they been more widely disseminated, the non-scientific writings would undoubtedly have been used to damaging effect by his critics, adding further to the hostility of the environment in which he operated.

Although Paracelsus displayed a shrewd instinct for self-preservation, in basic outlook he had much in common with other committed dissidents, including many who were exposed to active persecution. Such nonconformist activists were often young men and women drawn from the same age group as Paracelsus. Once converted to their new beliefs they displayed remarkable determination in pursuing their goals of self-improvement and furthering their message. They were well organized and energetic in their capacities, both as wandering preachers and as writers. This commitment was maintained regardless of adversity. The prison cell was often the source of their most inspiring writings.

Paradoxically, one of the mainsprings of radical activism was the early campaigning material of the Lutheran movement. Luther himself called for a decisive break with the past and he employed artists to embellish his message. The *Passional* woodcut sequence produced by Cranach was an early and effective example of the use of art for this propagandistic purpose.[69] The followers of Christ were instructed to reject the degenerate culture of the Roman church, which was luridly portrayed in some dozen scenes as the work of Antichrist.[70] In the evangelical alternative, Christ was represented as being decisively on the side of the common people. As indicated by Illustration 1, on the basis of the final verses of Matthew 16, especially verse 24, the followers of Christ were instructed to forsake everything belonging to the world, to take up their cross and choose the hard path to Jerusalem.[71] At this point the texts cited by Cranach underlined Christ's assurances concerning the guaranteed compensation of 'living water' and 'everlasting life'.[72] Cranach's woodcut depicts a disciple heeding Christ's message, accompanied by a group of common people, a man, woman and child, indicating the universality of the invitation to follow the evangelical path.

Enlarging on the imagery of Cranach, in his reflections on the birth of Jesus, Luther extolled, as representing the highest class of discipleship, the pious wise men who relinquished their country, home and possessions in order to set out on the arduous journey to locate the infant Christ.[73] Consistent with this view, in his depiction of the 'New Man' of the reformed faith, Valentin Krautwald outlined four main characteristics, one of these specifying that each aspirant should become a 'wanderer in this world'.[74] Such a model had venerable precedents, for instance the medieval mystic view that the attainment of true peace of the spirit and inner life was accessible only through extreme poverty, inward and outward, which implied a wandering existence without possessions, even the forsaking of marriage or parting from wife and children: sacrifices that signified surrender to Christ and commitment to tread in his footsteps. The philosophical and religious quest thereby became tied up with a decisive break with the established norms of life and a reversion to some kind of perpetual pilgrimage. Over the centuries this idea took hold among many types of reformers and it still retained its currency in the seventeenth century.[75]

At the time of Paracelsus radicals grasped the discipleship principle with great alacrity, and it was immediately applied for purposes well beyond the limits of tolerance of the Lutherans. In his famous letter to Müntzer, on the authority of the living Word of God invoked in John 6, Conrad Grebel demanded a more decisive break with the past than was being conceded by the Lutherans.[76] Consistent with the scriptural texts used as the basis for Cranach's *Passional*, in his exposition of the Schleitheim Articles, Michael Sattler cited Matthew 16: 24 to support the Anabaptist demand for total renunciation of civic office and powers of coercion.[77] Hans Schlaffer invoked the Matthew 16: 24–26 texts to demand the complete surrender of possessions as a prelude to wandering the world, preaching the gospel and baptizing all new adherents.[78] This preaching commission rested on further texts from the gospels of Matthew and Mark, which were taken as providing a definitive authority for all believers to adopt a high-profile role and preach the gospel, without regard to limitations such as holy orders.[79] The radicals derived a further boost to their confidence from associated verses describing the wider commission which referred to preaching the gospel to every creature, the baptism of believers, speaking with tongues, the casting out of devils and the healing of the sick.[80] Regardless of questions of interpretation raised by these verses, this wider framework must have struck a special chord with the young Theophrastus, since it added to the sense of the unity of the apostolic, magical and medical dimensions of the evangelical commission.

Naturally, the gospel commission galvanized lay preachers into action and contributed to their sense of broad purpose, including the understanding that they were contributing to the completion of the divine eschatological plan.[81] Characteristically, Jakob Hutter, addressing a patron and patient of Paracelsus, admitted that those who had achieved the status of true discipleship were few in number, but that they should try to grant every person the opportunity to know the true faith, so that there would be a chance that all war and all unrighteousness would come to an end.[82] As Sebastian Lotzer proclaimed, in these last times God would see to it that the common man would shake himself free of his clerical persecutors and the Word of God would then flourish without hindrance.[83]

In one of his early contributions on Paracelsus, Kurt Goldammer drew attention to the importance of the mission ideal of Paracelsus, using the as yet unpublished biblical commentaries to support this view. His long citations from Paracelsus's commentary on the Psalms indicate the importance attached to the mission injunction of Matthew and Mark.[84] This commission was invoked in many different contexts and was frequently reiterated. These same quotations not only justified some kind of mission role but almost imposed it on members of the laity in conformity with the apostolic example. Paracelsus obviously gave careful thought to the possibility of exclusive concentration on spreading the Word. He appreciated the attractions of the 'School of Pentecost' and the gift of the fiery tongue; also, he fully recognized the absolute primacy of the Light of the Holy Spirit in his own endeavours. However, he concluded that the gospels looked favourably on all useful vocations, since these involved commitment to the Light of Nature, which was a lesser, but still vitally important gift of the Father. On this basis, he was satisfied that a career as a natural philosopher and medical practitioner deserved to be valued as a worthy undertaking. Although vocational activities absorbed much of his energies, Paracelsus never lost sight of his broader commitment to furthering the gospel. This aspect of his mission assumed all the greater importance owing to the shortcomings of the clergy, whom he challenged to get out of their comfortable livings and recognize their responsibility to spread the Word in the real world.[85] Since in his eyes neither the old nor the new church fulfilled this mission, this weighty task devolved to lay persons such as himself.

As was consistent with his plan for the future blissful existence, prominence was accorded to the preaching commission. Preaching and teaching were proclaimed the leading priorities of the new order of society that he was unveiling.[86] The preaching commission was also cited in other locations to support his wider vision. For instance, with respect to his critique of the veneration of the saints,[87] he attacked the persistent obsession with dead saints. He insisted that the only legitimate source of relief for the needy was the living community of the saints. The latter were identified by their commitment to carry out the injunction to preach the Word; such persons would be richly rewarded, and even granted the power to purify the leper and awaken the dead.[88] This idea was similarly expressed in *De genealogia Christi*, where it was promised that those who followed the injunction and in Christ's name wandered the earth would be permitted to achieve as much as Christ himself or even more. If Christ served as their model, they too would be known by their fruits and works, which represented fulfilment of the Father's promised gift of works and miracles.[89] The potential rewards flowing from compliance with the evangelical commission and the workings of the spirit were therefore very considerable and not limited to the religious sphere.

The gospel commission possessed various points of relevance to the programme of Paracelsus. As far as he was concerned, the circumstances of the times imposed on him a solemn obligation to pursue his calling and spread the message of reform, regardless of adverse circumstances. Such a mission would inevitably involve self-sacrifice, but there was no choice but to press ahead rather than retreat to the option of the soft life to which the learned professions seemed to be irrevocably addicted. In view of his commitment to the apostolic ideal, it was inevitable that he should accept a transformation in the pattern of his life. His thinking closely followed the Anabaptist model with respect to personal and communal life. Paracelsus came to regard civic office, academic or court positions,[90] or even a settled career and marriage responsibilities, as encumbrances standing in the way of fulfilment of his mission.[91]

The unremitting criticism of the professions and universities that forms such a striking feature of the writings of Paracelsus was entirely consistent with his sense of mission. His mission values also suggest that he came to look on his brief tenure of an official appointment in Basel as a bad mistake that was instantly regretted. He much preferred the wandering existence which he extolled as a positive asset to both his spiritual and professional calling. His position as an outcast was therefore not entirely a matter of regret. As with fellow radical missionaries, it should perhaps be concluded that Paracelsus ended up with precisely the way of life he believed to be conducive to furthering his basic aspirations. Sacrifices were inevitable but he was confident that the relentless pursuit of his mission objectives would not only generate spiritual satisfaction but also yield benefits such as the enhancement of intellectual faculties and an extended capacity to exert power over nature. The apostolic path promised a new approach to natural magic and medicine, free from all the accretions of deficiency that undermined the credibility of existing systems. The arts and sciences were therefore likely to benefit as much as religion from the new freedoms issuing from the apostolic spirit.

The hardships to which Paracelsus became exposed, while not welcome and sometimes much regretted, were taken as necessary consequences of the way of life he had adopted, and were tolerated because of the tangible intellectual and utilitarian benefits that were in store. Notwithstanding all of his discomforts, his avoidance of sectarian associations and concentration on literary activity protected him from the cruel fate suffered by the Anabaptists. He nevertheless shared the sense of anguish of these radicals about the spiralling crisis in spiritual and secular affairs. Like the radicals or their medieval sources of inspiration such as Johannes Tauler, he often used terms such as *elend*, or *jammer* (indicating profound affliction and distress) in describing the current state of crisis. This language linked directly with *jammertal* (valley of tears, Ps. 84: 6–7) where the Psalmist gave the assurance that experience of extreme hardship carried assurance of reaching the pure springs and a life resplendent with blessings.

Jammertal was an image greatly favoured by leading opinion formers such as Sebastian Brant, Geiler von Kaysersberg and Martin Luther, but it was used with special feeling by the radicals. Schwenckfeld opened *Vom christlichen streit* with a long list of vilifications and persecutions that would be faced by believers as they passed through their valley of tears.[92] The community of saints would be exposed to the experience of anxiety, destitution and suffering. Patient acceptance of suffering in a spirit of humility was viewed by radicals as the expectation, test and common experience of the body of saints constituting the inner core of the regenerate church.

Although acutely aware of his exposed and vulnerable position, even in his earliest writings Paracelsus displayed unmitigated confidence that his persecutors would be confounded. *Septem punctis idolatriae cristianae* opened with an aggressive attack on his critics among the learned clergy, who were characterized as a den of thieves or pernicious weeds in the cornfield. The sterility of their religion was contrasted with the faith of the elect that was true to the spirit of the martyrs.[93] In his foreword to the four evangelists, he described his current experience in terms of *armut, hunger, elend* and *jammer*, which he stated had been the universal experience of those committed to the service of God.[94] In *De martyrio Christi*, in attacking both the Roman church and its reformist adversaries, he presented a lurid portrait of the mast swine who had infiltrated all parts of the church and insisted on reversion to the example of suffering laid down by Christ, in which case they should live in simplicity, fear and tribulation.[95] In *De genealogia Christi* he adverted to their current existence as a *jammertal*, but assured his reader that this was a transitory experience. The old, imperfect and mortal world, which to God was nothing more than foolishness or a child's game, was destined to melt away. By contrast, the regenerate were on the verge of the reward of a new birth, a new creation, a New Jerusalem, in which all things would be made perfect, and true wisdom would replace foolishness. In that new world everything would revert to its proper order. Enlightenment and peace would replace their present blindness and misery.[96]

With respect to his own vocational perspective, *jammertal* was depicted as a short time of trial. Those willing to make a complete break with the prevailing hegemony would be granted real understanding of the whole of creation; they would gain insight into the marvels (*magnalia*) of nature and hence become expert in all arts and crafts. This select group would exercise in their generation an effect equivalent to that of comets.[97] Since comets made their appearance at exactly the right and appointed moment, Paracelsus cautioned the elect to be patient. They would be unwise to act prematurely. Those who made haste risked falling into the hands of wild and dangerous spirits; they would sacrifice wisdom to supposition. With some prescience, he warned that aspiring authors should not worry about a delay of sixty or even seventy years in the production of their books.

As was consistent with his view that every being in nature was allocated its goal and time of fulfilment,[98] it was necessary to wait until their fruit was perfectly ripe. Recognition that fulfilment of his own literary ambitions required a lengthy period of gestation perhaps helps to explain why he avoided courses of action that would expose him to retribution from the civil and religious establishments. On this account he was fiercely critical of impatient religious zealots who courted martyrdom and thereby failed to honour their obligation to live out their particular calling. It was essential that everyone should await patiently until it was God's will that their suffering and labours were concluded.[99] In his case, he was sure that his patience was about to be rewarded and the time for recognition had arrived. The efforts of his learned rivals would be discredited, whereas his own work, informed by the highest of lights, would be revealed as appropriate to the spirit of the age. Accordingly, the long winter of his sufferings was over and he was sure that his generation was about to witness an enduring summer of fruitfulness.[100] Buoyed up by such optimistic projections, the seemingly thankless labours of Paracelsus were in practice conducted in the spirit of confidence that he was contributing to the shaping of an entirely new epoch, which he believed would witness the rebirth of knowledge, prepare the ground for widespread social amelioration and ultimately sweep away the burden of misery that was an all too prevalent feature of contemporary existence.

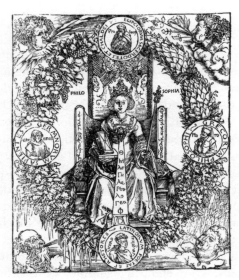

CHAPTER II

THE POWER OF PRINT

Anno 1517. Von diesem jahr hat Lichtenberger geschrieben, daß sich drey erneuerungen zu tragen werden, 1. mit D.Luther in dem Gottesdienst, 2. mit Theophrasto in der Artzney, 3. mit Albrecht Dürer in allerley künsten.[1]

Among the notable characteristics of Paracelsianism from its earliest stages was its effectiveness in presentation and promotion, essential to which was its success in exploiting the print medium. Since the humanistic establishment was bent on disrupting publishing efforts on behalf of Paracelsus, this breakthrough was no mean achievement. Sporadic obstruction continued for a short period after his death, but after 1560 the immediate followers of Paracelsus, led by Adam Bodenstein, the son of the reformer, Andreas Bodenstein von Karlstadt, proved adept at securing access to the printing presses in some of the key publishing centres. Quickly they gained and then retained the initiative. Thereafter the Paracelsian movement and its publishing arm experienced uninterrupted growth.

Paracelsianism was a significant publishing phenomenon. Building on the style of presentation developed by Paracelsus himself, the Paracelsians proved adept at packaging their ideas in a form that was attractive, marketable and serviceable. Their formula held good for a whole century. Paracelsian books occupied an important niche in the medical book market throughout Europe. Editions of the writings of Paracelsus remained the bedrock of this trade. They were supplemented by expositions and original works in the spirit of Paracelsus, including many spurious works published under his name. Most countries developed their own special variety of Paracelsianism, featuring many publications in the vernacular. The multiplicity of books covering the whole theory and practice of medicine, as well as allied subjects, enabled the Paracelsians to play a significant role in the European scientific movement.

Nearly a century ago, Karl Sudhoff, in his Paracelsus bibliography, provided a preliminary indication of the scale of Paracelsianism. His list comprised no fewer than 345 editions published during Periods III and IV, covering the dates 1560 to 1658.[2] Later studies of individual geographical sectors of Paracelsianism have added to this already formidable total.

The scale of the Paracelsian publishing operation underlines the limited nature of Paracelsus's own publishing achievements. The combination of logistical factors and an alien environment did of course preclude publication of more than a handful of his growing stockpile of writings. By the date of his death he had managed in the field of medicine to publish just one practical handbook of surgery, two short tracts on syphilis and one on balneology. In addition, he issued a series of astrological and prophetic tracts, most of them just a few pages in length. Sudhoff recorded only twenty-three editions for the period ending with the death of Paracelsus, of which only eight, representing just four separate titles, were outside the area of astrology and prophecy.[3] Least represented were the theological works, none of which was published during the lifetime of Paracelsus. Only a handful appeared in the period up to 1658, even though a recent inventory estimates that there were more than a hundred theological manuscripts in circulation. Among these, some of the fourteen biblical commentaries were impressive in their scale. Even specific topics such as the Eucharist attracted twenty-one writings, of which only six have ever seen the light of day.[4]

In compiling his biographical note on Paracelsus in 1545, Konrad Gessner experienced difficulty in locating the relevant evidence. Apart from the ephemeral broadsheet manifesto that Theophrastus rushed out in Basel[5] and a tract on the comet of 1531,[6] Gessner could only find evidence of one other publication, *Die Grosse Wundarznei* which, by 1545, had been frequently reprinted. This report by the assiduous Gessner suggests that most of the writings of Paracelsus had sunk without trace and that by 1545 he was known only by his surgery handbook. Just one other writing was seen by Gessner, the manuscript of *De gradibus, compositionibus et dosibus receptorum*,[7] which was in the hands of Christoph Klauser, the town physician of Zürich, to whom Theophrastus had made an abortive appeal for assistance with publication.[8] Gessner also knew that some kind of theological work was written in St Gallen, but he was unable to find out anything about its contents. The Klauser episode suggests that Theophrastus turned to Zürich in desperation owing to the recalcitrance of publishers in Basel. Gessner was supportive of Klauser's dismissive attitude to the threatening upstart. He must have taken satisfaction from his meagre trawl of Paracelsus publications, since this demonstrated the almost complete success of the campaign of suppression that elders among the humanist physicians had engineered. The evident popularity of the *Grosse Wundarznei* was a worrying sign, and showed that there were no grounds for complacency on the part of the establishment.[9] Gessner and his associates must have appreciated that it was quite likely that somewhere there existed an accumulation of unpublished works containing items that might become even more popular than the *Grosse Wundarznei*. Indeed, careful reading of the latter would have indicated references by the author to many promising titles.

The extent of the threat posed by Paracelsus is highlighted by the estimates of his pioneer editors, who suggested that he had produced upwards of three hundred non-theological works, of which about fifty related to medicine. A few editors mentioned theological manuscripts, but in the main these were ignored in their various enumerations and categorizations.[10] Such reticence undoubtedly reflected a continuation of the mood of caution exhibited by Paracelsus himself.

Despite his best efforts, inability to secure the publication of most of his writings was a major frustration, but he was not deterred by such disappointments. Fortified by his apostolic commitments, his literary energies remained undiminished. Paracelsus consequently retained confidence that his message and its packaging were exactly right for the special circumstances of the age in which it was his destiny to live. The campaign of suppression he no doubt viewed as a predictable and integral element of his *jammertal* experience and no more than a temporary setback. Even in his darkest hours, he was sure that the 'secta theophrasta' was destined to assume ascendancy. In the event, this audacious self-confidence proved to be well founded. His publications were only held back for a matter of some twenty years. Little disadvantage was incurred; if anything, the lurid rumours and greater notoriety surrounding the posthumous reputation of Paracelsus were a positive advantage to the promotional campaign waged by his followers.

Presentation and Promotion

Preoccupation with branding the person or product is by no means a recent innovation. In the age of humanism, for anyone launching a public career, especially if their name was to feature on title-pages, it was essential to give careful consideration to all aspects of self-presentation. A felicitous choice for name presentation was calculated to earn respect, enhance status and thereby assist the perennial preoccupation with finding avenues for upward mobility. This humanistic convention was not without pitfalls. Owing to the competitive and combative mood of the times, use of vernacular names or ill-chosen classical renditions might well lead to ridicule and humiliation. To avoid embarrassment, some kind of humanistic re-baptism tended to be conducted, often under the guidance of an experienced patron and at a stage in higher education when it seemed likely that the student would play an active role in the humanist community. Outsiders without these advantages of patronage imitated the conventions adopted by their better-placed competitors.[11]

In many cases, the humanistic name presented no problem; the first and family name in their vernacular form were often readily adaptable into a Latin equivalent. The Latin was, among other things, adopted to escape awkward letters like 'W'. Hence Joachim von Watt, the physician and reformer of St Gallen, in the humanist context was known as Vadianus. Sometimes the transition was straightforward, as with the distinguished Tübingen medical professor Leonhart Fuchs, who for literary purposes was Leonhardus Fuchsius, while his enemy and lower-level competitor, Walther Hermann Ryff, preferred Gualtherus Hermenius Rivius for his title-pages, even in his vernacular writings.[12]

With slightly greater complication, the family name of one of Paracelsus's main editors, Michael Schütz, mutated into Toxites.[13] Georg Tannstetter, the influential mathematician and physician from Vienna, was known as both Collimitius and Lycoripensis for literary purposes. Indeed, a leading humanist circle in Vienna was designated the 'Collimitiana'.[14] Reflecting the tendency of the Schmidts to elevate themselves into Faber (Latin 'blacksmith'), the physician Andreas Goldschmied, the son-in-law and political agent of Andreas Osiander (Andreas Hosemann), was known as Andreas Aurifaber. Often more ingenious devices were used. Thus Heinrich (or Ritze) Urban, a thirteenth child of peasant origin, studied at Erfurt University and entered the humanist circle of Konrad Mutian at Erfurt, who devised the name Euricius Cordus[15] at the launch of Urban's career as a medical humanist. The same name was then taken up by the next generation of Euricius's family, which included Valerius Cordus, another celebrated medical humanist and botanist.

For many Germans, the complexities and instability of their vernacular family names presented a problem. For instance Johannes Oecolampadius, the leading Basel reformer, derived this name from the Greek for 'house' and 'lamp' and thereby escaped the use of his German family name, Hussgen, Heussgen or Hausschein. Various ways to enhance common names were adopted. The prolific editor and translator Janus Cornarius inherited the family name Hainpol, Hagenbut and their variants, which were themselves related to *hag* or *hain*, variously denoting 'enclosure', 'hedge', 'bush', 'grove', or 'wood', and lending themselves to diminutive variants. Sensitive to this humble source, during his studies at Wittenberg Cornarius was advised to adopt his new name, using the association with the Latin *cornus*, or 'Cornelian cherry', no doubt partly to avoid the danger lurking in diminutives or 'dogrose', which was one of the variants of the original name. Another way to confer the name *hagen* with greater distinction was chosen by the respected Carthusian writer on divination, Johannes von Hagen, who built on the Latin *indago* meaning among other things 'enclosure', to become Johannes ab Indagine.

Inclusion in the name of some honourable place of origin was a commonly adopted device for the enhancement of status. Hence Henrich Loriti (Loretti, etc.), from Mollis in the vicinity of Glarus, at the end of his studies in Cologne adopted the name Glarean(us); and it was by this name that the versatile Swiss humanist and musicologist subsequently became known. Following the same convention, the reformer Andreas Bodenstein, born at Karlstadt in Franconia, became universally known by his place of origin. In Latin contexts, Karlstadt often called himself Carolostadius. Dirk van Ulsen spent much of his medical career in Nuremberg, but originated in Friesland. In his broadsheet on syphilis containing a famous woodcut by Dürer, Ulsen gave his name as Theodericus Ulsenius Frisius. At first sight it seems perverse to draw attention to this obscure place of origin, but it should be remembered that this usefully advertised his links with Rudolph Agricola, the leading Friesian of the day, and indeed other notable Friesians such Adolf Occo I of Augsburg, who was not only an influential humanistic physician but also an intimate associate of the Fuggers.

The new age of print was also a time for rough exchanges between rivals, sometimes involving lofty ideas but often exposing crude commercial rivalries or personal animosity. Beneath their thin patina of humanistic civility, scholars were adept at employing their sophisticated competence to humiliate their competitors. None was more agile than Ulrich von Hutten. Amid a torrent of invective, Ulrich von Hutten made a point of calling two influential Catholic dignitaries by the name 'Hans Schmidt' and then 'Hans' rather than by their preferred names Johann Fabri and Johann Augustanus Faber.[16] Hans was of course pejorative in itself, indicative of small fry or low grade, while in 'Grossen Hansen' it carried the connotation of 'big wheel', of course with negative connotations. Attempting a counter-offensive, one of Hutten's targets, Johann Faber, Vicar-General of Constance, attempted to turn his name to aggressive effect in his *Malleus haereticorum* (1524), written against the Lutherans.

The heated dispute that erupted between Cornarius and Fuchs in the mid-1540s involved probing all their weaknesses, including anything that might be dredged up relating to their names. This bitter exchange was conducted without reference to the suitability of the forum. For instance in 1538, in his edition of Hippocrates, Cornarius made a side-swipe at Fuchs, using the name *vulpecula*, the feminine and diminutive exacerbating the irritation of the slander. Cornarius liked to portray himself as a 'lion-hearted' defender of humanistic standards. Fuchs responded without naming his critic, but making the target identifiable as Cornarius. On the basis of wordplay on Cornarius's name in its Latin and German forms, Fuchs called Cornarius a rabid dog, distraught ox and dangerous fool.[17] Not embarrassed by these scurrilous exchanges, the two humanists indulged themselves in further mutual recrimination in pamphlets specifically devoted to the purpose, each with a title intended to ridicule the name of the adversary.[18]

'Paracelsus': Birth of a Brand

It is evident that the presentation of names was a veritable minefield, and the dangers were especially great for anyone with an instinct for controversy. This problem confronted Paracelsus at a decisive point in his career. Ostensibly, Paracelsus was in a strong position, in possession of a good name and honourable background. He belonged to the ancient and respected Swabian family of Bombast von Hohenheim and throughout his early life was known as Theophrastus von Hohenheim. Antiquarians are fond of reciting the fuller form: Philippus Aureolus Theophrastus Bombast von Hohenheim, although this was rarely used in practice.[19] Theophrastus von Hohenheim seemed sufficient to convey an appropriate sense of dignity and it required no interference for purposes of presentation. Fortunately for him, Theophrastus of Eressos was one of the few ancients whom he held in positive regard; indeed, from time to time he expressed satisfaction with this aspect of his inheritance.[20] Like Ulrich von Hutten, Theophrastus von Hohenheim seems to have regarded his name as a settled matter. It was consequently under this name that he drafted his early writings, both medical and theological.

No questions arose about his name during his early travels, or even during his stay in Salzburg or Strasbourg. The problems began in Basel.

His induction in the spring of 1527 went off quietly enough. In the official documents of the time he was duly known as *Herr Theofrastes von Hohenheim, der Arznei doctor, Stadtarzt zu Basel*, who was recorded as possessing a *doctorat der loblichen Hohen Schul zu Ferraria*.[21] Various official documents from this date record the frustrating attempt of Dr Theophrastus von Hohenheim to secure his position in Basel. The first serious blow to his reputation was the set of scurrilous verses that were publicly displayed at key sites around the city in the winter of 1527–28. These verses ridiculed the teachings of the new Stadtarzt and suggested that in view of his outlandish new medical terminologies he should be called Cacophrastus rather than Theophrastus, a suggestion that was conveyed by the title: *Manes Galeni adversus Theophrastum sed potius Cacophrastum*.[22] Of course, the victim complained, but the damage was done. The controversial town physician soon abandoned his post and retreated from Basel in a spirit of indignation.

The anonymous ghost of Galen had conducted its character assassination with devastating effect. The identity of the author has not attracted much attention, but the verses were clearly the product of an accomplished pen, perhaps that of a person familiar with the content of the lectures given by Paracelsus. In all probability, the author was a young medical humanist keen to improve his reputation by humiliating an ambitious rival.[23]

Although biographers of Paracelsus have tended to play down the significance of the *Manes Galeni* episode and its attendant barbs about Cacophrastus, from his subsequent reactions it is evident that this attack left a painful memory. This may help to explain why at the launch of his literary career he opted for a name change that shifted the emphasis to Paracelsus. In line with the precedent set by famous contemporaries such as Glareanus and Karlstadt, the initial intention seems to have been to introduce the name Paracelsus as a rough classical rendition and substitute for Hohenheim. Once discovered, the wider value of this new identity was appreciated; Theophrastus, with its pejorative connotations, was allowed to sink into the background, allowing the untainted name Paracelsus to predominate.[24]

Without any sound reason, it is nevertheless established as an almost indelible myth, especially at the popular level, that the name Paracelsus was introduced as a challenge to Cornelius Celsus, the well-known Roman medical encyclopaedist.[25] Such a claim was never mentioned by Paracelsus himself, and it does not seem to have occurred to his contemporaries. It is however worth noting that Theophrastus, at an early stage in his writing career, developed a taste for inserting the prefix *para* (indicating beside, past or beyond), as for instance in his writings entitled *paramirum* or *paragranum*. In calling for emancipation from the priesthood and relying on the guidance of the Holy Spirit, in his *De sacramento corporis Christi*, he alluded to his *paramirischen* writings and pointed out that these were supported by *parasagia* that would reveal profound secrets or *magnalia*.[26] It is arguable that this taste for the *para-* prefix was also a way of distancing himself from the groups that met his disapproval, especially the 'false priests' and 'false medics', to whom he tended to attach the prefixes *anti-* and *pseudo-*.[27] One further possible reason for adopting the name Paracelsus may be located in the strong taste of German mystics for the use of *celsus* and its compounds such as *excelsus* and *celsitudo* in their descriptions of God, or with respect to experiences calling for reference to height.[28] This was often linked to the use of *magnus*, as in *magnus est, Domine, et excelsus, et humilia respicis*, a sentiment that was congenial to Paracelsus and quite central to his thinking.[29] It is quite likely that some ancillary factors reinforced the preference for the use of the name Paracelsus, but the basic motive was to distract attention from the Cacophrastus affair by the simple device of throwing the emphasis on to a fresh name. As a classical rendition of Hohenheim, Paracelsus represented an obvious solution and this name proved so effective for its purpose that his original name ultimately became entirely superseded.[30] As a consequence, it is now almost forgotten that he was, for most of his life and for most purposes, known as Theophrastus von Hohenheim.

The absence of any medical association of the name Paracelsus is suggested by its first occurrence, not in a medical context, but in an astrological tract, *Practica D. Theophrasti Paracelsi gemacht auff Europen*, published in late 1529.[31] Thereafter, this name predominated in his many published astrological and prophetic tracts. As early as 1531, Sebastian Franck referred to him as *D. Theophrastus von Paracelsus, ein Physikus und Astronomus*.[32] It is evident that the new identification caught on quickly and was firmly established as the name by which he was known during the last decade of his life. The title-page of his first little medical publication, a short pamphlet on syphilis treatment by Guaiacum infusions, published in 1529, retained the original 'Theophrastus von Hohenheim'.[33] The same applied to his second medical tract, also on syphilis, published in 1530, although there is some evidence that 'Paracelsus' was suggested for inclusion at the draft stage.[34] At precisely this date, he also completed the first outline of his medical philosophy. This work, entitled *Opus Paragranum*, which survives in many drafts, remained unpublished until 1565.[35] The title-page gives the author's name as Aureolus Theophrastus Paracelsus. If the title-page of this edition is a reliable guide, this is the first of his non-astrological publications to carry the name Paracelsus. The various alternative versions of the Foreword contain a spirited denunciation of his critics in Basel. It is striking that they make specific reference to the 'Cacophrastus' affair, showing that this humiliation continued to rankle.[36] At one point he promised that the 'secta theophrasti' would triumph; then the ancients, beginning with Pliny and Aristotle, would have the prefix *Caco-* harnessed to their names.[37] As already indicated, the growing acceptance of the name Paracelsus was indicated by its inclusion as the sole name on the title-page of his comet tract published in the summer of 1531.

The sense of frustration experienced by Paracelsus about the failure of almost all of his writing ventures must have been all the greater as he lived at a time of unparalleled publishing opportunities. In Germany, the first thirty years of the century were marked by sustained expansion. Partly due to the impact of Lutheranism, a minor boom period occurred in the 1520s, coinciding with the early maturity of Theophrastus. Growth took place in all sectors of the market, but the pattern was uneven. The influence of Lutheranism on publishing gradually waned, but books relating to medicine and allied subjects remained in steady demand. In many respects the first half of the sixteenth century was a veritable golden age of medical book production. By locating himself in places like Strasbourg, Basel, Nuremberg and Augsburg, cities that accounted for the major part of German book production, Paracelsus undoubtedly hoped to facilitate publication of his bulging portfolio of unpolished drafts.

Given the increasing scale, evolving character and wide scope of the print media, the youthful Theophrastus was faced with some major decisions about the direction of his literary efforts and the location of his work in the book market. Although his energies continued to be spread across a broad front, for reasons already stated, he concentrated on finding publication outlets for his medical writings. No doubt he calculated that innovative, useful and accessible medical books would receive an enthusiastic reception, as well as generating some much-needed additional income.

Three sectors of the book trade, representing the humanist editors, the compilers of technical manuals and the authors of short tracts, were of particular relevance to the interests of Paracelsus.[38] The most prestigious publications were editions of standard medical authorities, especially from antiquity. For a person of the standing of the young Theophrastus, this was the most obvious and attractive avenue for establishing a reputation and gaining a foothold among the medical and social elite. Perversely, he rejected this alternative and instead was tempted to throw in his lot with the authors and publishers of vernacular medical manuals, who themselves represented a well-established and distinctive group experiencing notable commercial success. Although Paracelsus manifested some points of kinship with this sector, most of his writings were quite distinctive, and in the short term commercially less obviously appealing. Since he stood outside the mainstream, he sacrificed the opportunity to contribute to the ranks of the medical best-sellers. Finally, like controversialists in general, Paracelsus was attracted by the prospects presented by *Flugschriften*, or pamphlet literature. These cheap and ephemeral publications, sometimes comprising as few as four leaves, offered an entirely new avenue for dissemination, accessible to a wide range of writers and involving little risk to the publisher. Paracelsus both exploited this medium and drew upon its content for insights into the most effective means for the exposition of his ideas.

The Humanist Press

It was not easy to scorn the product of the humanist presses. As Paracelsus must have recognized from his visit to Basel, in taking issue with the humanist medical establishment he was confronting a veritable Goliath. The humanists were at the height of their productivity and influence. Early sixteenth-century German humanism was infused with all the enthusiasm of a new philosophy. Having previously learned to imitate, the German humanists aspired to equal and even emulate their Italian counterparts. On the model of the Italian academies, the Germans established their own informal humanistic academies or sodalities in many of the major academic and publishing centres. These pressure groups self-consciously worked to further the interests of the humanist fraternity. Illustration 2, the woodcut 'Philosophia', in which Albrecht Dürer represents the intentions of Conrad Celtis, aptly indicates the new spirit of assertiveness and self-confidence. The associated verses and four medallions depict the history of learning in four strategic stages. The Germans firmly occupy the culminating position. The tide of civilized values has moved from the south to the north and from the east to the west. The Germans had therefore taken over the baton of leadership from the Latins, and in particular were destined to make a decisive contribution in the field of philosophy. Albertus Magnus was portrayed as the figurehead of this new movement. This famous pioneer indicated that the Germans were by no means limited in their competence. Celtis believed that they occupied a place of distinction in all aspects of learning, and, to underline their supremacy in literary forms, his *Amores* was designed to emulate the Italian Neoplatonists in one of their main areas of creative writing.[39]

At the prestige end of the market, publishers linked up with teams of humanist scholars and technicians to produce impressive editions of classical texts, as well as original works with classical texts as their source of inspiration. Such volumes often included decorative and technical illustrations embodying the finest aesthetic and technical standards of the day.[40] The high estimation in which the artist–technicans were held was indicated by the expressions of admiration for Dürer in the work of Celtis. The Philosophia allegory of Illustration 2 was therefore the product of an equal partnership. Indeed it is sometimes suspected that the centre-left medallion 'Albertus', besides representing Albertus Magnus, was selected as a covert tribute to Dürer himself. The rising significance of illustration was evident in all parts of the book industry. Humanist–artist collaborations were expensive and not always unproblematical. The weighty authority of Sebastian Brant backed the use of illustrations for all classes of his writings. The success of his *Das Narrenschiff*, first issued in Basel in 1594 with its ambitious sequence of woodcuts, the majority by the young Dürer, left no doubt about the capacities of illustrations to reinforce the word of the poet.

At the end of his life Brant conceived the idea of an even more ambitious sequence of illustrations to accompany a German translation of Petrarch's *De remediis utriusque fortunae*, a work relevant to philosophy, medicine and many other subjects. After the failure of the initial publisher, who was an Augsburg physician addicted to alchemy, the project was picked up by Heinrich Steiner, who published the book in 1532 and again in 1539.[41] In the period between these two editions, Steiner had also become the main publisher of Paracelsus. The fine and well-illustrated editions of Paracelsus produced by Steiner confirmed the merit of opting for a publisher with experience at the prestige end of the market.

Reflecting the strength of the humanist involvement in medicine, this area captured an important share of the elite humanist book market.[42] Aware of the limited sales potential of their big folios, both publishers and their editors also produced more accessible digests and textbooks intended for a wider readership such as medical practitioners, students and the small class of well-educated lay people who dabbled in classical medicine.[43] The main labour was undertaken by a small group of medical scholars, but others participated in a minor capacity by locating new manuscript sources or adding commendatory verses or dedications. In addition, laymen such as Erasmus and Melanchthon produced orations or philosophical expositions touching on medicine.[44] Such contributions, like the wider literary activities of doctors, cemented the relationship of doctors with the wider humanist movement. By various means a stage army was assembled to support what was seen as a great civilizing mission.

The literary product of German medical humanism was impressive, even inspiring. Awkward for the ardent anti-humanist Paracelsus, Basel, at the date of his appointment as Stadtarzt, was emerging as an important location for medical humanist publishing. This was a logical development, since it was already one of the main European centres of scholarly and classically orientated book production and it preserved this bias, resisting the trend elsewhere towards concentrating on vernacular printing.[45] The medical side of Basel publishing had hardly begun at the time of the death of Johann Froben the elder in 1527, but in the next generation, under his son Hieronymus Froben, this publishing house became a leader in the medical field. Indicative of the attractiveness of medical publishing, the Froben business was joined, among others, by Johannes Oporinus. Collectively, the Basel presses made a substantial contribution to consolidating the authority of Galen and Hippocrates, whose influence was reinforced by expositions supportive of the Greek tradition. Such Greek bias was explicit and was furthered with evangelical, almost messianic fervour by the Basel editors.[46]

The humanistic medical enterprise in Basel was entirely new at the time of the visit of Paracelsus. A modest edition of Galen, translated by Erasmus, was published in May 1526, while a Latin translation of the works of Hippocrates was issued in August 1526.[47] Showing the vulnerability of the new enterprise, in his short introduction to the Hippocrates edition Andreas Cratander explained the relevance of his project to the furtherance of Greek medicine in a society where Greek was not widely known and where medical impostors were gaining a dominant voice. As already noted, Janus Cornarius was recruited by the younger Froben specifically to work on further editions of Greek medical texts, beginning with Hippocrates. The first fruit was a Greek/Latin edition of Hippocrates on airs, waters and places, which was published by Froben and Johannes Herwagen in August 1529, not long after the peremptory departure of Paracelsus from Basel.[48] Cornarius and Froben were embarking on a long-term and expensive commitment: in 1538 Froben published Cornarius's Greek edition of Hippocrates, which incorporated his emendations to the 1526 Venice edition; then in 1546 followed Cornarius's improved Latin edition of the complete works.[49] Cornarius and his collaborators established Basel as a key location in the development of Hippocrates scholarship. In the long biographical introduction to his Latin Hippocrates, Cornarius described his commitment to establishing the purified texts of Galen and Hippocrates as the basis for medical education. He believed that this reform was essential to elevating intellectual standards and reversing the decadent tendencies he had discovered on his first acquaintance with the German medical schools.

From the perspective of Cornarius and his collaborators, Hippocrates and Galen represented a massive intellectual endowment that had been inadequately exploited over the centuries. With the advantages of urbanization, printing and higher education, the opportunity emerged to capitalize fully on this system of knowledge. Hippocrates and Galen provided a chance for the doctor to reach the same intellectual and professional plane as the theologian and jurist, allowing the medical profession to occupy a similar place of dignity in both university and society. It was clear from the embattled spirit of Cornarius and other medical humanists that a whole century of dedicated endeavour by scholars had resulted in only limited gains. The enterprise in which the Basel publishers were engaged took on great symbolic significance in the battle to realize the exalted aspirations of the medical humanists. The pessimistic tone of the prefaces of Cornarius gave the impression that he was far from confident in the success of the humanist doctors in regaining the initiative from their multifarious enemies, who ranged from incompetent Galenic backwoodsmen to rampant empirics.[50]

The medical elite learned through daily experience that only by united effort would they be able to sustain their position of superiority against their competitors among the surgeons, apothecaries, and miscellaneous 'outsiders' who trespassed into their territory. The last thing they needed was the emergence of a charismatic and aggressive figure like Paracelsus, who seemed supremely qualified to assume a position of natural leadership over the rabble who stood to benefit from any weakness in the ranks of the physicians. The sense of fragility of their position explains the indignation and outrage with which Paracelsus was greeted. Just when the humanist physicians were in sight of the rebirth of the Golden Age that had taken generations to accomplish, an upstart emerged who threatened to undermine the entire edifice and destroy the credibility of the medical elite.

As already indicated, the medical humanist position was weakened by the increasing plurality of outlook among the educated public. Formally, the traditional pattern of education was maintained, with Galenic and Hippocratic theory retaining their status as the unchallenged paradigm of medical theory. However, among the intelligentsia Neoplatonism and Hermeticism exercised increasing influence, which led to importation of a significantly different body of theory that had the effect of bypassing, if not always confronting, established modes of explanation in medicine. Iconic figures such as Conrad Celtis, Johannes Reuchlin and Johannes Trithemius established Neoplatonism as the fashion of the moment and promoted the ideas of Marsilio Ficino and Giovanni Pico della Mirandola with enthusiasm. As indicated by their correspondence, their followers, who were often educated in Italy, were even more radical and intolerant of older philosophical orthodoxies. This helped to create a climate of opinion in Germany that eroded sympathy for Aristotelianism in particular and encouraged the broadest eclecticism, along the lines advocated by Pico in his famous Oration, usually called On the Dignity of Man. This trend inevitably generated a much greater tolerance of the arts associated with magic, and it created an audience that was intrinsically ever more receptive to ideas emanating from the likes of Cornelius Agrippa von Nettesheim and Paracelsus. Consequently, as far as the Galenic humanist elite was concerned, the philosophical tide was flowing in entirely the wrong direction.

The Popular Press

Even disregarding the threat posed by Paracelsus, an alternative to the product of the humanist presses was emerging from the lower echelons of the publishing industry. Newcomers within publishing gravitated towards practical handbooks, mainly written in the vernacular and addressed to a wide audience. Strasbourg was an especially important centre for this side of the market. At precisely the date of Paracelsus's stay in Strasbourg, three separate businesses were set up with the explicit aim of exploiting the popular market for medical and scientific books.[51] In Strasbourg, investment in technical publishing was an entirely new development, mainly the work of immigrant entrepreneurs.[52] This form of medical and scientific publishing was not only an immediate success; soon it became a staple of the market and more than most other subject areas turned out to be immune from downturns in the economy or changes in fashion. At first these publishers relied on bringing into general currency titles of medieval origin, but these were soon eclipsed by works by new authors, albeit frequently compilations, or even plagiarizations, of the work of more learned authors. One of the most successful publishers in this field was Christian Egenolff, who issued titles in Strasbourg between 1528 and 1530, and then mainly in Frankfurt am Main until his death in 1555.[53] Indicative of his commercial success after the bankruptcy of Heinrich Steiner, Egenolff bought up the greater part of his printing equipment and woodblocks, shortly after which he issued two editions of the surgical writings of Paracelsus with illustrations no doubt derived from Steiner's workshop.[54]

Egenolff was responsible for more than five hundred titles, the biggest category being herbals and medical handbooks, many of them richly illustrated. Egenolff also set up a successful type-foundry. No doubt reflecting market demand, Egenolff's first recorded titles were a prophetic and astrological tract commenting on Lichtenberger and a surgery derived from Lanfranc. Other notable successes of Egenolff in Strasbourg were his pair of handbooks on gunpowder and on mining techniques. Like his early medical titles, the technical handbooks were derived from manuscripts that had long been in circulation.[55] Among the successful and original Strasbourg handbooks were those by local medical practitioners, Hieronymus Brunschwig, Hans von Gersdorff and Lorenz Fries. The expanded edition of Brunschwig's handbook on distillation was issued by Mathias Grüninger in 1512, Gersdorff's *Feldbuch der Wundtartzney* was published by Johannes Schott in 1517, and Fries's *Spiegel der Artzney* by Grüninger in the following year.[56] Each of these books was successful and all were reissued during the 1520s.[57] Brunschwig and Gersdorff had died some time before Theophrastus's arrival in Strasbourg, but Fries was still active and for a short time was helpful towards his ambitious younger colleague. Practical handbooks issued by the Strasbourg publishers would have been congenial to the young Theophrastus. To the extent that he was reliant on published sources, these practical handbooks, rather than Galenic expositions, would have been valued for background purposes. Owing to the eclectic character of the popular handbooks, they were not disposed to identify their sources, and in turn they were not themselves identified when used by writers such as von Hohenheim.

Technical handbooks were an important addition to the print medium. They improved the level of knowledge across a wide spectrum of technical and scientific specialisms, including many areas relevant to health. Such sources helped to enhance standards among artisans, and they also made this knowledge available to a wider public. For the very first time, a wide range of technical information was available without restriction. Albeit without strategic guidance, the publishers specializing in the technical area managed to assemble an unpretentious but useful prototype of the *Encyclopédie* project of the French enlightenment.

Publishers like Egenolff created an opportunity for specialists of relatively humble standing to make a constructive contribution to the advancement of knowledge, gain access to a wide public and earn a degree of celebrity that in former generations would have eluded them. Given the buoyancy of the market for this important new genre of medical works, Paracelsus was no doubt encouraged to think of his own work as a logical progression from this trend. Lorenz Fries constituted a model of what could be achieved with modest capacities. During his short career, some sixty books were issued under the name of Fries, including thirty-two medical editions.[58] The full potentialities of the market for popular medicine were first revealed by Walther Ryff, who was probably working as an apothecary in Strasbourg in the 1530s but was active in publishing only for a short period between 1540 and 1548, during which years he was responsible for no fewer than 192 publications.[59] Equipped with a much stronger medical profile than either Fries or Ryff, Paracelsus must have been confident that he could at least establish a similar niche and then go on to make a more consistent and original contribution.

The shorter popular manuals shaded off into even more modest publications, the *Flugschriften*, tracts or pamphlets, and these in turn linked with the broadsheets, which often carried as much text as a small pamphlet. These cheap and accessible publications assumed enormous popularity in the first half of the sixteenth century. The rise in pamphlet production was spectacular, especially after 1517, with the peak being reached around 1524. The annual production of *Flugschriften* increased from about a hundred each year before 1518 to nearly a thousand in 1523; it is estimated that some 10,000 pamphlets were produced between 1500 and 1530.[60] Their main influence was exercised in the realms of religious and social affairs,[61] but their style and approach was adaptable to other purposes.[62] *Flugschriften* proved ideal for catering for the German obsession with events viewed as evidence of supernatural interference, such as monstrous births, outlandish celestial and meteorological formations, pestilence, episodes of extreme weather and associated phenomena such as floods and earthquakes, all of which attracted attention in the *Flugschriften* authored by Paracelsus.[63] Even local and minor incidents were sufficient to cause a flurry of pamphlet activity.[64] Any reports of topical interest were gathered up with relish by Paracelsus. He recognized that informed commentary from his pen would be valued and that timely interventions on such issues of the moment would be an ideal way of bringing his name to the attention of a wide public.

Reflecting the intensity of concern about celestial crises, the conjunction of Jupiter and Saturn in the sign of Pisces projected for 1524 attracted the attention of no fewer than fifty-six authors, who produced 133 separate publications, most in the form of *Flugschriften*, with Germany accounting for the lion's share of these.[65] Even broadsheets were brought into play in the medical and scientific sphere. The broadsheet was selected by Theodericus Ulsenius of Nuremberg as the vehicle for his astrological poem on syphilis published in 1496. The impact of this broadsheet was increased by the inclusion of a striking woodcut illustration, also making use of astrological symbolism and produced by Albrecht Dürer.[66] Woodcuts soon became standard ingredients in the published package and they were often vital to the success of pamphlets and broadsheets. Given the flexibility and popularity of the pamphlet medium, it was natural for Paracelsus to experiment with this form of expression. Pamphlets were not only one of his main sources of intelligence; they also presented a range of styles of popular exposition that were more appropriate to his purposes than standard methods of academic presentation. It is not surprising that he selected the pamphlet format for his very first medical publication. Pamphlets were in fact, in the course of his lifetime, the only medium in which he achieved any degree of success as a published author.[67]

The Paracelsus Book Club

Pamphlets, or short books that were in effect a collection of pamphlets, proved to be the literary medium in which Paracelsus excelled. Indeed, in view of his transitory way of life, this was the only realistic choice, since he lacked opportunities to engage in extensive periods of academic study or uninterrupted writing. Most of his writings bore the traces, and indeed often the scars, of the specific crisis he was experiencing at the time of authorship. The fact that so many of them are early and incomplete drafts suggests that his writing was interrupted and the opportunity for completion never again presented itself.

Notwithstanding such limitations, Paracelsus embarked on an ambitious and unusual literary exercise, involving the authorship of a series of popular writings covering the whole range of his speculations. At the core was a comprehensive outline of medicine, each element of which was employed to develop some aspect of his revisionist thinking. There was no realistic prospect of immediate publication, so the entire exercise was geared to a notional audience, a putative book club that was not yet in existence but was expected in the course of time to be constituted. This notional readership was expected to be persuaded by his new approach to medicine, but was also exposed to the wider social and religious programme that Paracelsus had in mind. On the basis of this wider frame of reference, the writing programme of Paracelsus was infused with a striking sense of purpose.

The abilities of Paracelsus as a communicator and polemicist were confirmed when his drafts were unearthed and published with very little editorial interference by the first generation of Paracelsians. His attention to elaborate prefaces or to the packaging of his writings into accessible formats seemed superfluous at the date of composition, but such considerations indicate that he was not deterred by the inhospitable environment in which he operated. Ever the optimist, throughout his depressing peregrinations he remained alert to the possibility of an imminent publishing breakthrough.

The most obvious and dramatic feature of the writings was their iconoclasm, as reflected in the almost blanket rejection of the dominant learned traditions in the various fields with which he was engaged. This seemingly intemperate response would have been recognized by his readers as entirely consistent with his critique of contemporary religious and social institutions. This wider perspective necessitated a general commitment to root and branch reform, and no other approach would have seemed appropriate in the light of his general mission objectives. Paracelsus was therefore liberated from the entanglements of the past, but the task of complete reconstruction that he set himself was mountainous in its proportions. He obviously appreciated the magnitude of this burden. He also resisted the invitation to take short cuts or adopt crude simplifications. His onerous mission was approached with the ominous sense of purpose that would be expected in the light of the gospel commission to which he subscribed.

Disruptions in the career of Paracelsus dictated the curious course of his studies and writing activities. His professional and technical competence was acquired in a haphazard manner from any source available in the course of his wandering existence. In practice he was more indebted to the standard literature of his main specialties than he acknowledged. He developed the art of acquiring information from written or oral sources until he obtained a working knowledge of the relevant specialist subject. His sources included practitioners and artisans of all kinds, which accounts for his facility in drawing on relevant analogies from almost any of the practical arts, especially those connected with mining, husbandry and agriculture.

Although his writings contain much material relating to theory that must have derived from his reflections on literary sources, even these parts of his work tend to be interspersed with data of a technical nature that could only derive from experienced witnesses. Taken as a whole, his writings are conspicuous for their high level of technical content, which on all fronts contains observations that still possess the capacity to impress the specialist. Our reformer accordingly approached the task of reconstruction from a position of strength regarding the depth and extent of his technical competence. His omnivorous search for useful information entailed an open-minded approach to the work of folk healers. For instance he reported on the work of a variety of dispensers of internal remedies or 'wound drinks', including a spirit conjurer and a gypsy from the Carpathians.[68] He was even rumoured to have spent substantial time among the gypsies.[69] Without expressing doubt, he accepted that the Wisdom of Solomon had been imported by gypsies from Egypt to the Alps and could still be found among peasants in many districts, especially around Entlebuch.[70] Frequently he drew on mythology, folklore and proverbial wisdom, all of which he regarded as a rich repository of information and insight, the influence of which is evident at many points in his writings.[71] One useful by-product of the search for the origin of the proverbial expression *alterius non sit, qui suus esse potest* was of the confirmation of his indebtedness to collections of animal fables.[72] Elsewhere I have drawn attention to Paracelsus's interest in folklore relating to spirit-beings located in forests, streams, the skies or mountain caverns.[73] In his writings, figures like Hansel and Gretel, Melusine, dwarfs inhabiting mountain caves, or exotic and dangerous beasts such as basilisks or crocodiles were treated with as much familiarity as any of the denizens of the farmyard. All of these beings were allocated to their particular functional niche in the plenitude of nature, which was portrayed in his writings as one of the manifestations of the Creator's rich endowment for human use and enlightenment.[74] Like Sebastian Franck, Paracelsus regarded fable and proverb as integral elements in the interpretation and deciphering of the living Word of God.[75] Anabaptist attitudes to such evidence were at this date greatly influenced by Hans Hut, who was struck by Christ's use of parables drawn from domestic arts and husbandry. As indicated in Chapter VI, animal lore was a basic component of the early Anabaptists' 'gospel of creatures'.[76]

Consistent with universally established cultural traditions and the expectations of his intended readership, Paracelsus drew freely on analogies from nature, on account of their relevance for explanatory purposes, but also for heuristic appeal.[77] Unlike those of Franck, Hut and most others, the analogies introduced by Paracelsus often injected an element of scientific understanding rather than reflecting the well-worn lore of fable. Indeed, the seriousness with which he regarded animal

lore was an inevitable consequence of his rendering of the macrocosm–
microcosm theory, which posited that, as the last created beings, humans
encapsulated the characteristics of all subsidiary forms of life. This
notion was developed at length with respect to both the physical and the
mental attributes of animals and humans.[78] It was therefore concluded
that animals were the mirror of mankind in which humans were able to
learn about themselves.[79] Animal life was also relevant to many other
biological problems. For instance, in concluding that various pathological
conditions could transmute themselves into epilepsy, Paracelsus likened
such spontaneous changes to the metamorphosis of an immature *lachs*
into an adult salmon.[80] The sudden appearance of shoals of fish in a
mountain stream was taken as a sign that poisonous emanations in the
vicinity were an imminent threat to human health.[81] When looking for
a felicitous way of characterizing the degenerate habits of the established
churches, he compared these institutions with colonies of ants, which
captivated their followers and then poisoned them with their acid
spray.[82] On the positive side, believers were cautioned to be patient and
to accustom themselves to the providentially determined cycle of their
fortunes. The whole of nature was subject to such a pattern of change, as
in the case of hibernating bears, whose summer of plenty was followed by
harsh winter, when they curled up and tended their paws and claws.[83]

Among his applications of the macrocosm–microcosm analogy,
Paracelsus underlined parallels between human and animal personality.
As we will see in Chapter VI, this subject assumed some importance,
since it was relevant to one of the gospel texts most favoured by both
Paracelsus and the Anabaptists. Animal behaviour was frequently held
up as an object lesson in vice. At one point, some twenty animal types,
ranging from the peacock to the snail, were cited to illustrate the
degenerate tendencies of the human personality standing in the way of
intellectual and moral enlightenment.[84] Readers would have been familiar
with his illustrative examples from their reading of fables and natural
histories, but the treatment by Paracelsus was noticeably more empirical
and philosophical. Some animals, especially dogs, were frequently
imported into his discussions.[85] The insatiable competitiveness displayed
among four named types of large hunting dog was cited to indicate the
base animal instinct prevalent among his academic competitors.[86] The
dog's habit of becoming angered into biting any person who twisted
its tail was taken as an understandable defensive response, suggesting
that righteous investigators should fiercely defend their rights against
ignorant impostors.[87] Just as the dog was instinctively the physician to
its own wounds, the heavens should be seen as the natural repository of

cures for human ailments.[88] Just as dogs instinctively knew the approach of the *Hundsschläger*, the slayer of stray dogs, Paracelsus observed that nature was alert to the shortcomings of delinquent practitioners of medicine.[89] With respect to the problem of begging, he noted the dog's instinct was to wag its tail to obtain the reward of food, but it never knew when to stop, with the result that it bolted food down until it was forcibly restrained. The dog therefore provided a warning against reversion to the practice of permitting unlicensed begging.[90] Dogs were endowed with tails to indicate their wants because they lacked an inner spirit with which to philosophize. Humans were thereby warned not to rely on their external faculties and neglect the development of their precious inner endowment.[91] The bloodhound was offered as a model for discovery in the arts. The medical practitioner was recommended to note the keen nose of the bloodhound, which led to remarkable finds of game. Medical investigators should learn, similarly, to sharpen their senses, in which case they would be rewarded by discovery of arcana in nature. The good doctor was analogous to a bloodhound and should faithfully imitate its behaviour.[92]

To illustrate the application of dog lore in the religious context, Paracelsus compared prophets such as David, even Christ, with a stray dog hanging around a pack of sheep. Such prophets were at first rejected, but then, just as the dog was recognized by the sheep, the suffering poor accepted David and Christ as their natural leaders, able to rescue them from their adversity.[93] On the other hand, the people possessed no confidence in their clergy, who were condemned for their loose living and avarice. Paracelsus warned these false apostles that, as punishment for hunting with hounds (also meaning engaging in trickery), they would end up being chased to a gruesome end.[94] It was also observed that the only way to select the best hunting dogs was to test their abilities in the most unpropitious circumstances, showing that personal faith was effectively put to the test only when the believer was exposed to the most demanding situations.[95] No doubt Paracelsus regarded himself as having equalled any hunting dog in his abilities to track down the truth in all of the capacities in which he operated.

The meticulous concern displayed by Paracelsus in mobilizing varied and colourful material to enliven his prose confirms his commitment to effective communication. In the attempt to evolve the most convincing manner of discrediting his competitors and enhancing his own authority, successive drafts of the same passage show evidence of careful reworking. Such complicated preparations demonstrate that he was not writing for his own private edification, either in the scientific or the non-scientific context. He was clearly framing his argument with the objective of undermining confidence in established authorities and substituting a blueprint of a totally different kind. The same target audience was being addressed in the medical and scientific writings of Paracelsus and by the propaganda of the various arms of the religious reform movement. Paracelsus geared his own reformation appeal closely to the mood of this larger movement. He was reasonably hopeful that the evident tidal wave of sentiment in favour of change would generate a positive response in his favour. In the circumstances it was not possible to test the audience response to his experiments in exposition, although the consistent demand for his astrological pamphlets must have been taken as an encouraging sign. Even more important, the major success of his *Grosse Wundarznei* indicated that even his more technical and ambitious writings were capable of finding a receptive audience.

Paracelsus never seems to have doubted his capacity to swim against the tide. Many obvious and successful models for his publications were available in the products of the humanistic and popular presses, but he adopted none without radical modification. While it was not remotely feasible to discard the classical system to the extent that he claimed, he decisively rejected the incrementalist approach to change favoured by his contemporaries, who predominantly believed that the antique system was sufficiently flexible to absorb any of the findings of modern investigators.[96] By contrast, Paracelsus regarded the old systems as an obstacle to progress and saw overt rejection as a basic precondition to evolving an alternative approach capable of absorbing the newer knowledge that was materializing in the medical sciences. He therefore saw no point in concentrating energies on editing ancient texts or producing popular expositions inspired by these sources. Sometimes he adopted familiar classical titles such as *De vita longa*, but his texts were distinctive in their approach, even at an early stage in his career, when his frameworks were constructed on more conventional lines.

The buoyant and diverse market in popular medical handbooks possessed greater appeal to Paracelsus. Whereas he rarely mentioned classical, Arabic and scholastic medical authors without derision, he was more tolerant of the late medieval practical handbooks, and no doubt his debt to authors such as Konrad von Megenberg or Hieronymus Brunschwig was more extensive than has yet been revealed. As already mentioned, at one stage he was on friendly terms with Lorenz Fries, but soon he rejected Fries and his *Spiegel der Artzney* as backward-looking, probably on account of the Colmar doctor's unquestioning acceptance of Galenic theory, his positive attitude towards the textbooks of Islamic origin, and also because he was unimpressed by Fries's adoption of crude schemes of anatomical illustration. The *Spiegel der Artzney* may have become a best-seller, but in the view of Paracelsus these simplistic encyclopaedias were just as pernicious as the summaries produced by the academic Galenists.[97]

In practice, the popular technical handbooks were taken by Paracelsus extremely seriously as a genre. Such sources demonstrated the potentialities of unadorned exposition and proved that the vernacular was capable of bearing the strain of discussion of any technical subject-matter. On the basis of such precedents, Paracelsus soon abandoned Latin and adopted German for every purpose. In his case, transition to the vernacular also signified a shift in ideology away from scholastic rationalizations and towards models of thinking more consistent with the dictates of his much-vaunted Light of Nature.

Paracelsus built on popular suspicions about the employment of foreign languages and recondite learning. Much of the practice of his competitors he dismissed as intentional obfuscation. They employed outlandish language to confuse their patients and extract larger fees. Such practices alienated patients from their doctors, in the same way that dog slayers were avoided by good citizens.[98] His stated objective was to make all aspects of natural philosophy and medicine accessible to the widest public and thereby open up the remarkable possibilities of these subjects. As far as medical professionals were concerned, they would only be able to make progress when they learned to collaborate with other specialists already converted to a more enlightened outlook.[99]

The wider ideological significance of the use of the vernacular by Paracelsus is confirmed by the description that he provided of his own professional aspirations. In the important *Prologus in vitam beatam*, he reported that he had given careful consideration to his vocation and had decided that it was better not to describe himself as an apostle; instead he wished simply to be known as a philosopher of the German type.[100] No other explanation was offered. Further insight into his expectations for philosophers (natural philosophers) of the German type is given at various points in his writings, among them the lengthy preface to his early *Herbarius*. Here he lamented the influx into Germany of ruinously expensive foreign medicines, most of which were completely useless in the German context. It was the purpose of his *Herbarius* to correct this situation and highlight the superior value of cheap, local products, including herbs. The blame was laid at the door of all those who profiteered from the pharmaceutical racket, but he was especially severe in his criticism of German doctors, who had become slaves to the writings of the Greeks and Arabs, thereby turning themselves into foreigners or aliens in their own land. His competitors were equipped with knowledge that was irrelevant to the circumstances of Germany. What Germans needed was their own medicine delivered by doctors who were familiar with their specific circumstances. On this basis Theophrastus was inclined to discard the whole of the ancient literature and restrict himself to information derived from German sources.[101] Thus, it was entirely appropriate that he should declare himself a natural philosopher of the German type.

Adoption of the German language for communication in medicine was entirely consistent with the broader ideological position of Theophrastus. German had been actively adopted as a favoured means of communication by the German mystics from the outset. Tauler insisted that plain German was the best means to communicate his message.[102] From the post-medieval perspective, although Conrad Celtis was steeped in classical culture, he wanted German humanism to possess a distinctive national flavour. The reformation movement proved a further boost to the vernacular. Among the radicals, the vernacular was a standard expectation. Humanistically educated figures such as Hutten and Karlstadt signified their drift to a more radical posture through adoption of German as their preferred means of expression. From the perspective of Theophrastus, if German was capable of articulating the deepest truths about faith, then it was without doubt adequate for all other purposes. Also like Celtis and Hutten, Theophrastus believed that his German cultural identity endowed him generally with superior credentials. For instance in the course of his defence against accusations of heresy, Theophrastus boasted that he wrote as a German and not as a foreigner (*ein Teutscher nicht ein Welscher*).[103] Just as German identity was taken to imply occupancy of the moral high ground, the clerical and medical establishment were portrayed as degenerates on account of their preference for heathen languages, likely subscription to alien values and unwillingness to come to terms with the demands of modern society. With hindsight, such zealous defence of German language and culture may seem rebarbative, but at the time it was essential for the purpose of establishing German as a viable language of communication in medical science, a possibility that most of Paracelsus's medical counterparts were unwilling to countenance.

Unconvinced by the spirited attacks of Paracelsus, the academic medical establishment remained doggedly rooted in the classical languages and culture. There was even a serious rearguard attempt to shift the emphasis from Latin to Greek. Except in advanced scholarship, Greek remained marginal, but Latin retained undiminished authority. As shown by the herbals of Brunfels and Fuchs, the anatomy of Vesalius, the natural histories of Gessner, or the mining of Agricola, leaders in their fields remained committed to Latin as their medium of expression, and indeed this was essential for any book hoping to achieve international distribution. Paracelsus was unconcerned about the continuing dominance of Latin in medicine or distributional problems associated with vernacular books. Indeed, the speed with which the herbals of Brunfels and Fuchs were reissued in German proved that there was already a decisive shift in favour of the vernacular.[104] For him, its advantages outweighed its disadvantages. On grounds of principle no alternative was conceivable. His primary concern was to gain the widest local audience, for which purpose he needed to employ the most accessible media and address the problems that were occasioning the greatest personal and collective anxiety. He was not deterred by diseases that were regarded as new or incurable, or by the bitter controversies surrounding such subjects. At an early stage in his career he plunged into the debate on syphilis, produced a review of the health problems of miners, now recognized as a pioneering work on industrial disease, and made the first of a number of attempts to reach a better understanding of the falling sickness. As his spirited efforts respecting syphilis indicated, the establishment was not welcoming to unconventional interlopers. Consequently, the Paracelsus book club was obstructed at its very launch.

When the obstacles were eventually overcome, the Paracelsus formula, comprising specialized monographs, or short books containing reviews of groups of related problems, proved to be highly marketable. There was no uniformity in the form of exposition Paracelsus adopted. Sometimes he focused on dispensing practical advice, in the course of which he exhibited a sure-footedness about therapeutics that suggested he was an experienced and conscientious doctor rather than a second-hand compiler. On other occasions he concentrated on theory, rendering his innovatory ideas more persuasive by the use of a philosophical, theological and ethical framework that was immediately meaningful and also congenial to the expanding constituency sympathetic to reformist ideas. Very often Paracelsus overreached himself and left behind drafts that were incomplete, which must have been irritating to the reader, but the fragments posed their own challenge to the reader's curiosity, for instance encouraging consultation of other examples of the same author's work in order to locate crucial missing links.[105]

The German Lucian

Expressions of scientific reserve or understatement were entirely alien to the Paracelsus method. With remarkable self-confidence and audacity, his works were artfully constructed to make a dramatic impact and to communicate an impression of originality and portentous importance. Given the revolutionary perspective of Paracelsus, his work called for something more than a dry academic presentation.

Since they are not entirely in tune with the early modern cultural context in which Paracelsus operated, modern analysts often express dismay about the colourful style, dramatic imagery and combativeness of his writing, which they feel is inconsistent with the measured standards expected from a scientist and member of a great profession. Even a friendly commentator such as C.G. Jung, although inured to squabbles among psychiatrists, was taken aback by the tendency of Paracelsus to let fly like a Swiss mercenary, leaving nothing to the imagination and treating his reader like an 'invisible auditor afflicted with moral deafness'.[106] An acquaintance with the conventions of literary exchanges among his contemporaries shows that Paracelsus was by no means exceptional in the robustness of his expression. Theologians and humanist scholars were apt to be drawn into literary brawls with one another, in which they resorted to the language of the lowest tavern. Virtuosi within the humanist medical elite appointed themselves the sole reliable arbiters of standards regarding the culture of antiquity. On this account they treated their competitors with condescension or ill-disguised contempt. The exchange between Fuchs and Cornarius, cited in Chapter I, constituted a typical example of this taste for polemic among the humanist doctors. In this case the quarrel exposed some deep personal jealousies, but it revealed real differences of outlook on important academic issues, as well as relating to rivalry between various co-operatives of publishers and authors.[107] As shown by his outbursts against competitors from humbler backgrounds such as Lorenz Fries and Walther Ryff, Fuchs was even harsher in his treatment of his commercial competitors than of Cornarius, his humanist rival.[108]

On the basis of his objective experience, it is understandable that Paracelsus possessed little sympathy for his medical colleagues. The Basel episode taught the young Theophrastus to expect pre-emptive strikes from his competitors. The *Manes Galeni* verses confirmed that the humanists were intent on ruining his career. He had experienced the same hostile reception from Klauser and Fries, both of whom had enjoyed success as popular medical and astrological authors. In Zürich,

Christoph Klauser passed a harsh verdict, probably indicative of his implication in sabotaging publication of Theophrastus's early medical writings. A display of animosity against Theophrastus might usefully confirm his own reputation for orthodoxy and thereby strengthen his case for promotion to the post of Archiater of Zürich, something that was achieved in the very year of his attack on Paracelsus. At exactly this date Lorenz Fries also attacked Paracelsus, no doubt attempting to secure his own professional position in Metz. Such experiences showed Paracelsus that he was likely to be abused from all sides.

Undaunted, he went on to Nuremberg and began the launch of the Paracelsus phase of his career. There he met Sebastian Franck, his prodigious younger contemporary, who commented on his strange but remarkable character, also on his striking tendency to deride and reject nearly all the practitioners and nearly everything written in medicine and astrology. On the basis of his sound humanist credentials, Franck added that this Paracelsus was reminiscent of Lucian.[109] This characterization is not inconsistent with the retrospective summary provided by Oporinus, which reported on the general dissatisfactions of Paracelsus and on his commitment to radical reform in both religion and medicine.

Franck's assessment of Paracelsus casts light on contemporary attitudes towards literary exchanges. There is no difficulty in finding literary sources supplying a precedent for our reformer's extensive and flamboyant critique of the existing social order, including its priests and doctors. The often ribald genres of the *Fastnachtsspiele*, other varieties of popular drama, as well as the *Flugschriften*, provide many of the basic ingredients of the wide-ranging critique mounted by Paracelsus. From the literary sphere it is also relevant to take account of the revival of interest in classical satire, especially Lucian of Samosata, the Greek satirist. Lucian was not only relevant as a literary model; on many occasions he ridiculed the doctors and philosophers of the establishments of his day in terms very reminiscent of Paracelsus. Lucian had already experienced a revival during the Italian Renaissance, but he was taken up with particular energy in the early sixteenth century, including in Germany. Translations of his work poured from the German presses. Just as important, his caustic style was a stimulus to the satirical writing of influential figures such as Ulrich von Hutten and Erasmus. Hutten himself was called the reborn Lucian by Johann Froben. In the introductory letter addressed to Thomas More in his *Moriae encomium*, Erasmus styled himself another Lucian on account of using the conventions of ancient comedy to 'snarl at everything'. This waspish approach seemed more effective as a tool of criticism than the crabbed and specious arguments of academic presentations. Agrippa von

Nettesheim is well known for experimenting with the Lucianic essay; it is even arguable that his *De incertitudine et vanitate scientiarum* (1530) represented a convoluted Lucianic exercise in which spirited satire was employed to defend what he seemed to attack.[110]

The dialogues of Hutten, or the *Moriae encomium* and *Colloquies* of Erasmus, contain extensive and effective use of Lucian for the purpose of propaganda against Rome and the subject clergy of the old church in Germany, as well as their allies.[111] As a form, the Lucianic dialogue caught on; around fifty examples appeared by 1525, some of them by authors who exploited this medium to highlight the superior acumen displayed by the lower orders. The best-known example was 'Karsthans', a literary figure accidentally brought to life by Thomas Murner, who in 1520 attacked Luther for inciting Karsthans types among the common people into disobedience. In return Karsthans was invoked as the leading figure in the Karsthans dialogue published in Strasbourg in January 1521, which had the purpose of vindicating Karsthans and his class.[112]

The writings of Paracelsus were rarely without their Lucianic elements. This style was especially evident in collections of short sketches, such as the *Sieben defensiones* and the associated *Labyrinthus errantium medicorum*. The latter was perhaps directly linked with *Moriae encomium*, which attacked many similar targets, at one point suggesting that it was easier to extract oneself from a labyrinth than from the entanglements of the philosophical 'sects' such as realists, nominalists, Thomists, Albertists, Occamists and Scotists.[113] These same groups were often the subject of attack by Paracelsus, and he also called them sects.[114] Franck may have drawn his conclusions from the personality of Paracelsus, but if he was granted access to any of his writings he would undoubtedly have regarded them as reflecting the Lucianic spirit owing to their 'snarling' style and portrayal of the medical profession as vain, ostentatious, hypocritical, avaricious and disputatious. Lucian conferred on Paracelsus the licence to elaborate on these themes at length and in a highly scurrilous manner. Paracelsus perhaps concluded that the Lucianic essay met the expectations of his intended readership and was consistent with the best literary practice of the day. He was happy to model himself on Lucian and Hutten, who between them had explored and exhausted the full vocabulary of invective. On the basis of such consistency with the successful Lucianic formula, Paracelsus had every reason to expect that his social criticism would fall on receptive ears and thus reinforce confidence in his scientific programme.

Magnus and Magus

Consolidation of the reputation of Paracelsus was reflected in changes in the rendition of his name. In his first medical publication, he was announced as Theophrastus von Hohenheim, doctor in both parts of medicine, a formula that was repeated in many later medical writings.[115] For the purposes of his first astrological tract, the same publisher, in the same year, announced him as 'Doctor Theophrastus Paracelsus'; this was commonly used on the title-pages of non-medical writings and increasingly for medical works as well.[116] The medical and astrological usages were commonly conflated, in which case he was called Theophrastus Paracelsus, doctor of the free arts of medicine and astronomy.[117]

As the first generation of editors entered the fray, yet further embellishments were introduced. He was soon described as the 'most learned prince of all physicians'[118] and *Paracelsi Magni*.[119] Lambert Wacker advised that he should rightly be called *Monarcha et princeps Medicorum*, as well as *theologorum Rex et Jurisconsultorum caput*.[120] Such representations, indicating depth of knowledge of nature, practice of the magical arts, but also sagaciousness in general, were implied in the characterization of Paracelsus adopted in the title of his most important book.[121] Accordingly, the title-page of this *Astronomia magna* or *Die gantze philosophia sagax* described the author as *hocherleuchten, erfahrnen, und bewerten teutschen Philosophi und Medici, Philippi Theophrasti Bombast, genannt Paracelsi magni*.[122] Not to be outdone by this elevated description, Michael Toxites described Paracelsus as master of the whole of philosophy and cosmology, the mysteries of the supernatural, the capacities of faith, and the powers of infernal spirits.[123] As these epithets indicate, through the efforts of his early editors Paracelsus became included among the select body of modern luminaries like Albertus Magnus for whom the epithet *magnus* was seen as appropriate. As suggested by Illustration 2, to the intellectuals siding with the construction adopted by Celtis and Dürer, affiliation with Albertus Magnus would have provided confirmation that Paracelsus was playing an honourable role in bringing to fruition the triumph of German culture to which the Neoplatonic reformers were aspiring.

As noted above, the promotional effort by the editors and followers of Paracelsus was a decisive success. Some impression of the standing gained by Paracelsus within a few decades of his death was given by Daniel Specklin of Strasbourg. In his chronicle of noteworthy events, he recorded that the prophecies of Johannes Lichtenberger concerning the year 1517 appeared to be fulfilled by the emergence of three important innovators, Martin Luther in religion, 'Theophrasto' in medicine, and Albrecht Dürer in the visual arts. Specklin knew that his readers would recognize this Theophrasto as Theophrastus von Hohenheim.[124] It is striking that Specklin includes Theophrastus in this distinguished company, especially since the medical reformer might have been regarded as something of a specialist. He was also much younger than both Dürer and Luther; the latter was exactly ten years older, while the former was more than twenty years his senior. By the date of Specklin's assessment, there was no doubting the impact of Luther and Dürer; Theophrastus was not in their league, but Specklin was right to detect the magnitude of his influence in the fields of medicine and in the scientific movement, and he may also have appreciated the broader ramifications of his appeal. Specklin was perhaps more prescient than he realized when he included Theophrastus among the Germans who were exercising a major cultural effect.

Specklin was an informed witness. He was a respected citizen, official architect and engineer of the city, and had plenty of first-hand experience concerning the impact of these three heroic figures. Strasbourg had been at the heart of the Reformation and indeed of the Radical Reformation. The town was also important in the applied arts, including publishing. After 1560, its editors and publishers had been conspicuously active in disseminating the work of Paracelsus who, it will be recalled, had briefly been a resident of the town. Paracelsus was a contemporary of the architect's father, Veit Rudolf Specklin, who was an eminent woodblock cutter, working in the tradition of Dürer. Veit may well have been a source of direct information concerning Paracelsus which he could have picked up from either Strasbourg or Basel, the two towns in which the older Specklin worked. Both towns were also main centres for the burgeoning Paracelsus publishing industry. In the famous herbal of Leonhart Fuchs, the elder Specklin was singled out for praise and he featured in a special portrait.[125] Fuchs himself would have been dismayed both by the spectacular rise in the fortunes of Paracelsus and by the collapse of the hegemony previously enjoyed by humanist physicians like himself.

The high estimate of Paracelsus by Specklin reflects the success of the Paracelsian editors in projecting the full range of his accomplishments and the revolutionary character of his contribution. The medical humanist leadership made a rather different estimate. They too came to concede the growing influence of Paracelsus, but by exploiting the deep-rooted prejudice against magic as an illicit and superstitious art inherited from the pagans they identified him as a dangerous soothsayer, which is how they regarded the magus of antiquity. Gessner and his associates drew on a long history of suspicion about magic, solidly backed by the authority of the church, which resulted in various degrees of prohibition over the centuries. By their emphasis on scientific procedures and positive utilitarian applications, such natural philosophers as Albertus Magnus, Roger Bacon and William of Auvergne helped to create a more tolerant attitude towards natural magic. Their efforts were reinforced by the Italian Neoplatonists, who in the late fifteenth century went on the offensive and endowed magic with the refinement of philosophical and theological respectability. Their exercise was at best a partial success and in some respects it was counterproductive. Even the elite among natural magicians remained exposed to suspicions of heresy.[126] Naïve expectations of tolerance were lacking in realism since they failed to reckon with the strength of the residual prejudice against magic, which was repeatedly exploited to their own advantage by social groups threatened by the activities of magical competitors. The papal witchcraft Bull *Summis desiderantes affectibus* (December 1484), the witchcraft inquisitors' handbook *Malleus maleficarum* (1486), and their subsequent high-profile impact were important straws in the wind, demonstrating the continuing risk of identification of natural magic with witchcraft accusations.[127]

Magical interests seemed even more suspect when they were associated with curiosity about the kabbalah, which attracted additional animosity on account of anti-Semitism and the accusation that the kabbalists were involved in a surreptitious campaign to 'judaize' Christianity. Such claims were nebulous, but many alleged dissidents fell foul of the judaizing accusation. The main attack on Reuchlin, produced by the inquisitor Jacob Hoogstraeten and published in 1519, was provocatively entitled *Destructio cabalae seu cabalistica perfida*. Accordingly, the controversy surrounding Johannes Reuchlin constituted a warning to anyone contemplating following the same path.[128]

Paracelsus may well have heard rumours about difficulties experienced by the Italian Neoplatonists on account of their pioneering labours in Hermeticism, kabbalism and natural magic. In a dangerous situation, they sought security in retractions or convoluted defensive exercises, as did Cornelius Agrippa von Nettesheim, whose adverse experiences on account of magic in Lyons ran parallel to those of Paracelsus in Basel.[129] Such examples constituted an object lesson that Paracelsus would have done well to observe.

In embroidering the case against Paracelsus, Gessner suspected that the reformer's blend of religion and magic was a pernicious combination. Paracelsus himself seemed to belong to the end of the line of the Druidic religion of the ancient Celts. Gessner believed that Paracelsus's astrology, geomancy, necromancy and other forbidden arts were kindred to the magical arts that the Druids learned in underground places from demons. From sources such as Nennius, Gessner knew about the authority exercised at the Celtic fringes of Europe by Druidic wise men or magi. He thereby concluded that the descendants of the Druids were the source of the arcane knowledge of Paracelsus, through whose work the Druidic religion and magic had become implanted on German soil in a new and dangerous form.[130] This line of attack is unlikely to have succeeded, partly because the Druidic religion was presented in an entirely favourable light by Celtis and his associates, for whom the Druids represented the aboriginal purity of the forest people to which the German reformers were aspiring.[131] According to this construction, the identification of Paracelsus with the Druids was a positive benefit to his reputation.

Unlike many of the other leading magicians, Paracelsus showed no tendency to vacillation or compromise. Magic, the kabbalah and their related disciplines were extolled at every opportunity from his earliest to his last literary efforts of all types, as is evident from the centrality of magic in all of his publications and also from his ambitious 'near misses' such as the Carinthian trilogy and the *Astronomia magna*. Paracelsus also differed from the Neoplatonic mainstream in his approach to the defence of magic. The Neoplatonists greatly depended on the *prisca theologia* and *prisca sapientia* argument, suggesting that their own conclusions derived from the insights of a lineage of incisive thinkers stretching back to the ancient Middle East. One of the variants of such an approach is implicit in the medallions and verses of the 'Philosophia' woodcut included as Illustration 2.

Paracelsus was disinclined to engage with the sources venerated by the Neoplatonists and he paid only perfunctory attention to non-biblical figures. His own historical justification of magic and kabbalah relied almost exclusively on biblical precedents and especially on the instance of the Magi who attended the birth of the infant Jesus in Bethlehem. When the magi featured in the speculative lineage of the Italian Neoplatonists, these were generally the Near Eastern magi, especially Persian magi, who were regarded as the ancestral and most esteemed of the type.[132] A short sermon was devoted to the Bethlehem episode by Ficino, but this was primarily intended to reinforce his argument about the veracity of ancient wisdom rather than isolating the adoration of the Magi as an event of decisive importance.[133] The Ficino sermon is additionally relevant since it draws attention to the popular Florentine fraternity devoted to the veneration of the magi. As a sign of the impact of the ceremonials connected with the Feast of the Epiphany, Giovanni Pico della Mirandola decided to stage his confrontation with his critics on this very date, presumably with the intention of demonstrating that his own new philosophy represented a decisive event in the apocalyptic cycle.[134] Paracelsus was no doubt unaware of this audacious act by his Italian counterpart, but he saw his own employment of the magi in the same momentous light.

Granting a positive image to the magi was not altogether uncontroversial. Ever sensitive to the dangers of magic, in their commentary on the opening verses of Matthew 2 or on the relevant aspect of the Epiphany, the church fathers were reluctant to acknowledge the virtues of the Bethlehem Magi.[135] The latter were even judged as reprobates who, on the impulse of divine guidance, abandoned their evil ways. The medieval period witnessed a relaxation of attitudes.[136] Germany was conspicuous for development of a more positive interpretation, as indicated by the popular pilgrimage to the relics of the Magi that were one of the prize possessions of the church in Cologne, or the *Historia trium regum* by Johannes von Hildesheim which established itself as a minor classic.[137] Reverence for these figures can be seen in the popularity of the Adoration of the Magi as a theme in the visual arts, notably the famous woodcut renderings by Dürer and the many imitations that they inspired. By the time of Paracelsus the Magi were well on the way to complete rehabilitation. Accordingly, Paracelsus could easily have claimed that his own attitude towards the Magi and the magic with which they were associated was not entirely at variance with the analysis of Luther.[138]

The Magi were exploited more actively by Paracelsus and adapted to the prerequisites of the spiritual reformers of the sixteenth century. The traditional view of the Magi as kings or princes was encouraged by Hildesheim but rejected by Paracelsus, who portrayed them as determined aspirants to the ranks of the spiritual elect according to his criteria for the apostolic mission. Owing to their receptivity to the Holy Spirit, the Magi were granted the massive reward of attending the infant Jesus. The example of the Magi and shepherds underlined the transformative abilities of the spirit even for those who were unacquainted with any part of the scriptures. For Paracelsus the Magi were too important to be co-opted as a minor addition to the stage army of the *prisca sapientia*. Rather, they possessed an importance of their own and constituted a model for those who aspired to a radical break with the past.

Given the exemplary value of the Magi, it is understandable that Paracelsus drew on their example for support on many occasions in his writings and in a range of contexts. In his various expositions on the second chapter of Matthew, Paracelsus emphasized the distinction between magi and astronomers. The knowledge of the latter was confined to natural regularities, but magi possessed deeper insights owing to their ability to interpret phenomena of supernatural origin. With the appearance of the star announcing the birth of Jesus, the Magi of Saba and Tharsis immediately recognized the limitations of their scientific understanding and turned for inspiration to the Holy Spirit. Owing to this higher enlightenment, the Magi realized that Jesus was separated from and elevated above the usual course of nature.[139] In one of his later commentaries, in accordance with the reference to signs and miracles from Luke 21: 25, the magi were defined as those luminaries who were equipped to understand, interpret and expound the meanings of all secrets and prophecies. By virtue of such superior insights, the competence of the magi greatly exceeded that of their rivals among doctors, priests or academics.[140] A remnant of his commentary on Isaiah was largely devoted to the contention that the star announcing the birth of Christ was a supernatural occurrence. On account of the momentous significance of this event, the star was only intelligible to a small elect of magicians, in this case the Magi of the Orient who, through their fear of God and upright behaviour, were privileged to be granted access to this remarkable secret.[141]

The Magi were invoked at important locations in the writings of Paracelsus. For instance they featured in the draft conclusions of the early *De invocatione beatae Mariae virginis*[142] and at many points in his last major book, the *Astronomia magna*, as well as in its abbreviated form, the *Erklärung der ganzen astronomie*.[143] These sources were broadly consistent with his interpretation of the Matthew commentaries. Paracelsus repeatedly insisted that the magi were not to be confused with astrologers or meteorologists. The competence of magi was not limited to natural regularities or oddities that preoccupied run-of-the-mill mathematical practitioners. The understanding of the latter was confined to externalities, which impacted upon human affairs but were limited in their effects. The magi were assumed to be competent in these conventional arts, but they were also able to probe into deeper secrets, phenomena involving an element of supernatural causation. Such direct interventions by God were designed to convey guidance to humans concerning their actions and destiny. The magi probed beyond the externalities of nature into the provinces of the 'inner heavens' and divine interventions. Such a level of understanding was confined to a select minority, who were receptive to the deepest inner experience. The wisdom granted to the Magi of the Orient, which drew them to the birthplace of Jesus, was then communicated by them to others and ultimately became the prerogative of the community of saints in later times. As confirmation that the magi were equipped with supernatural as well as natural powers, they were capable of conferring their virtues on others, for instance Muhammad and Hippocrates, both of whom, through this superior endowment, had come to be treated like gods by their followers.[144]

Paracelsus had no grounds to doubt the general opinion that God intervened actively in the physical world and furthermore provided omens intended for the guidance of troubled humanity. It was widely feared that the opening decades of the sixteenth century represented a significant and dangerous moment, indeed even a crisis point signifying the approach of the Last Judgement. Such fearful possibilities inevitably occasioned acute anxiety among the public, who naturally turned to their astrologers and theologians for guidance. Reflecting the seriousness of these issues, Ulinka Rublack recently began her review of Reformation Europe with a discussion of the interventions of Luther and Melanchthon in the seemingly curious backwater of monsters and omens. Deciphering the meaning of freak events not only offered an opportunity to capture popular attention. Such interventions also possessed the more serious purpose of providing insight into the workings of divine providence in order to determine what precisely was in store for the perilous future leading up to the end of time.[145]

Drawing upon his acquaintance with the *Flugschriften*, Paracelsus specially mentioned the meteorite that had descended to earth in ominous circumstances in Alsace, undoubtedly a reference to the large delta-shaped meteorite that fell at Ensisheim, Alsace in 1492. This event was put on the map by broadsheet commentary from the celebrated Sebastian Brant, and the meteorite was noteworthy enough to continue to attract comment in later decades. Paracelsus was categorical in his view that this stone was a supernatural occurrence, intelligible only through the application of magic.[146] Since the correct interpretation of such phenomena was the monopoly of the magi, this group was poised to make a decisive contribution to the understanding of the terrible times that were being witnessed. In view of the vital importance of their role, Paracelsus urged that the magi of later times should be regarded as the natural successors to the saints of old. In the past, the latter had performed remarkable things through their exercise of direct power derived from God, whereas the magi achieved their insights and performed remarkable practical works as a consequence of their inspired insights into nature.[147] Paracelsus was even tempted to conclude that the magi were born into their roles, elected by God to convey the secrets of the heavens and to explain the *mysteria* and *magnalia* implanted in nature by the Creator.[148] Given the intrinsic importance of magic and reliance on the elite cadre of magi for the mediation of this wisdom, it is entirely understandable that Paracelsus should make the outline and defence of magic one of the highest priorities of his literary endeavours.

In the embattled and disadvantaged position from which he operated, magic and the sense of belonging to the fellowship of the magi were important for the maintenance of his sense of self-esteem. Commitment to bettering the human condition was itself an honourable aspiration, but endowing this vocation with magic and kabbalah elevated the importance of this mission in the providential scheme of things. As a consequence of this ambitious conception, in his pursuit of the gospel commission Paracelsus could be satisfied that he was playing a fully proportionate part in the maintenance of demanding standards set by the luminaries of the prophetic and apostolic ages who constituted his models and inspiration.

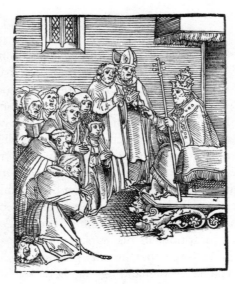

CHAPTER III

THE SOURCES OF DISSENT

meine junger seindt on gut, on reichthumb, aber es werden falsche junger khomen, die
werden mit behausung, weiber, frawen, zinsen, gutern, pfrunden prouision etc versorgt
sein, das sie nit mugen weichen, sonder werden predigen, was dem volckh angenem ist, [und
dann] jren schatz, steckel, seckel nit verlieren.[1]

Oporinus noted that Theophrastus, as a young man, had adopted an
analogous approach to the church and the medical profession. Our
reformer was equally critical of the classical influence in medicine and
the Roman hegemony over the church. On this account he maintained
an aloofness from both the religious and the medical establishments;
he struck out in an independent direction, pitting himself against the
medical and theological orthodoxies of his day, which was a formidable
and hazardous undertaking.[2] Although the religious and secular aspects
of his mission were promoted with equal intensity, as his remarks about
the Magi demonstrate, he insisted that spiritual enlightenment was an
essential precondition for the fulfilment of any other objective.

The Basel episode confirmed that he was well advanced in his
preparations for hostilities with the Galenic humanists, but neither in
Strasbourg nor in Basel was he inclined to reveal publicly his confessional
and theological alignments or his attitude to the religious power struggles
that were gripping the attention of the inhabitants of both cities.
Nevertheless it is evident that by this date he was completely familiar
with the key issues of contention among the theologians. Indeed he had
drafted a series of theological writings by the date of his stay in Salzburg.

The Marian essays produced at this early stage comprise one of the best-researched aspects of the whole of his literary output.[3] Biegger, Gause and others also touch on other writings stemming from this early date, notably his commentary on the first five chapters of Matthew and the *De septem punctis idolatriae cristianae*. Both are recognized as significant, but they have tended to be incidental to the main issues under consideration. As a consequence, these non-Marian early writings have still not received the attention they merit.

Paracelsus went on to produce a continuous run of theological writings, many of them of great length and interest. Notable among these is the ambitious commentary on Matthew, one of his largest undertakings, which has so far defeated even the most assiduous of his modern editors. Although the theological standpoint of Paracelsus, like that of many other radicals, was firmly based on the New Testament, he regarded the Old Testament as an indispensable source of witness. At one point he warned that proclaiming the gospel without an understanding of the writings of the prophets was the sure way to sectarianism. Among its various merits, the Old Testament provided insight into the commandments of God and into prophecies concerning the future messiah.[4] From an incidental remark in *Septem punctis* it is evident that Theophrastus had written by that date at least one study on the Old Testament.[5] He went on to produce a massive commentary on the Psalms, which has survived, and also what he called 'a comprehensive exposition of the Old Testament, line by line', which cannot now be traced.[6] The importance of the exegetic exercise was underlined by his belief that God had supplied the scriptures, together with the spiritual gifts requisite for their right understanding, to act as a guide to later generations, as something of a substitute for the direct authority exercised by the apostles at the beginning of Christianity. The scriptures represented protection against the witness of false prophets who would abound during the terminal crisis that he believed had already overtaken both church and state.[7] Such a situation was invoked in the quotation at the head of this chapter as well as that accompanying Illustration 3, in which Cranach firmly designated the papacy and the Roman church as alien forces and the root of Antichrist.[8] Commenting on the same text, Thomas Müntzer warned that 'this is a dangerous time and these are evil days'.[9] The present chapter deals with the response of Paracelsus to this perception of terminal decline within the church. Since the following pages are mainly concerned with the period before the idea of Paracelsus was conceived, for the most part it is preferable to call him by his original name, Theophrastus von Hohenheim.

Dangerous Associations

Collectively, his writings dating from his first stay in Salzburg confirm the high priority Theophrastus gave to his theological studies. All of the Salzburg writings contain polemical elements, but *Septem punctis* in particular makes no pretence at impartiality. The author maintained a consistently caustic and hostile tone, no doubt reflecting some background experience of harassment in the recent past. No doubt, he took limited signs of rebelliousness as an indication that liberty of conscience and free expression were on the horizon. *Septem punctis* seemed an appropriate response to this new situation, but it quickly became apparent that he had made a serious miscalculation.

The whole episode is intriguing and significant. *Septem punctis* constitutes an important milestone; it set the tone and established an intellectual orientation that became common to all categories of his later writings. Although this tract was an opportunistic intervention occasioned by circumstances particular to the eve of the German Peasants' War, it also provided insight into his more general intellectual alignments, confirming that he had already adopted much of the radical perspective that became more fully apparent in the course of his later writings. The importance of this first exercise in polemics is confirmed by echoes of its content in other writings from all stages of his literary output. Although *De septem punctis idolatriae cristianae* was one of his first polished pieces of writing, this tract was not published until 1986.[10] Before that date it was very little mentioned. Helpfully, Theophrastus indicated that this tract was written in Salzburg. In his edition, Goldammer favours early 1525 as the date of composition, that is just before the author's hurried departure to escape the escalating political crisis.

Septem punctis is a polished product that survives in no fewer than nine variant manuscript versions. Like the Marian tracts, it has all the makings of a publication. Possibly the author envisaged a substantial quarto pamphlet comprising some sixteen leaves, which would have been a commercially acceptable proposition. A publication on this scale would have been similar to many pamphlets covering similar ground, such as Haug Marschalck's *Spiegel der Blinden*, which had appeared in Augsburg in 1522. It is quite likely that *Septem punctis* was conceived as the author's first venture into the *Flugschriften* market. This was a realistic idea, since the tract was drafted at the peak of a veritable tidal wave of pamphlet production. Such publications provided unprecedented opportunities for participation in both religious controversy and social protest, as well as a chance to influence attitudes at what proved to be a decisive moment:

the wave of renewed unrest among peasants and their allies, which turned into open conflict in the spring of 1525.

Although evangelical preachers were making headway and Anabaptism was on the horizon, owing to the vigilance of the presiding authorities, in the run-up to 1525 Salzburg witnessed less overt unrest than occurred in many other parts of the German-speaking region. Thereafter the hold on events by the authorities rapidly collapsed. Theophrastus perhaps detected his opportunity to make his mark as a religious controversialist. *De septem punctis idolatriae cristianae* seems to have been framed with this objective in mind. In common with many other lay authors, Theophrastus opted for an assault on the corruptions of the clergy in the context of a general outline of the abuses and shortcomings of the established church. This formula for polemical tracts had proved successful elsewhere, but Salzburg had hitherto resisted the incursion of this kind of propaganda. As the seat of an unpopular and imperious archbishop and bloated clerical bureaucracy, it must have seemed an ideal location for conveying this message. No doubt, possessing some acquaintance with the trend in favour of reform in other cities, Theophrastus determined to try his hand with a similar line of attack in Salzburg.

Owing to the relative marginality of the reform movement and absence of a buoyant popular press, publication in Salzburg was not feasible. Discovering friendly publishers, in Augsburg or elsewhere, willing to take on this controversial manuscript also presented practical difficulties. Before such logistical problems were solved, the unforeseen escalation of political hostilities in Salzburg and its region seriously increased the risks to the author. It was further to his disadvantage that the peasant leaders, although extensively preoccupied with economic grievances, adopted a strong evangelical tone in the Salzburg area and indeed styled themselves 'brethren in Christ' to enhance the impact of their appeals for local support.[11] The local peasant leadership consequently appeared to identify with the message of *Septem punctis*, hence further tainting the reputation of the tract's author. *Septem punctis* accordingly became the first serious test of the prudential instincts of Theophrastus. Wisely, it was set aside and no serious opportunity arose again for its resurrection. By the date of his arrival in Strasbourg, his *Septem punctis* was no longer the viable publishing proposition that it might have been at the beginning of 1525. These few months represented a small window of opportunity coinciding with the culmination of the protest movement associated with peasant unrest. Soon the tide turned; by the end of 1525 expressions of radical dissent were completely out of place. A year later, in places favourable to reform like his new home of Strasbourg, many of the abuses highlighted in *Septem punctis* either had already been addressed or were ruled out as being unacceptable. From the perspective of an aspiring author, there was little point in courting notoriety by explicit identification with a programme that was rapidly becoming viewed as the province of dangerous dissidents.

Septem punctis

De septem punctis idolatriae cristianae is a rare case among the writings of Paracelsus where it is possible to ascribe a date of authorship with some degree of certainty. This tract was the product of an author in his early thirties. Considering that medicine had been his main source of income, the exercise shows an amazing degree of competence and confidence in this secondary field of activity. Indeed, Theophrastus confronts his brief like a seasoned religious controversialist. As a piece of writing, *Septem punctis* is accomplished and it maintains its high standard across a remarkably wide range. It is also evident from the text of *Septem punctis* that some of the important issues mentioned in passing were being subjected to more searching examination elsewhere.

The overt confidence displayed by Theophrastus in *Septem punctis* suggests that he was fully conversant with the theological and political debates that were raging around him at this date. Quite plausibly, this wider competence reflects experience gained in his previous travels, which might well have taken him to Augsburg, Nuremberg or Strasbourg, all of which were active centres of controversy and the popular press. He must also have been familiar both with the more accessible expositions of the leading controversialists and opinion formers such as Luther, Karlstadt and Zwingli,[12] but also with a sample of the tide of pamphlets by more marginal figures, including laymen like himself. *Flugschriften* produced at this date were often effective and commercially successful and they demonstrated the high level of ability of a substantial group of writers, who emerged not merely as minor exponents of the ideas of the religious leaders, but as able and independent thinkers in their own right. As a consequence of this capacity for initiative, these unknown figures from modest backgrounds were catapulted into positions of wider celebrity or notoriety. Theophrastus recognized an opportunity to make common cause with these interlopers, many of whom were, like himself, hard-working professionals, or even artisans. Although they came from the lower middle ranks of society and were known only within their particular callings, they possessed abilities that seemed more widely transferable. In particular they recognized the opportunity to make a mark for themselves and their class in the political and religious arenas. The 'revolution of the pamphleteers' thus created an entirely new situation; the pamphlet medium gave shoemakers, bakers, cooks, spoonmakers, bellsmiths, carpenters and hay reapers an unparalleled opportunity to disseminate their ideas and establish themselves as independent witnesses to the great and continuing revival of faith.[13] Such an historic opportunity to give practical expression to the freshly reasserted priesthood of all believers proved irresistible to the young Theophrastus.

As was his habit, in *Septem punctis* Theophrastus provided no insight into his reading and sources of inspiration. His debt to the Bible was obvious, but unlike most lay writers he inserted no explicit references to relevant biblical verses, or lists of parallel texts. Since *Septem punctis* addressed itself to major topical issues, tracts by many controversialists might have influenced the thinking of Theophrastus about presentation or interpretation. He would certainly have recognized that many new and untried writers were emerging as independent commentators deserving of attention in their own right. A good impression of the intellectual range and effectiveness of these contributions can be gauged from Berndt Hamm's recent analysis of some of the more important tracts produced in Nuremberg in the run-up to the German Peasants' War.[14] The leading name in this lay circle was the gifted and prolific shoemaker, Hans Sachs, who was particularly attentive to religious propagandizing at precisely the date when *Septem punctis* was being formulated. The four reformation dialogues and other writings produced by Sachs in 1524 contained many points of agreement with the position adopted by Theophrastus.[15] Although Sachs broadly maintained the Lutheran line, other artisans tended to radicalize the debate. On the pneumatological spectrum applied as an organizing principle by Hamm, it is evident that Theophrastus approximates most closely to the spiritualist party, for whom Luther was only one influence among many. The spiritualist position is outlined by Hamm with respect to Hans Denck as well as to the artist Hans Greiffenberger, who produced no fewer than seven pamphlets between 1523 and 1524.[16] Examples of such success in gaining a public platform for the articulation of radical ideas were by no means isolated and must have been an inspiration to the young reformer based in Salzburg.

By virtue of his self-confidence and honourable background, Theophrastus was in a position to assume leadership among the heterogeneous army of lay theologians. Certainly he showed no inclination to deference and every indication that he regarded himself as an authority on the same plane as the leading reformers of the day. *Septem punctis* well illustrates this position of independence. Although this tract possesses many points of similarity with other sources, it never descends to slavish imitation; indeed, it contains many expressions of radicalism that would have been disturbing to the Lutheran or Zwinglian camp. Confirmation of Theophrastus's sense of parity with the religious leadership is evident from a short letter that he addressed to Luther, Melanchthon and Bugenhagen (Pomeranus), which is undated but roughly contemporaneous with *Septem punctis*.[17] His letter drew attention to a commentary - preserved but never published - that he had just produced on the first five chapters of Matthew, and which advertised his intention of writing yet further biblical commentaries.[18] Such urge to enter into dialogue with other reformers was by no means uncommon. For instance Conrad Grebel announced to Vadian that he intended to make contact with Karlstadt, Müntzer and Luther. This same letter announced that he and his associates were currently studying the Gospel of Matthew.[19] Nothing is known of the Lutheran response to the little commentary and associated letter submitted by Theophrastus, but from the contents of the commentary it is evident that its overt radicalism would have alarmed the Wittenbergers and identified the author as a figure belonging to the company of Karlstadt, Müntzer and Grebel.

The opening lines of *Septem punctis* indicated that the exercise related to a campaign he had been waging in public using any platform at his disposal, including hostelries and taverns. He freely admitted that his demand for the abandonment of a wide range of cherished and entrenched devotional practices had brought him into confrontation with the local church establishment. The first salvo of *Septem punctis* outlined the full scope of his critique of questionable church practices, which he believed were against the spirit of the teaching of Christ as understood from the gospels. On the basis of the inescapable gospel criteria, he was distrustful of extravagant church festivals, pointless praying and fasting, the extraction of alms, offerings and tithes, burial customs such as those marking the first month and first year after death, confession and the administration of sacraments, and all other related priestly usages and means of extortion.[20] In case of any ambiguity about his intentions, using approximately the order of the opening statement, the seven sections of his pamphlet outlined his objections to these practices in greater detail. In the final two sections he recapitulated some of the earlier themes and added strictures concerning pilgrimages, the veneration of the saints, indulgences, religious orders, fraternities and religious images. The listing of abuses in *Septem punctis* was widely echoed elsewhere in the writings of Paracelsus, indicating that he remained unrepentant about his early radical critique and that he was not inclined to soften his attitude on most points of contention.[21]

The accretions of ceremonial that had been built up over the centuries, although in some respects superficially edifying, were regarded by Theophrastus as counterproductive and subversive to the true mission of the church. Such practices were either irrelevant or a positive barrier to genuine Christian experience among the laity. The extent of this abuse needed to be recognized before effective remedial action could be taken: hence the need for critical enumerations of abuses such as that offered by Theophrastus.

Of its type, *Septem punctis* was conscientious and remarkably comprehensive. In his coverage of detail the author left no stone unturned, as witnessed by his trenchant comments on subjects like clerical vestments, church ornamentation, and dangers posed by music and musical instruments. His tract was in effect a concise encyclopaedic guide to abuses within the Roman church, carrying to a logical conclusion the campaign that had been instigated a few years earlier by Luther and Karlstadt and which had already sparked off hundreds of pamphlets from every part of Germany. Illustration 3 reminds us that the primary objectives of the *AntiChristi* sequence of Cranach's *Passional* was to reinforce the early Lutheran portrayal of the vices of the papacy.[22] Even light-hearted smears, like those delivered by Erasmus, served to stoke up the fires of anticlericalism.[23] As itemized by Flood, the predominant targets for criticism in the *Flugschriften* of the 1520s were: the veneration of saints, penance, relics, indulgences, pilgrimages, masses for the dead, the Latin mass and liturgy, purgatory beliefs, clerical celibacy, monastic vows, clerical immunity from civil taxes and laws, traditional ceremonies and festivals, and mendicant orders.[24] Of this list, only clerical immunities were not mentioned directly in *Septem punctis*, although from the adverse comment about the privileged existence of the clergy it is clear what attitude would have been taken by its author. Other writers often included summaries of the type given by Theophrastus. For instance Wolfgang Capito listed objectionable practices of the papal church such as: 'the mass; singing, reading and piping the canonical hours; the consecration of priests, churches, salt and other sacramentals; praying for departed souls and seeking aid from departed saints; the veneration of images; going to confession; performing works of satisfaction for sin; distinguishing times, foods and places' – all items that were touched upon in *Septem punctis*.[25]

A further summary listing that might well have been familiar to Theophrastus derived from the rhymed couplets of *The Wittenberg Nightingale* by Hans Sachs, published originally in 1523 and many times thereafter. Sachs ridiculed the regular offices and canonical hours observed by monks, nuns and priests, which he denounced as useless blathering. Also disparaged were their posturing, scourging and prostrations, their use of bells, organs, candles, banners, lamps, and their blessings of wax, salt and water, their pursuit of works of satisfaction, pilgrimages and veneration of the saints, their exploitation of indulgences and ceremonies like the kissing of images of the Lamb during the mass, and in general their creation of new altars, the endowment of masses and obsession with the building of chapels at great cost owing to their lavish decoration, all of which required the extraction of revenues on a large scale. In the view of Sachs, this vast edifice of church practice was without scriptural authority; consequently it was a vain exercise and testimony to human excess.[26] The same themes were reinforced in a group of prose dialogues by Sachs, published in 1524 and reprinted on many occasions during the same year. The wide dissemination of the anticlerical propaganda of Sachs increases the likelihood that his work was accessible to Theophrastus. In view of the success of Sachs as a writer, inevitably his work contributed to building up a core imagery that was widely drawn upon by reformers such as Theophrastus. Yet it is noticeable that the common line was not followed in all respects. Sachs closely identified with Lutheranism, with the result that Luther's name was repeatedly and favourably mentioned in his writings. Despite the obvious opportunities for Theophrastus to follow suit in *Septem punctis*. Luther was never mentioned, and when he was invoked elsewhere this was almost invariably with the purpose of entering some strong note of reservation. This instance confirms that, from the outset of his career as a religious activist, Theophrastus was determined to maintain a position of resolute independence.

Articles and the Art of Remonstration

Little attention has been paid to the title and organization of *Septem punctis*.[27] Such questions are well worth considering because they connect with the issue of designing petitions of remonstrance, at a date when these experienced a massive leap in numbers and when they were becoming radicalized in content. *Septem punctis* ranks among the most pungent critiques in a class of pamphlets that was generally notable for its asperity of tone. It is helpful to establish precisely where *Septem punctis* fits into this niche in the *Flugschriften* market.

Goldammer speculated that the seven-article format was adopted because of the prevalence of number seven symbolism both in the folklorist and Christian contexts.[28] The popularity of this symbolism with radical thinkers is confirmed by its use as an organizing principle in a famous tract by Jörg Haugk von Jüchsen.[29] Theophrastus could draw upon support for seven symbolism on many fronts.[30] Both the German mystics and Anabaptists made reference to the seven gifts of the Holy Spirit.[31] Of equal relevance were the variant imageries of the seven holy virtues and their counterparts, the seven deadly sins.[32] Theophrastus may well also have had in mind the seven works of corporal mercy, as defined by Lactantius, since these would have been a natural complement to his seven categories of sinful practices, his own list of deadly sins, which in one place he calls 'the book of the seven damned works among Christians, devised by the earthly Lucifer, and through which the people are misled'.[33] It was also impossible to escape the impact of the altars devoted to either the seven joys or the seven sorrows of the Virgin Mary, the most elaborate and famous examples of which were among the outstanding products of devotional art of this period.[34]

In view of the predominance of seven symbolism, it is hardly surprising that, when the Swiss Anabaptists finalized their Schleitheim Confession in February 1527, it was expressed in the form of seven articles.[35] At this point it should be indicated that structurally *Septem punctis* was very different from the Schleitheim Articles and indeed the other confessions of faith, or the many statements of basic political objectives expressed in article form at the time of the German Peasants' War. Articles of this type were all products of careful deliberation and signified some kind of statement of agreed principles drawn up between the parties involved. By contrast, the seven sections of *Septem punctis* raised miscellaneous issues, great and small, and were discursive, unstructured and polemical. The aim was to deploy the materials to maximum rhetorical effect rather than draw up a legalistic framework for specific operational purposes. Despite this obvious structural difference, the concerns raised by Theophrastus overlapped with a great many of the statements of protest on religious and secular issues that reached their height at precisely the date when *Septem punctis* was drafted.

The habit of expressing grievances or aspirations in the form of lists of articles (often called theses) was extremely common. Precedents for these forms of representation went back well into the previous century. Such articles took many different forms, ranging from raw lists of complaints to set-piece scholastic presentations.[36] From Luther, Zwingli and the Anabaptists to the various camps among the peasant leadership, lists of articles were adopted for considered presentation of remonstrations and objectives to local or national rulers. Among the writers of successful *Flugschriften*, Otto Brunfels adopted the article format for his *Von dem*

Pfaffen Zehenden, which included various themes also touched upon in *Septem punctis,* but Brunfels was not a direct model for Theophrastus since, like many others using this formula, he opted for a long list of short articles, in his case nearly 150, whereas Theophrastus consolidated similar materials into seven omnibus articles.[37]

Theophrastus must have known about the increasing social activism of the citizenry and peasantry in the Salzburg area and the Tyrol. In this area, activists' concerns reflected a mood of discontent that had been simmering for a long time in many parts of Germany; by the autumn of 1524 formal statements of grievance were making their appearance. It was evident that embryonic lists of articles were being circulated, but most of the many variant lists of articles of the German peasantry were only finalized after Theophrastus had completed his *Septem punctis.* He may also have known about the lists of articles presented to the meetings of the Reichstag, which were widely circulated in association with the Reichstag at Worms in 1521, as well as in later meetings of the same ruling body. The two best-known types of demands for reform were the 'Hundred Gravimina' and the 'Neun Artikel', both of which touched on many themes developed by Theophrastus. Similar complaints were even more widely publicized in the pamphlets of Hutten, which were a further alternative source of inspiration for the young Salzburg reformer.

As is evident from his social-ethical writings, Theophrastus was sympathetic to the grievances articulated by the peasant leadership. Sets of articles emanating from the peasants also tended to have an evangelical and anticlerical slant that he would have found congenial. It should however be noted that classic statements like the Twelve Articles of the Upper Swabian Peasants, which were disseminated throughout Germany in many editions, were predominantly concerned with immediate economic grievances. Such issues were incidental to *Septem punctis,* which only touched on economic questions to the extent that these were within the orbit of the offending practices of the church. Nevertheless, in statements of grievances, the linkage between the evangelical and the economic was sometimes close and explicit. The final text of the Twelve Articles was thick with biblical citations and the whole remonstrance was presented as a natural corollary of the evangelical message.

More relevant, in view of their likely accessibility to Theophrastus, were the expressions of grievance emanating from Salzburg. These demands must have been in circulation for some time before they were formally sanctioned. The best-known version was the twenty-four Salzburg articles, completed at the end of May 1525, which was exceptional among the articles of the German Peasants' War in the prominence it gave to the evangelical theme and to complaints about abuses within the church. Not only were these articles furnished with a long and aggressive theological preamble, but the first nine and longest of the articles were concerned with the misdemeanours of the priesthood and extortionate practices within the church. Their tone of passionate denunciation left no doubt that the local archdiocese was regarded as a profiteering tyranny, which is exactly the impression communicated by *Septem punctis*.[38] The rest of the Salzburg articles focused on grievances against all classes of landlord, among whom ecclesiastical bodies occupied a place of special prominence.

Unwittingly nor not, *Septem punctis* constituted an obvious complement to the twenty-four Salzburg Articles, and the two documents should be seen as sharing a similar perspective. Theophrastus must have been familiar with the lay dissident movement that was taking shape in the Salzburg area among miners, peasants and citizens. The degree to which he had any foreknowledge of the twenty-four articles, or of related expressions of grievance, must remain a matter of conjecture.[39] However, it is safe to speculate that, in the heat of the moment, both friends and enemies of reform were likely to conclude that Theophrastus was a fellow-traveller, and indeed perhaps an ideologue of the wider reform movement.

A further instance illustrating the appeal of the article format is provided by Conrad Grebel. In September 1524, Grebel opened up a correspondence with Thomas Müntzer by setting down a list of twenty-five articles addressing issues of common concern.[40] Grebel intended to launch a dialogue, but owing to the instability of the times his letter was lost from sight and perhaps was not even delivered to Müntzer. The first nine articles addressed issues concerning music in church services; many of the remainder related to reform of the Eucharist; others touched upon themes such as idolatry, church buildings and vestments; while as an appendix he raised the issue of taxes and tithes. The parallel with *Septem punctis* is therefore perhaps closer than is superficially evident, indicating that Theophrastus shared many of the same preoccupations as his Anabaptist contemporary.

Perhaps the closest parallel to *Septem punctis*, among the great variety of article formats, was provided by Jörg Vögeli, a town official, soon promoted to become city clerk of Constance. Vögeli's *Schirmred ains layeschen burgers zuo Costantz* was completed in February 1524, published shortly afterwards in Constance, and a year later in Basel.[41] Vögeli's *Schirmred* owes its origin to the mounting problem of indiscipline among priests and preachers. The growing number of priests displaying evangelical sympathies provoked punitive action from local disciplinary bodies. Commonly, complaints against preachers were expressed as a list of articles to which the offender was expected to reply. Penalties ranged from expulsion to execution. Arraignments of suspect priests took on the character of test cases, as for instance the twenty-four articles aimed at Matthias Zell in Strasbourg in late 1522. The accusations were eloquently defended by Zell himself, thereby enhancing his standing and further weakening the position of the already declining old church party in Strasbourg.[42] Zell's lengthy *Christliche Verantwortung* (1523), although nothing like *Septem punctis* in format, in the course of its diatribe drew attention to very many of the same abuses, and it criticized them in the same manner. When the authorities in Nuremberg became concerned about the views of Hans Denck, their famous schoolmaster Andreas Osiander was commissioned to deal with him. In January 1525, Osiander drew up seven articles seeking clarification mainly of Denck's views on the Eucharist. After a brief exchange of views, the spiritual reformer was expelled from the free imperial city.[43]

Disciplinary controversies in Constance were influenced by events elsewhere, perhaps mostly by the arraignment of Martin Idelhuser of Ulm in 1522, who faced charges summarized in twenty-two articles.[44] The Idelhauser case set a precedent for a more concerted attack on indiscipline in Constance itself. Here, thirty-four articles were drawn up against Bartholomäus Mätzler. The latter was a minor figure, but his problems were elevated into a test case by the *Schirmred* produced by Vögeli, which was an ambitious, polished and radical statement amounting to some 20,000 words. This statement represented the views of the growing faction favouring a distinctive Constance conception of reform. Accordingly, the *Schirmred* was immediately circulated to the civic authorities to stir up support for this campaign.

Like Theophrastus von Hohenheim, Vögeli prominently styled himself a layman, but neither of them allowed this limitation to inhibit their criticism of the clerical hierarchy. Vögeli's tract was somewhat longer than *Septem punctis*, but it was similarly organized under seven headings. The first dealt with tithes and the removal of treasures and decorations from local churches. The second was concerned with clerical vows, civic oaths and masses endowed in memory of the dead. The third section listed objections to canonical hours, alms, anniversaries, candles, masses, bells and vigils for the dead. Like Theophrastus, Vögeli produced a long list of objectionable practices, ranging from many of the existing sacraments to specific traditions such as the blessing of monastic orders and their members, the consecration of churches, cemeteries, chalices, vestments, crucifixes, lights, salt and water, the use of special altar cloths or vestments for priests celebrating mass, feasts and fasts, and other practices lending themselves to superstition such as the baptism of bells. The fourth section was concerned with the sacrament of holy orders and the question of clerical marriage. In the fifth section Vögeli challenged the hierarchy of the Roman church and called for power to be transferred to a devolved 'universal Christian church'. Such changes inevitably envisaged strengthening the position of the laity and reducing the authority of the priesthood. In the sixth section, Vögeli argued for narrowing down the sacraments to three: baptism, marriage and the Eucharist. In the seventh section he attacked practices associated with the veneration of the saints and the Virgin Mary. It was accepted that all saints should be held in respect, but not to the extent of elevating them to threaten the unique mediating role that belonged solely to Jesus Christ.

The content of the seven sections of the *Schirmred* and *Septem punctis* was differently distributed, but it can be seen that they cover the same ground, at similar length and from a broadly compatible perspective. Also, as confirmed by other writings produced at this date by Vögeli, his theological perspective was remarkably in tune with Theophrastus. Both were primarily concerned in their tracts with the problem of abuse in the old church, but both authors developed a sense of the way forward for an evangelically inspired church in which the authority of the laity would predominate. The need for the intervention of Theophrastus was highlighted by the direction of events in Salzburg, where Archbishop Lang and his advisers were actively tightening up ecclesiastical social discipline in exactly the opposite direction to that advocated in *Septem punctis*. The declaration summarizing the pre-emptive strike of the Catholic hierarchy dates from May 1525, and coincidentally was also divided into seven sections.[45]

The Assertiveness of Commodification

Adverse commentary on many church practices in *Septem punctis* was conducted within a wider framework of criticism. Theophrastus fully reflected the mounting sense of grievance at all levels in German society concerning the financial burdens imposed by Rome, which seemed to have expanded to the point where the system represented a thinly disguised system of extortion. This issue elevated resistance to Rome into a major political crisis upon which there was a consensus extending well beyond the embryonic reformation movement. The complex and grinding system of levies, including the bizarre devices associated with indulgences, occasioned a tide of popular resentment and indignation that was exploited by religious reformers, who were not slow to recognize an opportunity for advancement of themselves and their causes. Demands for redress were expressed in different ways by Hutten, Karlstadt and Luther, while the same complaints were given colourful expression by writers who were even more in touch with popular opinion.

Reformers believed that the papacy presided over a system that was corrosive in its effects and embodied corrupt practices that had infiltrated all of the institutions of the church. Everything going on in the church was suspect on account of the prevalence of monetary transactions. Over a long period, by slow accretion but recently at an accelerating rate, the church had become subject to the same process of commercialization or commodification that was prevalent in the civil sphere, but without the attendant advantages of normal commercial transactions. Church and state were two arms of the same economic system, geared to exploit the poor and concentrate wealth in the hands of the few. Instead of acting as a vehicle for refuge and protection, the church had been transformed into an exploitative system that was more obviously offensive and offered fewer powers of redress than the rest of the commercial system. This outcome seemed completely incompatible with the principles of Christian liberty that were taking root at this date.

The fear of the growth of usury and commercialization in general was deep-rooted among medieval thinkers. Tauler described covetousness as the worst of the seven deadly sins and the cause of the greatest evils in every sphere of society. He complained that all creative endeavours were corrupted by covetousness. The church, and indeed the whole of society, was accused of being in the grips of simony, the sin to be abhorred by the church more than any other.[46] Condemnation of the practice of purchasing the remission of penalties, especially the remission granted to souls in purgatory through papal indulgences, was central to Luther's Ninety-five Theses. In response to the popular proverb 'As soon as coins ring out in the collection box, souls spring out of purgatory', Luther complained that the only effect of these offerings was to augment profits and feed the avarice of the church.[47] Luther concluded that the whole ecclesiastical hierarchy had abandoned its vocation to preach the word and was instead preoccupied with the accumulation of material possessions.[48]

Commodification was elevated into a prominent theme in the early writings of Karlstadt. He complained that empty words were the only benefits derived in return for the huge payments made to Rome. The papacy was in major respects a mechanism for cleaning out the purses of the Germans.[49] Such faults were repeated at every level in the system. Karlstadt pointed to the indignity of foundations, monasteries and collegiate churches competing for the bag of money supposed to be devoted to the care of souls.[50] He took exception: first, to obligatory tithes, rents and other levies demanded on a regular basis, secondly, to further exactions obtained through moral leverage exercised by the mendicant orders, and finally, to the fees charged for the whole range of services provided by the priesthood. Collectively these exactions constituted huge gains for the priesthood and were looked upon with total distaste by the reformers. Any asserted benefits, such as the maintenance of church fabric, the provision of clergy, or charity to the sick or poor, were regarded as minimal compared with the extravagant resources devoted to ostentatious decoration or the personal gratification of the priesthood. Karlstadt drew the contrast between the ignorance and negligence of the priesthood and the extravagance of their style of life.[51]

In the very first of his works written in the vernacular, Hutten issued a powerful call to the German nation decisively to reject all forms of profiteering by the church.[52] In his advocacy of Luther, Sachs expressed outrage that the sacraments of the church were riddled with charges; he pointed out that priests displayed great ingenuity in evolving devices for extracting fees in connection with every aspect of their work. The church was thus reduced to a body of tradesmen. Since priests habitually cheated their flock, they were no better than wolves in the sheep-stall, while Rome, as the head of their hierarchy, was the presiding genius responsible for this skinning of the innocent.[53] The same message was conveyed in the woodcut illustration accompanying this poem, which shows a flock of sheep standing at the mercy of a pack of wolves and other voracious predators. Reflecting the popular indignation occasioned by the commodification of religious practices, this theme was actively exploited by the pamphleteers, many of whom unearthed curious examples of ingenious devices for extracting money for services undertaken by the priesthood. Collectively the *Flugschriften* built up an impression of scandalous practices that were out of control and which were undermining the credibility of the church.

From the above remarks it is apparent that leaders of opinion such as Luther actively connived with a growing tide of criticism of questionable church practices. In writing *Septem punctis*, Theophrastus von Hohenheim must have appreciated that he was adding his voice to a strand of anticlerical agitation which commanded a wide consensus of support in many parts of Germany and even existed as an undercurrent in Salzburg. The accumulated evidence presented in *Septem punctis* was used to build up a picture of the overwhelming materialism of the church. In his own lively manner, Theophrastus dwelt upon the preoccupation with

monastic and church buildings and their embellishment, the multiplication of endowments, the elaboration of church practices and corporate
developments, all tending to support a massive body of functionaries
who served no useful purpose and whose ill-gotten gains were used to
pay for an artificially affluent lifestyle. At the same time less glamorous
yet essential functions such as preaching the gospel, care of the sick and
support for the poor were seriously neglected. He discussed almsgiving,
pilgrimages and indulgences at some length to indicate the extent to which
the priesthood was involved in the exaction of money, which brought little
benefit to donors or the needy and instead was diverted for the purpose
of enhancing the comfort of the priesthood and their dependants.

Theophrastus employed the Magi attending the birth of Jesus to
reinforce his message. The Magi presented the Saviour with the most
valuable gifts, but these were of no consequence to the child, since
neither Christ nor the Father recognized any merit in material offerings;
yet it was evident that the Magi aspired to the true faith and were worthy
in their hearts. On this account the Magi were confirmed as a model of
exemplary practice for later generations of believers. On the other hand,
Herod and his legion of imitators in later generations were obsessed by
materialism. Money was no more than a superficially tasty titbit (*helkückle,
höllküchlein*) in the eyes of God. Although the goodwill of priests and
magistrates might be purchased by such offerings, their materialism was
offensive to God. Such practices needed to be completely eliminated,
since they reflected obsession with the values of the natural world and
were a barrier to the Holy Spirit and to the operation of divine grace.
Theophrastus saw no evidence that the 'new Herods' or 'new jerusalamite
hypocrites' who sat on the Roman throne were alert to the need for
emancipating the church from this endemic materialism.[54]

According to his estimate of the alms given for the purposes of the
poor and sick, only one heller out of each gulden reached the intended
recipients.[55] Charities for the poor were an ostentatious swindle.[56] On the
basis of this misappropriation of alms, the priests and their dependants
lived like lords, while the poor were fed on kitchen waste.[57] The egregious
avarice of the priests at the expense of the poor led Theophrastus to draw
liberally on the rich treasury of relevant pejorative epithets assembled in
the *Flugschriften* of his allies.[58]

His anger was all the greater because this situation was so obviously
contrary to the example of Christ and the apostles, who placed healing the
sick and help for the poor at the centre of their commitments.[59] Despite
this scandalous situation, Theophrastus noted that the abuses remained
unchecked; hence the weeds flourished in the cornfield. The so-called

Christian priesthood continued to enjoy their well-endowed benefices, being supplied with possessions, accommodation, ample rents and rich offerings, which conferred on them high prestige, dignity and authority. On that account they enjoyed ample opportunity to satisfy their appetites for food and drink, all of which served to maximize their profanity, luxury and impurity.[60] Noticeably, in *Septem punctis* Theophrastus downplayed the sexual relations issue, which was uppermost in the expositions of most other critics, but this was not an oversight. The habit of the priesthood in consorting with prostitutes and keeping mistresses was prominently mentioned elsewhere in his consideration of abuses by the priesthood.[61] As indicated by the epigraph on page 70 above, ten years after *Septem punctis*, when he was becoming known as Paracelsus, it seemed that things had changed very little. He concluded that the priests were willing to make any concession which might enable them to hang on to their material possessions. In particular he mocked their liking for luxurious clothing, labelling them *belzpfaff*, indicating the wearing of furs, with undertones about their habit of fleecing their communities and their reversion to being false shepherds or ravening wolves in the clothing of sheep.[62]

Against Commodification

Septem punctis not only contains a lively portrayal of the decadence of the church, but also conveys a positive message. Already at this early stage in his writing, Theophrastus was committed to combating the seemingly inexorable spread of commodification throughout the Christian church. In the first place, he proposed to reform the sacrament of penance, which was scarcely an original idea, since penance was one of the first targets identified by many other reformers, including Luther; however, the approach of Theophrastus had some differences of emphasis.[63]

On account of offering remission from the temporal and purgatorial consequences of sin in exchange for money, the 'trade' in indulgences, which burgeoned in the early sixteenth century, seemed to exemplify the dangers of commodification. As Erasmus observed, it seemed as if the Philistines were in the ascendant, fighting for the earth, preaching earthly rather than heavenly things, advancing material values rather than those appropriate to divinity. The modern Philistines detracted from Christ's message in the interests of the many who stood to gain from the traffic in indulgences.[64] In his *Moriae encomium*, Erasmus denounced the pope and the bishops for neglecting the harvesting of souls and, as a result of their obsession with harvesting money, for turning the church into a sea of profiteering (*mare bonorum*).[65] On the basis of concerns of this kind, in

1517 Luther issued his famous Ninety-five Theses on Indulgences which, although in many respects tentative, gave palpable encouragement to anti-papal agitation. Luther soon concluded that, on the right understanding of the sacrament of penance, works of satisfaction demanded as a penalty from the contrite were inconsistent with faith and incapable of gaining merit in the eyes of God. Accordingly, such expensive exercises as indulgences served no helpful purpose; indeed, on account of their materialism, they were a source of harm. As a consequence of this line of argument, works of satisfaction in general stood to lose their value. As a consequence of the debasement of this currency, a lucrative part of the income of priests stood to be liquidated; in the process their power was likely to melt away.

Zwingli and Grebel also adopted this line of argument. They regarded indulgences as the worst of all the abuses that had been multiplying for a thousand years; they pointed to the fright and despair generated by misuse of the sacrament of penance; indulgences were characterized as the selling of rights that should be freely given. Papal authority over the keys of the church was thereby transformed into a vehicle for maintaining the priesthood in luxury, which was incompatible with the principle of simplicity that was essential to the teaching of the gospels.[66]

Matthias Zell drew upon his first-hand experience as a professional *penitentiarius* to condemn penitential practices. The penitential system was operated by priests who were no better than 'robbers, thieves, usurers, simonists and benefice-eaters'. These functionaries liked to be called 'gracious sir, high and worthy lord', but were no better than foxes in a hen coop. Owing to these depredations, not only were the people being robbed, but Zell insisted that priests controlling these practices were guilty of acts of callousness in their impositions of penance, with the result that they were responsible for much personal grief and suffering.[67]

Theophrastus appreciated that, since a substantial number of the church practices to which he took exception were undertaken in the context of works of satisfaction, reappraisal of the sacrament of penance was unavoidable. He immediately opted for a more radical solution than was proposed by Luther. For fulfilment of this sacrament, he insisted that nothing was needed other than an expression of remorse, which echoed the call in his Matthew commentary for elimination of the greater part of the sacrament of penance. The only essential components in preparation for new birth were remorse and sorrow, which were sufficient protection against sin to maintain regard for the truth, absolving any need for constant reference to past sins or for the payment of penalties. Confession, fasting and absolution were dismissed as useless externalities.

Furthermore, he regarded the modern emphasis on the sacrament of penance as distasteful and entirely inconsistent with the New Testament. Neither Christ nor the apostles shared this concern; their emphasis was on faith, hope and love (the three virtues of medieval piety that were viewed as an exclusive gift of God) rather than on penance.[68] According to Theophrastus, penalties or works of satisfaction were otiose. Contrition was conceived by him as an entirely private act, not conditional on oral confession to a priest, or indeed on any act of public contrition as favoured by some of the radical groups. His further discussions of this sacrament were not always so radical, but in general Theophrastus was consistent with his instinct for eliminating ceremonial and enhancing the freedom of the laity from controls exercised by any priesthood.[69] Attack on prevailing practices associated with the confessional and the call for contrition both featured prominently in *Septem punctis*. Such an approach to repentance was regarded as essential for the restoration of the 'catholic' church in accordance with its original apostolic aspirations.[70] As he proclaimed elsewhere: where there was no true contrition and suffering, then there was no true love, and those who could not love God were not capable of loving their neighbour, hence not capable of fulfilling the basic commandments of Christ.[71]

Rethinking the sacrament of penance provided an opportunity for decisive reversal of the commercialization of church practices and a return to greater consistency with the spirit of the primitive church. The ideas of Theophrastus about renewal ran through the text and provided a unifying principle for *Septem punctis*. By a process of accretion over the centuries, the 'catholic' institution formed by the apostles had been turned into what he variously called *ecclesia*, *menschen ecclesia*, *maurkirche*, or *tempelhaus*, terminology indicative of a man-made edifice corrupted by ceremonial and dogma unsupported by New Testament authority. Only radical reversal of these changes would bring about a church organization that was again infused by the grace of God, consistent with the message of Christ and genuinely open to inspiration by the Holy Spirit.[72]

Betraying his debt to the antitheses much utilized by the mystics and Neoplatonists, in *Septem punctis* and widely elsewhere Theophrastus conducted his exposition according to a series of interconnected polarities such as the distinction between material and spiritual in the macrocosm, flesh and spirit in the microcosm, and generally between the outer and inner, or old and new, in each case the former being inferior to the latter. The Roman church was portrayed as being preoccupied with the material, the level of the creature, the outer ceremonial, most of which was attributed to the sin of pride. Its whole edifice was noisy, sterile, fruitless and symbolic of death. On the other hand, the true believers cleaved to the religion of the Holy Spirit, requiring the qualities of humility and the inner faith of the heart, which were silent yet truly fruitful and indicative of life. As an unregenerate body, the old church knew only the light from artificial sources such as candles and oil lamps, while true believers belonged to a different kind of church, in which they were enlivened by the inner light of the Holy Spirit. The existing system was organized so that material products of the church might be engrossed by the rich and powerful, whereas the new faith was open to the weak and the poor, who more readily understood and accepted Christ's commandment to love their neighbours, allowing benefits to be distributed in accordance with need rather than on the basis of avarice.[73]

Theophrastus characterized his revised ideas about the sacrament of penance, including the idea of contrition as stemming from the heart and being inspired by faith, as the sound fruit of a healthy tree rather than the worm-eaten fruit of a rotten tree. The sacrament of penance was a worthless externality, an *auswendig* practice, whereas personal contrition touched the inner being and was *inwendig*, and thereby conducive to salvation.[74] Precisely this distinction was the main point of the eleventh antithesis of Cranach: in the first part (with reference to Luke 17: 21, counteracting warnings of Matthew 15: 8–9 and Isaiah 29: 13), Christ insisted on the '*innerlich*' faith, whereas in the second part, indicated in Illustration 3, the papacy was displayed as being entirely preoccupied with '*äußerlichem*' functions. Consistent with his concern with this outer/ inner distinction, the short essay by Theophrastus on righteousness was entirely organized around the *inwendig/auswendig* dichotomy. For true righteousness it was necessary to follow the path of inner faith and the rule of the heart rather than the materialistic, outer legalism of the existing church.[75]

The *Schriftgelehrten*

From the perspective of Theophrastus, the priesthood presented an almost insuperable obstacle to the transformation of values that was needed in the church. This class had a vested interest in the maintenance of the status quo, acting as if the institutions with which it was engaged would suffer a loss of legitimacy if any concessions were offered. Responding to this intransigence, Theophrastus turned his criticism on the entire clerical profession.

The introduction to *Septem punctis* fastened on two priests, to whose names Theophrastus attached all the characteristic weaknesses of the contemporary church. Perhaps these were functionaries with whom Theophrastus had conducted real disputes, but it is also possible that they were literary constructs, invented for the purposes of the diatribe of Lucianic proportions that ensued in the body of the text. His two opponents alleged superiority on account of their academic credentials. They regarded it as an affront to be challenged by a person lacking standing in the field of academic theology. Like other radicals, Theophrastus was undaunted by such criticism and pointed to the precedent of Christ and his disciples, who laid down the foundations of the faith without having had any formal education and confidently confronted the scribes and Pharisees. These persecutors of Jesus Christ were identified as the forerunners of his academic critics.[76] Theophrastus retorted that he knew all about universities, indeed in many parts of Europe. From this position of strength, as well as on the basis of his professional involvement with natural philosophy, he declared that the training offered by the academies was an impediment to evangelical faith. He concluded that the authorities most highly regarded by theologians, from the ancient philosophers to the church fathers, were of dubious value, their writings better regarded as a kind of poetry rather than theology.[77]

As Biegger points out, *Septem punctis* represented an extreme expression of sentiments found elsewhere in Paracelsus's earliest writings. Priests were denounced as learned pedants (*schriftgelehrten*), whose effect was to concentrate attention on the dead print (*buchstab*) of the scriptures and so undermine the message of the living word.[78] Once framed, this radical critique of the clergy, with its overt distaste for scholasticism, was never seriously modified; if anything, it became more strident and more widely applied in the later writings.[79] In reaching this conclusion, Paracelsus was by no means isolated. Educated minds among radicals such as Grebel, Karlstadt and Müntzer, at a similar date and reflecting the same motivations, suddenly and vehemently turned against scholasticism. The humanism of Erasmus was associated with a distinct distaste for Aristotle and it embodied a sharp assault on the aridity of scholasticism.[80] In sermons and popular writings such as *An den christlichen Adel*, Luther too was prone to scathing verdicts on the deficiencies of the universities, Aristotle and the scholastics.[81] Such sentiments were immediately picked up and given wide publicity in *Flugschriften* by many different hands.[82] Consequently, the expressions of reservations about the learned clergy and scholasticism contained in *Septem punctis* were not unrepresentative; rather they reflected a mood that was becoming widespread and being encouraged by opinion formers.

Given his declarations concerning the intellectual bankruptcy of the priesthood, it is understandable that Theophrastus displayed a distaste for their whole mode of behaviour. He looked on their vanity and status consciousness with particular disfavour. The passion of the clergy for ceremonial splendour, ostentatious dress and exhibition of their jewellery only served to underline the endemic materialism of the system. Ever sensitive to the prevailing habit of using headgear to denote status and drawing on the bawdy of the *Fastnachtsspiele*, Theophrastus could not resist ridiculing the bishop's mitre, the two points of which he likened to the horns on the caps of fools. This comparison was reinforced by a passing reference to Kunz von der Rosen, the court jester to Maximilian I; the reader was no doubt expected to remember that in 1488 Kunz had disguised himself as a priest in order to assist his master out of an embarrassing situation.[83] In his commentary on Matthew, Theophrastus ridiculed the cowls and hats that were worn as status symbols. The former was no doubt specified because each order was associated with a characteristic cowl, and because the Latin term also meant fool. He drew attention to the two red silken cords that ended in a pyramid of tassels, which belonged to the red hat worn by cardinals and featured prominently on their coats of arms. These silken cords were also likened to the horns of the fool's cap. In other words, the chosen dress of the priesthood, intended for outward show, in fact indicated that they were no more than fools, who contrasted with persons of inner faith, whose hearts were preserved in purity.[84] The rich vocabulary relating to doltish stupidity was energetically exploited throughout the writings of Paracelsus, usually with the aim of deflating the rich and powerful both in the church and in secular spheres. His readership would be completely familiar with these associations, both from popular entertainment and from the more refined tradition exemplified by *Das Narrenschiff* of Brant and the *Moriae encomium* of Erasmus.[85]

It is striking that Paracelsus drew on exactly the same literary conventions to imply exactly the opposite connotations for *Narrheit*. In his *Prologus in vitam beatam*, he equated the idea of foolishness with the simplicity and purity found only in those who, through earnest sacrifice, were content with a life of complete poverty. He appreciated that such people were likely to be dismissed as complete fools, but only by adopting such extreme simplicity was there any chance of achieving inner contentment. In their case, foolishness was seen as great wisdom in the eyes of God.[86] From this perspective, the fool of Paracelsus was the equivalent of the *idiota* in Cusanus or in the *Moriae encomium* of Erasmus, able to apply the penetration of insight that was denied to the scholar.[87]

Paracelsus was deeply suspicious of the affluent classes and their academic coteries, warning that such groups were by their nature inclined to fall victim to wild fantasies and ultimately satanic influences. He told them to follow the example of children, simple people and disabled groups such as the deaf, all of whom, he believed, were blessed by God with uprightness, foresight and true wisdom.[88] Such conclusions were developed at some length. Society had a strong preference for the beautiful and perfect physical form and held that anything else was inferior. Paracelsus insisted that God was not misled by such superficial understanding. In the judgement of God, the misshapen person was not necessarily inferior, and indeed stood a much greater chance of escaping corruption. Wisdom was more likely to reside in the fool rather than in the guildmaster. Paracelsus advised villages to cherish the mentally handicapped, since only they were likely to preserve an uncorrupted mind.[89]

Paracelsus made active use of New Testament imagery derived from husbandry in his accounts of the depredations of the priestly class. Priests were like barren fields, unfruitful trees, or pernicious weeds in the cornfield;[90] they were the equivalents of *ratten* (*kornrade*, corncockle, *Agrostemma githago*); they corrupted religion and fabricated an idolatrous *rattengott*.[91] With respect to their function as confessors, Theophrastus played on the pun between confession (*beicht*, *peücht*) and stomach (*bauch*), which gave plenty of opportunity to dwell on the theme of the idleness and gluttony of the clergy.[92] He held that the clergy were no more than a bunch of parasites, guilty of the sin of pride which, as already noted, he accepted as the most intractable and serious of the deadly sins.[93] In reaching such a depressing conclusion, Theophrastus found himself in the broadest company. Notably, avarice and pride had also been attacked by mystics and radicals, including Johannes Tauler, who expressed similar thoughts in analogous troubled circumstances some two hundred years earlier.

False Apostles Ascendant

Owing to the political sensitivity of their position, Tauler and his confederates expressed themselves with reticence and calculated restraint. Nevertheless, it was evident that their sophisticated imagery was calculated to convey a strong sense of disapproval of the superficiality and inappropriateness of the religious practices of their day. In their eyes, the church had connived in the erosion of spiritual standards and had resigned itself to the growing tide of materialism that the mystics regarded as a menace to state and church. Such ebbing away of spiritual values signified the dominance of malign, creaturely instincts reflecting the recidivist tendency of human nature against which it was necessary to show continuous vigilance. Any concession to such inherited weakness of disposition was likely to obstruct the hard ascent to spiritual enlightenment that the mystics tirelessly preached.[94]

Similar disquiet was evident within many strands of medieval piety. Among these, mystical sources, such as the sermons of Tauler and the *Theologia Deutsch*, are known to have made a direct impact on Paracelsus and many others in his generation, ranging from Luther to the Anabaptists.[95] *Septem punctis* contained distinct traces of the influence of the mystics, and this bias persisted into Paracelsus's later writings. As already indicated, Theophrastus also expressed the more assertive spirit of indignation that became prevalent in his generation, and especially around 1525, when anger boiled over into social unrest.

The critical tone was set by Ulrich von Hutten, who mercilessly attacked the papacy for turning the church into a body of unscrupulous tradesmen. Instead of being the shepherd to his sheep, the pope was guilty of butchery (*schinderei*), submitting his flock to flaying and scarification (*schind und schab*).[96] Hutten issued an urgent call for the German nation to throw off the Roman yoke and rise up against the papal tyranny.[97]

From the adulation he received, it was evident that Hutten was expressing widely felt resentment. His sentiments spread like a forest fire through the medium of the popular protest literature to all corners of Germany. Luther allowed himself to be carried along with this tide in his early writings, and even when he became more cautious he occasionally lapsed into loose radical talk. In framing a political philosophy that was self-evidently conservative, he still managed to reflect some of his earlier dismay about the shortcomings of both secular and spiritual leaders.

In the first extended statement of his political philosophy, Luther followed Augustine in designating the prince and the bishop as the two arms of the modern state. But he was not particularly sanguine about the record of either secular or religious rulers. Princes and bishops were both derogatively likened to minor *junkers*. In fact they were fools, who liked to kick people around and interfere with matters of conscience. Unworthy rulers included popes and bishops, who were fatally misguided (*verkehrten, verkehrt bösheit*), perhaps a thinly disguised reference to the proverb *je mehr gelehrten, je mehr verkehrten*, which was employed by reformers of every colour at this date.[98] The priesthood had turned everything upside down. Reflecting one of his favourite themes, already noted above in a different context, Luther complained that they neglected their responsibilities of preaching of God's Word and failed to concentrate on 'inner' matters concerning the soul. Instead they were preoccupied with 'outer', secular adventures involving palaces and territorial gains. Owing to such obsessions, they indiscriminately flayed and scarified their subjects, imposing customs duties on some things, taxes on others, and even turning bears and wolves loose among the population to facilitate their pleasure in hunting. In the corruption of standards there was nothing to choose between secular and spiritual tyrants.[99] Despite such strong language, when it came to church practices Luther, notably in his *Invocavit* sermons of 1522, sheltered behind his principles of evangelical freedom and objection to the use of coercion, in order to support the status quo and impede the pace of change. He urged that caution was not only a necessary concession to the secular and religious establishment, but that it was essential to 'spare' the population from the cultural disorientation that would be occasioned by radical alterations in their patterns of worship.

The erstwhile allies of Luther responded with exasperated rage. Thomas Müntzer, employing the selfsame imagery of flaying and scarifying, conducted an inflammatory attack on Luther for tolerating a political situation that allowed for the continuation of abuse and exploitation.[100] The same position was adopted by Karlstadt, who attacked Luther for disingenuity in claiming that it was necessary to slow down the pace of reform for the sake of sparing the weak. Karlstadt regarded it as intolerable to accept any further continuation of practices that were self-evidently inconsistent with the Word of God. Accordingly, it was wrong to perpetuate a situation where the churches had been turned into houses of spiritual prostitution and adultery. If church practices were offensive to conscience and the Word of God, then nobody could possibly benefit from the continuation of such abuses. It was necessary to accept that any decisive act of betterment required immediate and complete elimination of such discredited practices.[101] Grebel's break with Vadian and Zwingli followed the pattern of fellow-radicals' disenchantment with Luther. Grebel agreed precisely with Karlstadt. The latter's idea of disingenuous compromise (*falsch schonen*) was seized upon by Grebel and made central to the articles he submitted to Müntzer, whom he suspected of backsliding, especially on the question of music in churches. As far as Grebel was concerned, there was no excuse for departing from the Word of God, which he believed provided definitive guidance on how to teach, govern, direct and make devout and improve the devotions of all manner of humanity.[102]

The outlook of Paracelsus, aptly summarised in the quotation at the head of this chapter, coincided precisely with the position taken by Karlstadt and Grebel. All of them blamed the crisis of the times on the interference of false apostles. A God-given opportunity for betterment in spiritual and secular affairs had been presented, but by 1525 it was evident to the radicals that a successful outcome had been prejudiced and the reform effort had been dissipated owing to disingenuous concession to biblically unsanctioned practices on the part of the politically astute, unprincipled careerists in the reformist camp. Paracelsus regarded their motive as naked greed. Their Christian teaching was adapted to the tastes of whatever sectional interest would least threaten their material well-being.

Throughout the writings of Paracelsus, the church was ranked first among the agencies of economic exploitation. The economic motive was regarded as basic to the manifold corruptions that were endemic both in the old church and among the rivals locked in contest over its replacement. His attraction to the Psalms of David was partly due to their sensitivity to issues of this kind. With reference to Psalm 139 (140), Paracelsus declared that David appealed for God's protection of the poor against their wicked exploiters, the powerful and the rich. Paracelsus's list of offenders was headed by priests and monks, but went on to include the nobility, all manner of profiteers and exploiters, including merchants and tradespeople. Like other critics, he used the terms *zins, zehnte* and *opfern,* as his favoured shorthand to describe the spectrum of dubious and unbiblical impositions on the poor. The whole establishment was engaged in cheating the poor, who were consequently reduced to humiliating ruin and martyrdom. Flaying and scarification well described their predicament. The priests were among the worst offenders; through their masses for the dead and purgatorial myths they exploited both dead and living indiscriminately. As a consequence of such abuses, Paracelsus accepted that the poor had been pushed to the limits of their patience. Yet he pleaded with them to be patient and await the justice ordained by God, which he assured them would surely come to their aid.

The objections of Paracelsus to resistance and resort to the sword were a firm matter of principle, but this could not be taken as acquiescence to the settlements proposed by Luther or Zwingli. Since rich and poor were irreconcilable, the confrontation between them represented an impasse that was likely to continue for a further brief interval of time. Paracelsus offered little expectation of change for the better in the short term. In the medium term, he held out distinct hopes for amelioration and reconciliation. God would see to it that the poor would witness retribution against their oppressors and then enjoy the benefits of universal betterment. In the meantime the oppressed classes needed to exhibit the greatest alertness to invitations to self-destruction by false prophets in their midst, the preachers, visionaries and sects who invited futile displays of force. No doubt such entreaties against rebellion were expressed more sharply on account of the recent disasters of the German Peasants' War. Patience was not presented as part of the experience of humiliation but as evidence of compliance with the single true spirit of righteousness or pure intent that could only hold sway among the weak and oppressed.[103] Such sentiments are reminiscent of Hutten, who promised that whoever joined him in good faith and pure intent in rooting out evils among the priesthood would be helped by God to achieve a real betterment in the affairs of the German nation.[104]

Disadvantaged groups were warned by Paracelsus to expect harsh treatment that would tempt them to relapse into fatalism. But they were assured that, on the basis of scriptural promises, all those who successfully preserved their integrity could look forward to a secure subsistence. With respect to his own situation, Paracelsus was confident that his chosen mission possessed firm scriptural sanction. After all, for those who were faithful to the example of Christ and the apostles, giving direct relief to the poor and attending to the sick was a major priority, the value of which could not be contested.[105]

Concentration on such practical objectives was designed to avoid any self-defeating confrontation with the authority of church or state. Adopting the high moral ground also placed envious competitors at a distinct disadvantage. Through the display of shrewd calculation, it seemed possible for the architects of change to enjoy a wide sphere of discretion, enabling them to contribute actively to immediate amelioration as well as engaging in planning for a better future: for Paracelsus, through such ambitious undertakings as his *vita beata* sequence of writings. In the light of such an analysis, notwithstanding the constraints of the system or the vulnerability of his own situation, Paracelsus was not overawed and remained convinced that the false apostles would be confounded and the corruptions of the system would melt away. He was therefore emboldened to join the ranks of the select circle of thinkers who addressed themselves to important questions concerning social and intellectual reconstruction. In the case of Paracelsus and others such as Michael Gaismair, their speculative plans were remarkably comprehensive in scope and audacious in character.

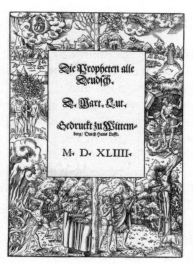

CHAPTER IV

CALL OF THE NEW

Im alten Leib aus Adam können wir nicht wandeln zu guten Werken. Der neue Leib muss den alten regiren, dann sind wir eigne Hausleute bei Gott, dann wächst aus dem alten Leib die edle Anthos.[1]

The escalating confrontation of Paracelsus with his antagonists in Basel forced him into a public defence of his position. He openly attacked the Galenic establishment and stumbled into a premature declaration of his own alternative thinking about medical theory and practice. The Basel episode was scarcely a textbook public relations exercise, but at least it demonstrated that Paracelsus was serious about his reformist intentions. Although he had published nothing at this stage, he had already drafted a handful of medical writings that tentatively pointed towards the ideas unveiled in his Basel lectures. In addition, he had produced some theological writings that provide insight into his basic motivations and general orientation regarding the reform imperative. This wider framework of ideas had the effect of reinforcing his doubts about the credibility of the prevailing beliefs and practices of the medical profession and it strengthened his resolve to strike out in a new direction.

His new outlook on medicine and natural philosophy never strayed far from the language and concepts evolved in the religious sphere of his work. He generalized his anticlerical critique and argued that in every significant respect the medical profession merited exactly the same damning verdict. In the spirit of the quotation at the head of this chapter, and consistent with the message of the New Testament, Paracelsus believed that reconciliation with God required rejection of the old and full embracing of the new.[2] Since Christ was the new supreme ruler representing the new dispensation, his injunctions concerning a complete reappraisal of traditional values had to be observed. Under the new law, it was necessary in every sphere of life to dispense completely with old ideas (*das alt is alles aus*). Such a complete reformation was the only course open to those aspiring to share in the life of the heavenly flesh of Christ.[3] As shown in Illustration 4, the dichotomy between the old and new was represented in the most dramatic forms in the propaganda emanating from the Lutheran camp, which underlined its own special perspective on the saving power of the blood of Christ.[4] Among the Florentine Neoplatonists, on the basis of his own apocalyptic fervour, Giovanni Pico de Mirandola had attacked the limitations of learning and called for a radical reappraisal, which he launched as his own new philosophy.[5] Innovation was therefore demanded from many directions, but Paracelsus was determined to be in the vanguard of this call of the new.

The Learned Professions under Siege

Most of the anticlerical diatribe embodied in *Septem punctis* was obviously more widely applicable. In particular it was transferable to the learned professions as a whole. Since the professions shared a similar background, education, training and cultural outlook, and occupied neighbouring niches in the social structure, they were subject to analogous shortcomings. Indeed, the professions had many points of direct contact. Lawyers commonly worked on behalf of clerical clients, while medical practitioners were employed in religious foundations. As their numbers and status increased, medical doctors aspired to privileges formerly exclusive to the clergy. On the basis of their long years of training, technical expertise and ethical standing, the three professions demanded, and largely received, a special place in society, which conferred on them immunity from taxes and civic duties and freedom from controls affecting other trades.

The advantageous position enjoyed by the professions was at the expense of their neighbours, whose taxes and civic responsibilities were proportionately increased. Adversely affected citizens inevitably wondered whether the professionals compensated the community with benefits proportional to the costs entailed. As major players in the local economy, religious institutions were the focus of most critical attention, and duly became a main target for reformers. When the latter gained the ascendancy, the whole system of clerical institutions was remodelled; in the process the monastic system was largely dismantled. Reformers promised that the reconstituted church would be better placed to perform its traditional office. The Reformation had the effect of buying time for the clerical establishment, although in the eyes of radicals the new was apt to be regarded as little better than the old.

Lawyers, as the second most numerous group among the professionals, were also in the firing line. They were intrinsically unpopular; the growth of their power, occasioned by the ongoing modernization and centralization of legal administration, deepened resentment among the many classes who suffered at their hands. The resentful populace appealed first to ancient rights and then to the gospels to support their grievances. Roman law was distrusted and was represented as a vehicle for the aggrandizement of lawyers who were depicted as aliens or intruders. Indeed they were often foreigners, or were portrayed as such. Modern law was criticized for its asymmetrical design; lawyers were recognized as facilitating exploitation by the church and big financiers. In the light of these tensions Strauss describes the situation in the early sixteenth century under the rubric: 'Lawyers: A Profession under Indictment'.[6]

Reflecting this state of siege, the legal profession was subject to a campaign of 'ridicule, abuse, rage, and scorn', in which opinion formers like Luther were pleased to engage for their own benefit.[7] On account of the high profile of grievances that had a legal dimension, reform of the legal system featured in the more deliberate plans for constitutional reform of such authors as Michael Gaismair, Johann Eberlin von Günzburg, Hans Hergot, Wendel Hipler and Friedrich Weygandt. The constructive interventions of such authors were broadly consistent with the mood of popular social resentment.

The *Moriae encomium* of Erasmus directed characteristic waspish comments against the clergy, who were abused at length, but he also made a point of indicating that lawyers and physicians were guilty of similar vices. Lawyers were accused of manipulating their work to maximize their profits. On physicians, in a way reminiscent of Paracelsus, Erasmus noted that 'the more ignorant, reckless and thoughtless the doctor is, the higher his reputation soars, even amongst powerful princes'.[8]

In his Latin dialogue *Praedones*, Hutten marshalled the full range of invective from Lucian to vent his anger on merchants, lawyers and priests. The complaints about priests and lawyers were analogous. Hutten was clear about the priorities of lawyers: they were bent on self-enrichment and would serve any agency, including tyrants, in order to further this objective. They pretended to be learned men and hence paraded about in costly robes as if they were scholars of standing, whereas in fact they neglected the sound arts and serious disciplines. The legal system was a sham that could be bent to any purpose.[9]

The part played by administrators and lawyers in adding to the burden of perceived disadvantage in town and village accounted for the prominence of grievances with a legal dimension in the petitions associated with the German Peasants' War. In the Tyrolean revolt a major target was the removal of Gabriel Salamanca, long-time Habsburg bureaucrat, *Generalschatzmeister* and *Hofkanzler*, who, among other things, was seen as a symbol of foreign domination. As a consequence of widespread animosity, Prince Ferdinand was forced to dispense with Salamanca and his entourage.[10] Not surprisingly, the misdeeds of lawyers were included in the social commentary of the *Flugschriften*. Typically, Sachs portrayed law as a snare liable to reduce laymen to poverty without producing any meaningful redress for their legitimate grievances.[11]

Paracelsus frequently attacked the legal profession, but his comments were usually made in passing. He was in no doubt that the law was subject to the same vices as the church and medicine. Law headed the list of professions (called by him 'religions') that were subject to corruption and were practised against the spirit of the scriptures. All of the professions under review were regarded as decadent (*tödliche*) and their works were depicted as pernicious foolishness (*narrenwerk*).[12] In another of his commentaries on corrupt branches of learning, he concluded that the relevant practitioners artificially generated divisions among themselves to communicate a spurious impression of healthy dialogue, but in fact this was intended to disguise their conspiracy to cheat the public.[13] As an example of the delinquency of lawyers, Paracelsus cited their tendency to advise rulers to adopt courses of action that were calculated to stir up conflict rather than peace, with the aim of enriching themselves and their clients regardless of their contravention of the commandments of God and the teachings of Christ.[14] He ended another commentary by denouncing in turn priests, medical doctors and jurists for displaying similar weaknesses. The first two were accused of slavish dependence on their learned authorities, whereas lawyers were attacked for slavishly following the orders of their princely patrons.[15]

The campaign by physicians to elevate their own status by improving their humanist credentials and identifying with the more established learned professions was largely successful. Such shrewd manoeuvres were not, however, an unmitigated benefit. Inevitably, physicians came under the same shadow of suspicion as their fellow-professionals, especially at the time of the German Peasants' War. Of course, since classical times, the medical profession had been the subject of adverse jibes, and this was evident in popular satirical dramas and *Fastnachtsspiele* of the early sixteenth century,[16] as well as in more extended presentations, the most famous example of which was Brant's *Das Narrenschiff*.[17] Medical practitioners also became caught up in the tide of social criticism associated with peasant unrest. The propaganda of the Reformation and peasant movements drew upon the established satirical tradition. Ancient and modern critiques were combined in the writings of Ulrich von Hutten. Following the Lucian precedent, Hutten readily linked physicians and lawyers. He declared that in olden times Germans had no time for physicians or lawyers; their affairs and health were in better order as a consequence.[18] Physicians also featured to some extent in the *Flugschriften* of this period. Citing the proverb that the biggest cheats were taken to be the cleverest citizens, Marschalck lamented the prevailing spirit of materialism, which induced the habit of exploiting even closest neighbours. The illustration that came most immediately to his mind was that of the medical practitioners who peddled potions and syrups, the cost of which was likely to ruin even their prosperous patients.[19]

Given the multiplicity of grievances upon which urgent action was demanded, abuses relating to medicine and the medical profession tended to constitute such a low priority that they were unlikely to capture much political attention, except perhaps temporarily, for instance at times of major public health crises. Physicians themselves stood to be disadvantaged by some of the changes associated with the Reformation, such as the loss of offices associated with religious foundations that were abolished. On the other hand, any adverse effects were offset by gains stemming from secularization and the evolution of civic structures. Such incentives help to explain why humanistic physicians quickly and contentedly blended in with the religious and social arrangements in centres where Protestantism took control.

Doctors under Indictment

Any complacency among the humanistic physicians was shattered by the activities of Paracelsus. Even though almost all of his writings were prevented from reaching the printing shops, his ideas spread around the many places that he visited in the course of his travels, while the content of his growing stockpile of draft writings was known to contain an explosive indictment of the medical establishment. In the short term, the damage from this critique was curtailed without difficulty, but at the cost of trauma which stretched out for a whole century.

The impact of the attack mounted by Paracelsus was amplified by its reference to the wider context. Naturally, he exploited all the traditional criticisms of doctors and the practice of medicine and he was able to make more effective use of this ammunition because of his personal engagement in the medical profession. But the traditional formulas were only part of his armoury. The line of argument pursued by Paracelsus was more damaging because of his thesis that corruptions of the medical profession were part and parcel of the general pathology of church and state that was the dominant preoccupation of contemporary social criticism. Accordingly, the faults of the medical profession were not ascribed to limitations in technical competence that might be easily addressed or become self-correcting over the course of time. Instead doctors were viewed as agents of the vices that were endemic to the system as a whole, in both its spiritual and secular dimensions. Unless they could prove otherwise, the medical profession was assumed to share the same shortcomings as the other professions, especially the priesthood. If medical practitioners rejected this analysis and refused to implement root and branch reform, then Paracelsus believed that they should face appropriate sanctions from their communities and expect in the course of time to be subject to the more serious sequel of divine punishment.

By habitually melding together his treatment of medical, theological and social issues, Paracelsus made sure that the medical establishment faced the true seriousness of its situation. Such a mode of attack allowed him to reiterate and amplify his religious message while at the same time stigmatizing his medical competitors, whom he characterized as embodying the worst excesses of the priesthood. For instance, in the opening and closing sections of *De caduco matrices* he assessed the performance of priests and doctors in the light of Christ's instruction to love one's neighbour and give aid to the sick and poor. Like the radicals in general, Paracelsus attached profound importance to these particular commands. By his own actions, Christ demonstrated the priority that should be accorded to these humane practices and expressed his dismay at the refusal of priests and others to respond to cries for help from the sick. According to Paracelsus the church and monastic orders were quite as delinquent as the priests and Levites at the time of Christ. The extravagant liturgical and ceremonial practices of the church were calculated to overawe the people, distract attention from their neglect of the poor and give the appearance of caring, while in practice the clergy siphoned off as much of the proceeds as possible to support their own private comfort.

It was concluded that medical doctors shared these same vices. The books produced in their high schools equipped them with an elaborate body of useless knowledge, derived from lifeless print. Such fabricated learning gave no reliable insight into the appointed order of nature or into the principles of medicine; that could only derive from direct experience and required the motivation of the heart. Out of false theory the medical doctors generated incompetent practice.[20] Their professional work was no better than the 'sweet words' emanating from priests. The mainstream of this profession was therefore no better than apostates, scribes and Pharisees. The offenders artfully disguised their shortcomings and consequently were able to continue to extract generous fees from their patients, although, in reality, like priests and monks, doctors neglected their duty to Christ and served the purposes of the Devil. Because they spurned gifts dispensed by the Holy Spirit and were obsessed by pride, doctors became victims of their materialistic instincts, inducing a general corruption in values as a result of which, although medicine was full of opportunities for improvement, it was dominated by error.[21]

Paracelsus played on popular sentiment by drawing the comparison between medical treatment and indulgences wrung out of peasants to support the endowment of churches. Both were expensive and produced no beneficial result for the people; both priests and doctors rejoiced at their good fortune, while their victims were left to lament their ill health and suffer anxiety about the fate of their souls.[22] In redrafting this comment Paracelsus introduced the equally explosive comparison between medical practitioners and mendicant monks. The latter were called by their customary derogatory labels which denoted pestering parasites (*clamanten, geilern, parfotten, holzschuern*). Also, medical practice was lumped in with the veneration of church images and therefore judged to be a variety of idolatry (*kothauer und contrafeit ölgözen*). Both professions were attuned to be superficially appealing to the common man, but their services were of no more value than piles of rubbish.[23]

Such colourful invective, dominated by caricatures of the various offending parties and sometimes approximating to dialogue form, were characteristic of many contributions likely to crop up at any point in the writings of Paracelsus, but especially at the beginning and end of books and chapters. Such satirical digressions became an even more evident feature of his writings after his experiences in Basel. An early example was provided by *Bertheonea*, his first significant surgical work, which survives in incomplete form.[24] This compact but ambitious book was intended for the technical market, perhaps designed to supersede the compilations from medieval sources that were at that date the dominant available product. Following the usual pattern, publication was long delayed; *Bertheonea* finally appeared in print only in 1563. The Foreword, in its variant forms, as well as other sections of this work, retailed frank admissions about the standard of the available technical literature and the level of competence of Paracelsus's competitors. The technical sections were introduced by a sustained comedy, quite up to the standard of the contemporary stage work of Pamphilus Gengenbach of Basel and Niklaus Manuel of Bern and obviously intended to entertain, but also with the serious purpose of heaping ridicule on the entire medical profession and deriding their standard professional procedures as activities more fitting for the province of the pantomime.[25]

Characterizations of medical practice by Paracelsus were never formulaic; their continuing prominence in his writings testifies to their propagandistic value; but they also provide a reminder of the overriding relevance of ethical and religious considerations. This element in his writing also confirms the high priority attached to communication with the widest audience. His readers would immediately recognize parallels with the satirical literature or the *Fastnachtsspiele*. Paracelsus made sure that medical doctors retained their reputation as prime candidates for the ship of fools. It is unlikely that he drew directly upon Lucian's satirical depiction of medical practitioners; he was more likely to be familiar with echoes of the classical author in the essays of Erasmus and Hutten, both of whom prefigured the sharp criticism and boisterous style adopted by Paracelsus in dealing with the professions, although neither they nor any other contemporary German author developed the critique of the medical profession with anything like the intensity found in Paracelsus.

The spirited satire on the vacuous learning of his opponents in the *Paragranum* made extended reference to the comparison between medical practitioners and the minor clergy. Both classes were accused of being engaged in practices that were of no more worth than the antics of actors participating in *Fastnachtsspiele*. Their academic or liturgical posturing was designed to deceive their clients and extract from them the maximum fees. In the case of medicine, patients risked their lives by falling into the hands of these academic impostors (*bacchanten*, meaning wandering scholars but also blockheads). Such practitioners were so incompetent that any artisans, even humble leather tawers, were likely to be superior in their abilities in medicine. Because of the protection of God and the wonderful self-healing powers of the human body, recovery often took place. As a consequence, the peasantry were apt to be deceived into thinking that learned doctors were in possession of real skills, although all of their actions stemmed from foolishness (*narrheit*).[26] In practice, the peasantry was not entirely deceived. Reflecting the low estimate of medical practitioners, in popular parlance these money-grubbers were caricatured by coarse nicknames like Dr Kelberarzt, Dr Starwadel and Master Gimpel, the apothecary.[27] Elsewhere Paracelsus held this Dr Starwadel and his apothecary, Master Hemmerlin, responsible for embezzling the charitable donations to hospitals and thereby turning these institutions into dens of thieves (*spelunca latronum*).[28]

The medical schools at Freiburg, Erfurt or Vienna appeared to be producing competent doctors, but the fictions of their teachings were so easily mastered that a fool (*gul*) could readily be turned into a doctor.[29] Like the faculties of theology, the medical schools were no more than peddlers of *narrheit*, which represented the path taken by the humoralist, pseudo-medicus or other uncritical minds who placed themselves at the mercy of the will-o'-the-wisp.[30] In the case of Basel, for which Paracelsus developed particular enmity, its teaching represented both foolishness and cheating (*narrheit, bescheißerei*).[31] Their association with medical faculties gave doctors the chance to parade about in their academic dress, in gowns decorated with embroidered buttons and wearing doublets and berets, for which purposes they had developed a taste for red fabrics, all of which, Paracelsus speculated, was calculated to deceive the peasantry.[32] Their pretentiousness was reinforced by the habit of wearing jewellery featuring many kinds of precious stones. The whole effect was likened to fool's gold. On account of their underlying incompetence, they and their precious Aristotle and Avicenna deserved to be dragged into the mud, which was appropriate because of the taste of pigs for wallowing in mud. They ought also to be chased after by children in the street and be called '*narr, narr*'. The medical faculties were labelled *narren faculteten* and their ostentatious dress *narrenzeichen*, signs of their function as breeding grounds for modern Pharisees. Their ignorance of the Light of Nature was destined to be exposed, causing them to be recognized as unmasked fools (*entloffene narren*).[33]

Paracelsus obviously had personal reasons for wanting to turn the tables on colleagues who enjoyed greater worldly success. He asked who deserved to be regarded as play actors in medicine: the town physician (*stattarzt*) and others of the medical elite, or himself, slandered by them as a fool? There was no doubt that he would be vindicated and they would be exposed as frauds. On any correct understanding, court physicians deserved to be known for their flattery and thirst for money, while town physicians should be renamed as *statnarren*.[34] Predictably, Paracelsus concluded a similar characterization of the idle incompetence of his rivals by suggesting their eligibility for the ship of fools (*narrenschiff*).[35]

As his attacks on medical faculties and town physicians indicate, our reformer was not hesitant about insulting his better-placed contemporaries or their most cherished sources of wisdom. In calling for a wider frame of reference for medical theory, with respect to Aristotle's *Meteorologica* and its commentators, he called these works a great polyphemic fantasy. Those commentators who heaped artificial praise on their master were dismissed as *gugelhanen*, on which basis he relegated their work to the level of the pointless chanting of monks.[36] He took exception to such habitual deference to authority, which he viewed as a sure sign that the commentators were unconcerned about truth or utility in the matters upon which they commented, providing that their twaddle continued to bring in the money. The medical elite were engaged in an elaborate deception. They were nothing more than *buzi* or clodhoppers of the *Fastnachtsspiele*, whose destiny was to be unmasked, when they would be exposed as impostors. In the hands of such corrupt and undiscriminating intellects, medical practice possessed no firm basis or truth.[37]

The basic problem with the medical establishment was that medical training had not been revised to take account of the changing times. It was foolish and completely unrealistic to think that a system of medicine more than a thousand years old could be applied to the entirely different conditions of the day. As a consequence, doctors of medicine, despite all their finery, were less competent at medicine than the unlettered peasant. When the doctors realized the magnitude of their incompetence, they should learn from the example of the king of Nineveh, who ordered general resort to sackcloth and ashes as an act of remorse and sign of last-minute repentance.[38]

Underlining the seriousness of his indictment of the medical profession, Paracelsus found little to differentiate doctors from murderers. He alleged that they generated so much trauma that large amounts of useful agricultural land had been turned into graveyards to receive the victims of their mistakes.[39] He likened doctors to rampaging armies or hangmen.[40] Clerics and doctors alike were attacked for making their professions into dens of thieves (*spelunken*).[41] What kind of justice was at hand, he asked, when a petty criminal was punished with execution, whereas murderous doctors were rewarded with advancement in status? Such a double standard had made a mockery of civic values.[42] Civic authorities were blamed for closing their eyes to the mischief of physicians. By sycophantic means the latter had inveigled themselves into court circles in order to secure immunity from censure. Again, Paracelsus underlined the double standard of justice in action when the authorities pursued the lowest members of society to extract taxes on such things as caraway seed while allowing doctors to prosper on the basis of general professional incompetence and menace to the lives of their patients.[43]

A major priority for Paracelsus was detailing how the commercialization that was endemic in the church was equally rife throughout the
field of medicine. His concern about this problem is evident from his
Bertheonea. The tenor of the Foreword was determined by the author's
distaste for what he perceived as the dominance of commercial considerations in medicine. At the very outset he pointed out that in their
professional work doctors were faced with balancing considerations
of payment and health. Righteous doctors were preoccupied with the
fruitful work of healing the sick; for them payment was no more
important than chaff produced in winnowing. Only a practice conducted
in this spirit was capable of yielding the attention to detail necessary
for curing the patient and for gaining the level of understanding that
was freely available under the agency of the Light of Nature. His own
work was intended as a lifeline to practitioners and patients who wanted
to base their treatment on a more authentic understanding of nature.
Contrary to this proper, ethical standpoint, the normal course of practice
was preoccupied with filling the purse; hence the doctor was tempted to
bamboozle and cheat the patient.

Since they represented the most pernicious combination of arrogance
and incompetence, the worst offenders were found in the higher echelons
of practitioners. This elite was the equivalent of the vain and idle monks
in their alien monastic environment. The knowledge of these academically
trained doctors was at best derived from dribs and drabs of second-hand
information. They divided up into warring sects; pretended to follow
some favourite authority, ancient or modern; claimed to possess special
knowledge; and were inclined to make up elaborate recipes containing
mostly useless ingredients for which they claimed exalted properties.
Such types had become 'recipe makers', who had no real experience or
knowledge upon which to ground their prescriptions. In reality they
were idle dependants of apothecaries. Since they had no interest beyond
their comfortable world of cosy kitchens, their work was best described
as kitchen skivvying (*küchenarbeit*), everything being dictated by the
wish to scrape up bits of money, and certainly not according to criteria
relating to health.[44] The combination of idleness, vanity and avarice of
these self-appointed *hochgelehrt* added up to the sin of pride. Accordingly,
the academic doctors were at home among their own type, monks and
nuns, in foundations associated with the nobility and in the courts of
princes.[45]

Even the most learned physicians, who faithfully imitated Hippocrates
or Galen, were on the wrong course, since their knowledge was abstract
and at best only relevant to a distant place and time. The Greeks and

Arabs expected to force nature into their system rather than to base their ideas on nature. All the vain effort expended on the study of such irrelevant sources would have been much better applied in the direct investigation of diseases and cures. The medical faculties or 'High Schools' and their professorships or *stul* were condemned as the equivalent of the papal or *römisch stuhl*. On account of their exclusive concentration on the ancient authorities, such schools were only suitable for functionaries who were content to remain ignorant of the truth. Just as Rome was insensitive to spiritual health, so the medical faculties were unconcerned whether the sick lived or died.[46] In the end the doctors could not disguise the fact that they were unaware of the realities of nature. Their polypharmaceutical remedies were artful compositions, like impressive symphonies, but the sound was no more significant than the noise of a bee in a beer mug. His critics would no doubt dismiss him as a fool, but, Paracelsus insisted, they were guilty of rejecting the Holy Spirit and of turning their back on the dictates of nature.[47] The shortcomings of medicine and the natural sciences seemed all the more tragic because God, out of His mercy, had in His creation made generous provision for every need. All the professions seemed to share in the same tragic misjudgement. By depending on Aristotle, Albertus and Avicenna and their like, they had turned their back on the works of the Creator, which were the only legitimate basis for knowledge. They had opted for the tares rather than the productive fruit. As a result their practice was lacking in firm empirical support and their outlook was contrary to the Light of Nature. Since they had squandered their inheritance and were in thrall to the Devil, it was not the alleged dissidents such as himself but members of the sophisticated professional establishment who should be identified as enthusiasts (*schwermer*), sectarians or false apostles.[48]

Alluding to his important maxim, *alterius non sit* ..., Paracelsus pointed out that professional incompetence was an inevitable product of the economic system in which physicians worked. By reducing themselves to the position of servants to the rich, they sacrificed their basic freedoms. In order to support this kind of lifestyle, entailing maintenance of costly households and silken clothing, their judgements were dictated by the motive of economic gain. The only means to escape from this slavery and regain professional freedom was to revert to the apostolic way of life, and become like a totally unencumbered pilgrim (*lärer pilger*).[49] Paracelsus was therefore driven to the conclusion that commodification was subversive of the freedom essential for the effective practice of medicine.

The Labyrinth of Error

The powerful indictment of the old and of the strength of commitment to the new, although initially developed in the religious context, were generalized to the entire field of interest covered by the writings of Paracelsus. He believed that only absolute confidence in the providence of God would enable progress to be made in any sphere of human existence. The wilful failure of human beings to trust in God had led them into a labyrinth from which no escape was possible without a complete transformation of values. His medical and scientific writings were littered with lamentations about the error (*irrung*) that he believed was the hallmark of the traditionalists. For instance, in *De causis morborum invisibilium*, he underlined his own commitment to first-hand experience of nature, which he contrasted with the fantasies contained in the writings of his humoralist rivals. They were warned that their work would remain groundless unless they acted out of a genuine yearning for eternal bliss.[50] In his *Labyrinthus medicorum errantium*, Paracelsus spelled out this same message with respect to what he called the 'religions' of medicine and natural philosophy. Similar conclusions were applied to every aspect of his mission.[51]

Being consistent with his verdict on academic theology, in view of the depth of corruption and intrinsic intellectual limitations within the medical profession and all parts of academic institutions relating to medicine and the sciences, he was driven to favour root and branch reform. Such a radical course would involve writing off almost the entire literary inheritance and starting again from the beginning. As already pointed out, such a revolutionary approach represented an action of remarkable audacity, particularly considering that the humanist doctors believed they had already embarked on a massive and comprehensive task of reconstruction that seemed to be nearing its completion and was looked upon by its adherents as a proven success.

Paracelsus seemed to take little interest in this great and productive labour of his rivals. Since, from his perspective, classical sources were misguided and largely irrelevant to later circumstances, the humanists had embarked on a futile exercise. It is not surprising that he showed little acquaintance with humanist authors, even with the recent Neoplatonists, whose basic worldview was broadly compatible with his own. Although he displays obvious generic affinities with figures such as Marsilio Ficino, Giovanni Pico della Mirandola or Cornelius Agrippa von Nettesheim, there is surprisingly little evidence of specific reliance on their writings in the work of Paracelsus.[52] Of course, such authors may well have exerted influence without being cited, but as yet nobody has succeeded in making a convincing case for direct borrowing with respect to the authentic writings of Paracelsus. It tends to be categorically stated that Paracelsus was indebted to the *De vita* of Ficino and the *De occulta philosophia* of Agrippa,[53] but the only evidence of direct reference to these works is in spurious writings attributed to our author. In fact, of all the writings of Ficino, only the third part of *De vita* impinged directly on the specialist interests of Paracelsus. The accounts of magic in *De vita* and texts of Paracelsus possess some broad similarities, but these are perhaps best explained by their reference to common Neoplatonic sources. Even more obvious common characteristics were shared by Paracelsus and Agrippa, but it is unlikely that our reformer had access to *De occulta philosophia* before the publication of a full edition in 1533. Since the sprawling handbook of Agrippa was itself a compilation, Paracelsus may well have drawn upon similar antecedent sources such as medieval encyclopaedias, bestiaries and technical handbooks.

On closer inspection, most cases of alleged direct influence proved difficult to substantiate. For instance, Paracelsus seems to make two separate mentions of Techellus, a medieval author of great obscurity. It turns out that both citations occur in writings of contested authenticity; one possibly reflects a doubtful reading of the manuscript source. The more reliable instance located in the *Liber principiorum*, may well derive from a section on Techellus in Megenberg's *Das Buch der Natur*, which had been available in print since 1475.[54] Such use of Megenberg's popular medieval natural science encyclopaedia comes as no surprise, but it is nevertheless consoling to have some direct confirmation of the reading habits of Paracelsus. It is already evident that the Techellus instance is not unique and it may be that Paracelsus derived a fair amount of information from this source, which provided convenient indirect access to material from earlier medieval encyclopaedic surveys used by Konrad. Naturally, the complicated relationship between late antique and medieval encyclopaedias and bestiaries creates daunting problems for determining the definitive background source for the host of medieval transmissions that found their way into the publications of Renaissance authors.[55] Sources such as *Das Buch der Natur* possess the advantage that they were readily accessible and compact vehicles for the transmission of practical information. They were also relevant because of their broader speculations – for instance, in the case of Konrad, through exploring the macrocosm/microcosm analogy and through providing insight into the natural philosophy of Albertus Magnus.[56]

With respect to the broader philosophical orientation of Paracelsus, the following two chapters elaborate on his Neoplatonic worldview and its theological dimensions. Some of this grounding was obtainable from sources such as the late medieval German mystics, who exercised a major influence on Paracelsus and his contemporaries. Such writers provided a congenial general framework, but Paracelsus must have been familiar with some authors who addressed more specific natural philosophical issues. Of course, Ficino was an obvious source, but in practice his writings were an inconvenient point of access with respect to the particular requirements of Paracelsus. Perhaps a more likely candidate is Giovanni Pico della Mirandola, especially his famous Oration and his more expansive *Apologia*, both of which were accessible in the widely distributed 1504 Strasbourg edition of his *Opera omnia*. Paracelsus would have been attracted by many features of the presentation by Pico in the Oration, especially his exposition of Neoplatonic philosophy, but also by some idiosyncratic points such as his apocalyptic fervour, his appeal to the audacious instincts of youth, his advocacy of a new philosophy and his tendency to regard magic and the kabbalah as a joint endeavour, accorded the highest priority in his system of knowledge.

Although on grounds of principle Paracelsus was broadly dismissive of the standard authorities of antiquity, he found some of their basic ideas difficult to replace completely and they sometimes assumed prominence, especially in his early writings.[57] Later, his criticism hardened and the humoral system was attacked as an impediment to understanding, incompatible with the explanatory categories he was evolving.[58] Humoralism was even seen as a sinister influence. For instance, in calling for a new approach to the physiology and pathology of excretion, he firmly concluded that humoral theory was a barrier to understanding. A more accurate interpretation required attention to the seats of deposition of excrements and to their characteristic and diverse chemical compositions. The whole system and its limitation to four humours seemed inconsistent with the approach that Paracelsus was advocating. A better basis for understanding was the macrocosm–microcosm theory, which he believed would immediately expose the humours as irrelevant. This approach was helpful because it allowed for an idea of human anatomy comprised of many definable organ sites, each corresponding to an equivalent location outside the human frame.

Paracelsus never tired of drafting lurid caricatures to communicate the pernicious weakness of a medical practice based on humoral theory. He pointed out that in the treatment of a fever lasting for twelve weeks his own direct approach would be to complete the treatment in ten days, whereas the Galenists would stretch treatment out over the whole term of the fever. In the course of this time they would use syrups, laxatives, purgatives, a great variety of special foods, and temperate drinks such as julep (rose water), much theorizing and many soothing words, without exercising any effect before the disease had run its natural course; in effect, this allowed the patient to recover autonomously.[59]

Humours had been made into a 'profession'. In fact they were nothing more than an arbitrary construct without legitimate philosophical foundation. Such fictions stood in the way of the aspiration to turn doctors into *medicis naturalibus*. According to the reformist conception, doctors should only adopt ideas consistent with the course of nature. Such reorientation would establish a sound grounding in philosophy, astronomy and other natural principles. With such understanding they would appreciate that the four humours were a fiction and no basis for their profession. Humoral theory was an alluring piece of sophistry adopted by the medical faculties to give the aspirant doctors a command of clever-sounding doctrines, enabling them to claim some exclusive expertise. It suited the system to leave these assumptions unchallenged, but support for this artificial construct had the effect of separating doctors from more discerning minds. The only way to reintegrate doctors into the intellectual community was for them to abandon their current ways and rehabilitate themselves according to entirely different standards.[60]

From the earliest stage of the medical writings of Paracelsus, represented by sketches such as the *Volumen paramirum*, the great luminaries of antiquity were generally subjected to blanket condemnation. He appealed to his contemporaries to grasp the chance to transcend the false teachings of the Aristotles, Platos, Virgils, Catos and all of their type.[61] Generally he indiscriminately lumped in masters with their interpreters and treated all as equally pernicious in their influence. For instance, he warned his reader not to fall into depending on books produced by the 'Tantalorum', a category that included a diversity of types such as 'Galeni, Avicennae, Averrois, Drusiani, Guidonis, Rogeri'; instead he appealed for serious students to turn directly to the books that God the Creator had written.[62] To call the traditionalists creatures of Tantalus was not without its point, since this mythical figure, although the son of Zeus, was addicted to self-indulgence and betrayed the trust of his father owing to his unbridled tongue, for which he was cruelly punished in the afterlife. This representative list of culprits was appropriately headed by Galen; after him, the next obvious candidate for dismissal was Avicenna, author of the most authoritative textbook used in the medical faculties, with Averroës meriting inclusion on account of his role as a leading interpreter of Aristotle. Whereas the humanists drew a sharp distinction between the Greeks and the Arabs, Paracelsus saw both as expressing the same vice.

Three successful medieval medical authors were also lined up for criticism. Guy de Chauliac was author of the most competent and widely used surgical handbook; and Rogerius had produced an older surgery in the tradition of the School of Salerno. The final author was Pietro Torrigiano (Drusianus), a notable and productive early fourteenth-century commentator on Galen. As a selection, the authors included by Paracelsus constituted a fair representative list of the standard authorities of his day. Such compilations were therefore not haphazard or eccentric, but confirm that he was well informed about the tastes of his contemporaries in the medical faculties.

Judgements on suspect authorities by Paracelsus were not confined to predictable candidates and they were not limited to a few names mentioned repetitively. In the course of his writing Paracelsus made occasional, but always casual, reference to a wide range of medieval sources. Such famous collective works as the *Articella*, or popularizations such as the *Viaticus*, seem to be mentioned only rarely in his writings.[63] It is difficult to draw conclusions about such citations, but it may be that the close proximity of the references to the *Articella* and to Jacobus de Partibus (Jacques Desparts) indicates that Paracelsus was familiar with Desparts's *Collecta in medicina* from the version included in recent editions of the *Articella*.[64] Following a similar line of thought, it is notable that in two separate places Paracelsus condemns an identical list of five medical authors on surgery, Guy de Chauliac and Roger Frugardi (Rogerius) together with Leonardo da Bertapaglia, Lanfranc, and Teodorico Borgognoni.[65] At first sight, such citations suggest that Paracelsus had access to a good range of standard books. In fact all of these authors were collected into one of the standard editions of the surgery of Guy de Chauliac. Other texts included in this collection were criticized elsewhere in the writings of Paracelsus. Accordingly, he may have derived his seemingly extensive knowledge of sources from just a few collective volumes. In some cases his familiarity with specific authors may not have extended beyond acquaintanceship with their names as they were listed on title-pages. A commentary on Galen by Symphorien Champier listed half a dozen commentators on Galen among his sources, including Torrigiano and Gentile da Foligno, both of whom Paracelsus cited occasionally and condemned without showing any evidence of having read their actual writings.[66] Similarly, it is possible that a couple of passing references to Abulcasis, an important Muslim medical authority, were made because of the inclusion of his work in the surgery of Pietro d'Argellata, which was mentioned often by Paracelsus.

Following the above line of argument, a case could be made for the very limited reading of Paracelsus, but this would be undermined by his reference to some authors who were not widely anthologized, such as Johannes de Garlandia, the supposed author of alchemical works more widely ascribed to Martin Ortolan or Hortolan. Not surprisingly, Paracelsus showed ready familiarity with the major names of medieval alchemy. Just as in the case of surgery, he displayed confident command of standard alchemical practices. Considering the importance he attached to the chemical arts, it is striking that, as with surgery, he gave few specific references to the relevant literature and almost invariably wrote disparagingly about the leading authorities in this field such as Ramon Lull and Johannes de Rupescissa.[67]

In alchemy as in other aspects of his work, Paracelsus's reading may not have been as extensive as he insinuated, but the confident way he handled the subject-matter of most branches of medicine indicates that he was writing from a position of strength. His command of technical subject-matter was quite up to the standard of the best among his contemporaries. The extent to which this competence was the result of dependence on specific literary sources has not so far been demonstrated and must therefore remain a matter of conjecture.[68]

Although Paracelsus was unhesitant about his negative verdict on the standard authorities of medicine, it is noticeable that he was sparing in his remarks about some of the leading figures, particularly from distant antiquity, some of whom were of mythical origin. Hermes Trismegistus was sometimes mentioned with respect, although he was blamed for burdening medicine with the fallacy of the four humours and the chemical theory that metals were derived from mercury and sulphur. Hermes and most of the late classical authors were blamed for slavishly imitating previous authors.[69] This endemic weakness in the literature of medicine was judged to replicate the damaging sectarianism that had affected religion. Too readily authors divided up into factions, which then proceeded to enter into bitter conflict. Then, instead of seeking knowledge from its source in nature, they were satisfied to imitate their masters and keep on chewing over the same old and unreliable information.[70]

When examining the historical record for untainted sources of inspiration from the past, Paracelsus found it difficult to locate any figures worthy of respect outside the confines of the Bible. In their various ways the patriarchs and prophets of Israel seemed estimable prefigurations and were represented as embodying inspired practices. As a direct link with the early church, the Magi from Saba and Tharsis or the apostles and Dionysius the Areopagite were also aptly venerated. Of the figures from the more distant past, Plato was rarely included among the most malign influences. Hippocrates was sometimes criticized, but more often absolved of blame, which counts as a rare instance where Paracelsus was in accord with the humanists.[71] At one point he wondered whether Apollo, Machaon and Hippocrates were in their localities responsible for all the wonders that were attributed to them. He concluded that in their case the legends were correct. Figures from Greek mythology, such as Apollo, Asclepius, Machaon and Podalirius, were also just as real to Paracelsus as the sages of the Old Testament or the Magi from the Orient recorded in the gospels. The Magi reminded Paracelsus that the arts of magic originated in the Orient and that nothing good had come out of the west. Tragically, these fertile ancient traditions had gradually become corrupted and extinguished. He presented his select spiritual elite from among the ancients as exemplars of sound practice, in contrast to the useless sophists who succeeded them. These in turn spawned an even worse tradition of charlatans, mercenaries and hirelings, with whom Paracelsus was in competition. As a self-proclaimed representative of the *Hippocratorum*, he expressed gratitude to the authorities of Carinthia for according him respite and asylum, which was a belated and rare privilege in his life.[72]

As is evident from the above remarks, Paracelsus was not predisposed to a positive assessment of the philosophical legacy of anitquity. He neither shared the prevailing optimism about the classical past that took root among his contemporaries nor subscribed to their idea of a *prisca sapientia*, thought by the humanists to account for the faultless transmission of philosophical wisdom from the distant past to the present. In line with the dichotomy between the old and new represented in Illustration 4, he regarded the entire intellectual legacy of classical antiquity as suspect. Whereas the Renaissance thinkers placed a high value on the widest spectrum of ancestral writers, Paracelsus was inclined to discard all types, including the poets who exercised particular appeal on his Neoplatonic contemporaries. Their estimate is reflected in the Philosophia woodcut shown in Illustration 2, where prominence is given to the medallion featuring Cicero and Virgil as the joint representatives of Latin culture. Contrary to this construction, Paracelsus frequently inveighed against the intrusion of poetry into theology and natural philosophy. The poets and the mythology they elaborated only rarely featured in his writings. The only parts of the pagan tradition that were tolerated by him were those that could be readily integrated into the honourable traditions of the patriarchs, who were accorded a prominent role in the origination and transmission of magic. For example, in Illustration 4 Moses, their leader, is shown at the top performing magic and at the bottom leading the patriarchs, shown as an embattled group huddled into a defensive corner.[73]

The idea of a disjunction with the past was reinforced by observations about the completely changed environment of the modern world. The population of the earth had expanded, but the wisdom implanted by God had not prospered; it had survived for a time in its ancient centres, but then it had gradually been corrupted and lost. In all spheres of life and learning there had occurred an apparently irrevocable process of decay. Wisdom seemed to have reached a climax at the time of Solomon, while medicine prospered most under Hippocrates. Since then civilization had gone into a downward spiral, not arrested by the advent of the Christian message. In the light of such irrevocable decline, Paracelsus concluded that his own times represented a crisis of depressing proportions.

The only possible relief was offered by the rediscovery of the message of Christ. Only this offered a means of sure salvation and general restitution. It was at last possible to envisage liberation from the burdens of oppression. Reflecting on the depth of transgression into which western Christianity had sunk, Paracelsus regretted that his contemporaries still wilfully rejected the courses of action that were acceptable to God.[74] He lamented that his times were dominated by false witnesses and malign forces that exercised unrelenting control over the legions of the blind that continued to dominate his age. Since such reactionary groups had invested heavily in their baseless knowledge, seekers after the truth were likely to face a hostile environment and were destined to be locked in contest with enemies inspired by *fliegenden geister*.[75] The hazardous circumstances of modern times were also a reminder of the incremental alterations that had taken place throughout the cosmic system. Among the adverse effects were new environmental threats and entirely new diseases, requiring new names, new modes of explanation and new forms of treatment. It was obviously absurd to expect that medical writings originating a thousand years earlier would be remotely suitable to meet the needs of such a dangerous situation.[76]

Radical Renewal

The above exposition aims to communicate the depth of anxiety of Paracelsus concerning failings that he feared were endemic to both church and state. Those in power abused their privileged position and abandoned their duty of care for the poor. Many of the basic functions of society were subject to distortion and malfunction because middling groups such as tradespeople and the learned professions were permitted to neglect their callings in the interests of the pursuit of avarice. Germany enjoyed neither peace nor social harmony, while the gathering pace of growth in the economy produced only unrest as a response to perceived inequities in the distribution of wealth and anger at the large extent of unaddressed poverty.

Deliberations concerning their troubled times drove critics to the conclusion that current corruptions were deeply rooted. Central to their experience and analysis was dissatisfaction with the church, both in its religious role and in the exercise of its power over secular affairs. Unimpressed by the dominant streams of influence within the church, many critics concluded that fundamental changes were required in order to restore Christianity to the practices of the primitive church. The individuals and miscellaneous groups who rebelled against the old church were equally disenchanted with the formulas adopted by the magisterial reformers.

Consistent with his general disposition, Paracelsus demanded the rejection of centuries of degenerate church practice and he even largely discounted the huge patristic legacy. With regard to written authority, the New Testament assumed paramount importance. Identifying with the theology of the New Testament, he blamed the excesses of the churches on their preoccupation with inappropriate laws and precedents from the Old Testament, which he represented as distortions that were the work of the Pharisees, Sadducees and Levites. Reaction against the modern Pharisees encouraged the explicit New Testament bias in his theology that was already evident in 1525 and continued throughout his career.[77] However, he retained respect for the Bible as a whole and drew liberally on books of the Old Testament, especially the Psalms, but many of his main propositions were exclusively derived from the New Testament; where it was a matter of contradiction between the two books, he firmly rejected the Old Testament option. With respect to the authority of the two parts of the Bible, he felt the Old Testament deserved to be treated with reverence, since it contained 'shadows', 'figures' or 'signs' premonitory of the content of the New Testament. The New Testament possessed higher status since it was the fulfilment of these earlier signs, on which account it represented the perfect 'light', rather than insubstantial shadows.[78] Paracelsus's conclusion was reflected by Cranach in Illustration 4, where the observer was directed towards New Testament images on the right as indications of the way forward, but on the left-hand side Moses and the prophets were also depicted in a most positive light.

Adoption of a scriptural orientation for belief was not without its problems, since it risked delegating control of interpretation to churchmen, theologians and university faculties, whose judgement and loyalties were suspect and whose interests were served by maintenance of the status quo in church and state. The interests of these *schriftgelehrten* as a social group were so bound up with the various establishments that they were unable to disentangle themselves from the traditions of authoritarianism that had brought ruination to Christianity. Accordingly, one of the hallmarks of the radical position was its stigmatization of the professional theologians, who, it was asserted, propagated a sterile philological understanding of the dead print of biblical sources, whereas what was required was a living understanding obtainable only through the free operation of the Holy Spirit.[79] The radicals held up the prospect of real rather than nominal application of the principle of the priesthood of believers, which involved investing complete responsibility in any person who displayed remorse and fear of God, demonstrating heart-felt faith, opening themselves to the guidance of the Holy Spirit, and pursuing the path of suffering as exemplified in the life of Christ. By bringing these new freedoms into full operation, it seemed possible to evolve religious tenets that were clear and universally acceptable to true believers. With regard to the scriptures, there was confidence that the meaning of impenetrable texts would be revealed by a process of independent diligent enquiry that was within the capacities of every person of normal aptitude; the 'common man', in the parlance of the times. Paracelsus drew upon a biological analogy to describe this process. The Word of God was like a seed, which in the care of the believer would grow to become a wonderful bloom, but in the care of the unregenerate this seed would wither away and produce no benefit.[80]

In the 1520s, the radical standpoint was shared by a wide coalition of reformers. Radicalism was at its height during the impressionable early maturity of Theophrastus, and therefore just before his reincarnation as Paracelsus. The radical perspective provided a lifeline and indeed inspiration to a wide social spectrum that perceived itself as undervalued and exploited. Radicals promised a genuine shift towards the democratization of faith. In its secular dimension, this outlook gave grounds for the optimistic belief that a great diversity of unheard grievances would become fully articulated and then be addressed. The radical movement accordingly helped to unleash capacities that had not previously been able to find expression. Given this new situation, many critics of the current state of affairs concluded that they were living at a turning point in history, when the old order had run its course and had nothing further to offer except the continuing erosion of Christian values and escalation of social injustice.

Radicals such as Paracelsus were confident that there was no inevitability about the continuing hegemony of the forces of Antichrist. Under the divine plan, as they interpreted it, the regenerate had been granted a decisive opportunity to intervene and change the course of events in the precious but limited period before the Last Judgement. This challenge was interpreted in many different ways. Reformers competed to evolve programmes for a decisive measure of betterment. The first priority was religion, but their schemes also implied a wider cultural reorientation. They envisaged immediate action with respect to pressing economic grievances and basic constitutional issues. As a consequence, their programmes often affected many areas of social life. As indicated earlier, in more radical circles there was a determination to root out the old and, without delay or concession, install a new order of religious and secular life based on strict adherence to the values of the gospels and the primitive church. Paracelsus powerfully expressed these radical aspirations, and his special mission was to point out the possibilities of their application in the field of medicine and the sciences. The previous section briefly summarized his conclusions concerning the dismal state of the medical profession, which accounted for the failure to unlock the enormous potentialities of knowledge vested in nature by a benevolent deity. In line with reformers acting in other spheres, although Paracelsus was depressed by the current state of affairs, he was confident that a better future was in prospect.

It is quite possible that the activism displayed by figures like Vögeli and Theophrastus von Hohenheim in the mid-1520s represented attempts to encourage the newly assertive civic leadership in both Constance and Salzburg to confront their respective ecclesiastical hierarchies and demand consistency with evangelical standards. Although this was not their primary intention, their programmes also had the effect of reinforcing the demands made by the peasant movement. Theophastus and Vögeli shared the widespread belief that they were on the threshold of fundamental change in the order of state and church. Vögeli repeatedly insisted that the time for change was 'now'.[81] In the introduction to *Septem punctis*, Theophrastus pronounced that the young represented truth, while the old stood for fabrication. In the terminal struggle between the two, the new was bound to succeed because it carried the stamp of genuine Christian inspiration.[82] At the beginning of his short commentary on Matthew, Theophrastus portrayed the recent history of the church as a Babylon and time of imprisonment. In his own times, he predicted, new and false prophets would arise, but the agents of falsehood were about to discover that their tenure would be short-lived.[83] Whereas Vögeli, like Sachs, deferred to the leading reformers of the day and was content to represent their thinking, Paracelsus was more self-reliant. Already in Salzburg he inclined to rank the magisterial reformers among the false prophets.

The antithesis between old and new was reiterated with great frequency by Paracelsus. The old/young distinction was in turn linked with other antitheses favoured among the radicals. The old/young symbolism was perhaps particularly attractive to Paracelsus on account of its links with biological symbolism. The new stood for fresh generation through the cyclical process of procreation, or for the regular pattern of seasonal rebirth operating within nature. On this basis he concluded that the party of the young represented the truth and the spirit, whereas the old guard were representative of fabrication and materialism. The latter would therefore be impotent to hold back the young. The failings of the old church reflected its slavish dependence on the Old Testament and its failure to understand the need for renewal. Paracelsus's critics were identified as the followers of Cain, a category which included the church fathers, bishops and theologians, whose knowledge was better classified as poetry rather than theology. By contrast, his own declared formulations were based on the inspiration of the Holy Spirit and the gospels.

Utz Rychsner, the Augsburg weaver and radical, attacked precisely the same targets as *Septem punctis*. Rychsner stigmatized existing ceremonials as discredited relics of the old law which were now exposed as intolerable under the new law that was gaining the ascendancy.[84] As attested by Illustration 4, which itself was widely known in many variant forms produced by the Cranach workshop and numerous imitators, the old/new antithesis was widely employed. The approach adopted by the Cranachs, Paracelsus and Rychsner was increasingly dominant, but it is worth pointing out that many of their allies expressed the distinction the other way round. Since they were engaged on the mission of reviving the early apostolic church, the old represented the traditional, unchanging and eternal values, which had been subject to corruption at the hands of the medieval church. As a consequence, innovations had been imposed that were contrary to the spirit of the apostolic church. From this perspective the new was rooted in original sin and reformation was needed to revert to older apostolic principles. This latter construction coincided with much of the social agitation emanating from local communities, who saw their ancient customs being undermined and replaced by new codes of law, enforced by university-educated lawyers who were seen as an alien force operating on the behalf of distant commercial interests. The preceding view was already evident in the Middle Ages among traditionalists who were alarmed by the incursions of new thinking.[85]

The above argument was developed at length by 'Judas Nazarei', a significant figure, albeit one who is still not identified with certainty.[86] The woodcut illustration on Nazarei's title-page aptly summarized his view of the basic divisions of society. On the left stood the pope, surrounded by the symbols of his authority and supported by a cardinal, Thomas Aquinas and by Aristotle, and below them stood their later adherents. To the right were located the icons of reform, headed by Moses and Aaron representing the Old Testament, an evangelist, Paul and Luther, together with other representatives of the church militant, who were ready to engage in the contest in support of the gospel.[87]

As a major influence on Nazarei, Luther, in the introduction to his edition of the *Theologia Deutsch*, also dissociated himself from the innovators and stressed that his exercise was intended to promote the return to older, more authentic values. Even Paracelsus occasionally remarked on his distaste for the *neotericus* or *modernischen secten*, including the influential *devotio moderna*. Notwithstanding the pretences of these groups to be reformers, in the view of Paracelsus they represented the spirit of the *stülen oder schulen*, so reminding the reader of the association between the Roman throne and the university faculties.[88] Elsewhere he attacked the pretentious *neoterici* or *moderni* for cobbling together their herbals from unreliable sources. On investigation, their information was found to derive from monks, nuns and old women; accordingly it was as worthless as tittle-tattle, no more robust than a church built on foundations of sand.[89] Of course both of his old/new usages had the same targets of criticism in mind and both embodied commitment to the complete overhaul of current practices. In the case of Paracelsus, as for other radicals, the call for reform possessed a distinct apocalyptic frame of reference, aiming to buoy up morale by arousing dramatic expectations of improved fortunes at some time in the foreseeable future. Paracelsus was more unusual in that he stressed the possibility of imminent amelioration, which prompted him to develop provisional ideas on a broad range of measures for social betterment. As indicated by the quotation at the head of this chapter, this optimistic prospect was offered as serious incentive to all believers who accepted the full discipline of the Christian message.

Works, Wonders and Signs

Already in 1525 Theophrastus recognized that it was possible to escape from the labyrinth of error represented by the confected, man-made systems contained in the doctrines of the old church. The New Testament offered the community of believers the promise of access to a higher plane of secure understanding (*rechter erkantnus*).[90] His heartening message concerning the imminent demise of the old and his almost utopian prospects for the new introduced a distinct ray of hope for the oppressed classes, who were promised relief after what seemed to be an endless experience of despair. Indeed the gospels seemed to contain firm assurance that there would be improvement in human affairs. His own programme was conceived as an appropriate response to this gospel message of hope, and was seen as laying the foundations for immediate, tangible and striking advances in all spheres of practical endeavour.

Paracelsus's analysis of the contemporary predicament had much in common with the dominant anthropology among his fellow radicals and their mystic precursors. In the first place, the long experience of degeneracy of the human condition was seen as a necessary consequence of material existence, inevitably reinforced by the disobedience of Adam and Eve, whose sinfulness had occasioned their expulsion from paradise. Siding with the mystics rather than the mature Luther on sin and justification, Paracelsus placed the emphasis on the positive and realistic prospect of redemption and reconciliation with God. Notwithstanding the transgressions of Adam and Eve, God, in His boundless grace and mercy, permitted all subsequent descendants of the original sinners to enjoy a life of spiritual and material fulfilment, in return for which all true believers accepted an unrelenting ascetic regime as a necessary expectation. The comprehensiveness of the endowment from the Creator was indicated by such testimony as the availability of herbs and medicines, that were provided for every eventuality. Such ready assistance was symbolically important and denoted that God, ever mindful of having created humans in His own image, retained an irrepressible instinct to provide for all conceivable contingencies of human existence.[91]

On the above analysis, all the descendants of Adam and Eve were granted ample inducement to strive for their salvation and for their subsistence. Naturally, figures like Paracelsus and Sebastian Franck placed their greatest emphasis on rewards offered for compliance with the message of Christ; they also conceded that the illumination offered by the Holy Spirit and Light of Nature had exercised a proportionate effect in Old Testament times. As the example of the patriarchs and prophets indicated, primitive piety was richly rewarded by religious insight, philosophical acumen and practical attainments.[92] On the other hand, the Old Testament also told the story of the depth of the penetration of evil, the dire results of which were evident by the time of Christ, as indicated by the malign reputation of the Pharisees.

Through the example of Christ's life, the sacrifice of his death, and glory of his resurrection, the prospect of regeneration was made available to his disciples and later generations. For Paracelsus and his radical contemporaries, Christ was the archetype of the new creature. Faced with choice, the unregenerate opted for the easy course, continued to take their nourishment from Adam and remained at the level of the creatures. By contrast, as indicated by the quotation at the head of this chapter, believers who opted for the more demanding path of renewal were eligible to reap the full benefits of transformation offered by divine grace through the agency of the Holy Spirit. No easy course was available to sincere believers, who were expected to observe profound contrition and take on a regime of humility and sacrifice following the example of Christ. By displaying commitment to Christ and fear of God, they might participate honourably in the sacraments of baptism and the Lord's Supper, signifying that they were free of the limitations of the flesh of Adam and eligible to become translated to a new level of kinship with the Creator and with Christ. All sincere believers thereby joined the communion of the prophets, apostles and saints. On the basis of ample authority drawn from the New Testament, such believers were allocated the status of a new birth, new body, new creation or creature, new world and New Jerusalem; they would transcend the limitations of blood and flesh, and would ultimately be enabled to defeat both disease and death. The Holy Spirit granted that the mean limitations of mortal existence would be replaced by a more noble alternative, variously characterized by Paracelsus as being like a quintessence, 'heavenly flesh', 'clarified' existence, or status akin to that of angels. Hence the new cadre of convinced believers were infused with confidence that ultimately they would achieve a state of perfection. Their new birth placed within human reach the possibility of salvation, redemption, resurrection and transfer into the realm of eternity. Such exceptional rewards were of course not to be fully realized until after death and the Last Judgement, but even during life they offered tangible opportunities for amelioration through their partial fulfilment.[93]

Optimistic expectations were obviously a great consolation to believers. It was also comforting for the oppressed to know that those who had prospered in this life were likely to come to a dismal end. The programme of writers such as Paracelsus possessed special additional salience on account of its direct relevance to the current condition of society. He reinforced the radical social critics' negative projection of the way of life and values of the privileged classes. Their vices incurred the penalty of exclusion from the ample rewards anticipated from the process of renewal. Those persisting in their life of luxury and wantonness fatally impaired their capacity for accessing the truths of nature and could not be trusted to handle such knowledge with responsibility. They were the equivalent of adulterers, who would pay the full penalty for their greed, betrayal of honour and abuse of their calling. The full benefits of amelioration would be allocated only to the poor and oppressed, whose condition of life and experience of sacrifice furnished them with the intellectual capacities appropriate to meet the challenges of renewal.[94] God would see to it that the select body of believers was rewarded in their arts and labours, which would duly flourish in the building of a New Jerusalem or earthly paradise. Compared with this utopian prospect held out to the suffering poor (*armen und elenden*), the proud social elite and followers of Mammon were promised harsh retribution, including the prospect of eternal punishment.[95]

Thanks to God's mercy, sinners were temporarily spared the consequences of their folly, although Paracelsus warned them that they had no grounds for complacency. The wonderful works of God had remained accessible during every single period or 'monarchy' in the history of civilization. On account of this predestined order, the current monarchy would be treated in the same way. As history had richly confirmed, the degenerate helped themselves to the lion's share of the secrets of nature, which Paracelsus presented as an unwanted dysfunction within the system. Such apparent injustice was an inevitable consequence of the operation of free will, which involved temptation and, on the part of the majority, the choice of evil and succumbing to the seductive lures of the Devil. The righteous seemed to be disadvantaged by their regime of humility and sacrifice. Paracelsus pointed out that the example of Moses and many other Old Testament exemplars of righteousness demonstrated that, when it came to confrontation with reprobate rivals, ultimately the righteous were convincingly justified. As indicated by the vignette in Illustration 4, the patriarchs were often obliged to draw upon magic in confounding their critics within and enemies without.[96] Believers should be confident about their prospects in the new situation of spiritual and material renewal that was on the horizon owing to the collapse of confidence in all the existing structures of authority.

There was, Paracelsus believed, an unparalleled opportunity for inventiveness and a complete reconstruction of knowledge.[97] History demonstrated that there was a continuous history of renewal in all of the arts, but the possibilities for transformation were insignificant until the full dawning of the religion of the spirit and inner experience. The moment had arrived for this full exposure to the joint action of the Light of Nature and the Holy Spirit, which would make evident the full bankruptcy of all old regimes. All previous knowledge would look like gross stupidity and be discredited owing to the failure to transcend materialistic values. Only those willing to reject the old leaven (*sauerteig*) inherited from the Pharisees, completely shake off the old dust from their feet, reject the old birth and embrace the eternal light of the Holy Spirit would enjoy the full benefits of the new birth.[98] Scholars, rulers, warmongers and merchants were warned that they all faced fearful consequences owing to their neglect of the inner spirit and inability to rise above the corrupting influences of their animal nature.[99]

Whereas most other radicals limited themselves to questions relating to religious experience or ethical issues arising directly from these considerations, Paracelsus made it his business to work out more fully the secular dimension of the argument about renewal. To amplify his forecasts about expectations, Paracelsus naturally drew on medicine and the sciences as his main examples, although it was evident that similar ideas were applicable also to other aspects of civil affairs. Relevant biblical texts, especially from the New Testament, were marshalled to provide convincing underpinning for his conclusions. As a consequence, many passages in the writings of Paracelsus are little more than strings of biblical quotations and short glosses. Such sources were not identified, partly because this was not his habit, but also perhaps because his intended readership was expected to be familiar with the same texts. No doubt he was confident that this mode of argument would be found both congenial and convincing by readers accustomed to the reasoning employed by reformers drawing on the medieval mystic tradition. Paracelsus artfully played to their favoured imagery and he made repetitive use of the scriptural quotations and proverbial expressions that they found most salient.

The following example illustrates his use of this approach with respect to a couple of short paragraphs drawn from the *Labyrinthus medicorum errantium*.[100] Paracelsus decisively sided with the advocates of free will. His astrology was strongly tempered by the insistence that every person was endowed with freedom of choice, a conclusion articulated in one of his most memorable proverbial expressions of biblical origin: *Der geist geistet, wo er will; ist niemands eigen.*[101] Given the corrupt disposition of humans and the wiles of the Devil, there was of course every incentive to opt for the *fliegenden geister* and fall back into traditional habits of thinking, which were suspect and led to all manner of erroneous conclusions. The only escape from this labyrinth was to banish the old creature and aspire to the new.[102] Such an exercise would involve a challenging act of discrimination if the pearl of wisdom was to be snatched from under the sow.[103] First it was necessary to be willing to pray, seek, knock and take the right door.[104] Only the discriminating believer would recoil from the allurements of the flesh and opt for the more arduous route of the spirit, and then reject the lifeless dead print communicated by the authority of learned pedants. Under the inspiration of the Holy Spirit, knowledge would be transformed and revitalized.[105] Only the path of spiritual enlightenment provided access to the highest forms of wisdom and secrets, denied to all those who failed to emancipate themselves from conventional values.[106]

More than his other radical counterparts, Paracelsus extended his message to consider the practical advantages stemming from spiritual enlightenment. Since the Creator was the source of all wisdom and yearned to restore humans to His own image, it was emphasized that the process of renewal would prompt the spontaneous flow of generous benefits to address all human needs.[107] Just as ordinary sinners knew how to meet the requirements of their children, God understood precisely how to respond to every need of society.[108]

The above extracts are characteristic of the thinking of Paracelsus, and the various components were reiterated with great frequency in the course of his writings. One further typical element, missing in the above passage, was the biblical promise concerning signs, wonders and works (*zeichen, wunder, taten*). Numerous biblical texts alluded to signs and wonders; especially prominent were episodes attributed to Christ and later, by the transmission of authority, to his apostles.[109] On the basis of a powerful impression gained from many texts, signs, wonders and works were recognized by Paracelsus as basic to the experience of the early church.[110]

Naturally, the thaumaturgical aspect of the primitive church was deeply appealing and it was taken as decisive evidence that replication of the same feats would accompany the process of spiritual renewal that seemed to be approaching its zenith. Signs, wonders and works were held out as a real expectation, but, in consistency with New Testament precedent, Paracelsus insisted that the full understanding of such phenomena was a privilege reserved for the congregations of true believers (*auserwählten*), who were joined by spiritual bonds and qualified to participate in the sacraments as outlined in his writings.[111] This represented a major qualification, but it was a further consolation to the long-suffering and oppressed believers that full participation in their congregational way of life would bring about tangible benefits denied to outsiders. Whatever the level of understanding granted to the normal run of society, Paracelsus wanted believers to understand that their special position of enlightenment through the Holy Spirit granted them the prospect of superior fulfilment, not only in the exercise of spiritual insight, but also with respect to an ability to exercise command over nature.

Paracelsus believed that the realization of heightened expectations for future amelioration depended on the initiative of an elite cadre drawn from the ranks of the community of true believers. Since such activists required very special aptitudes, they would be few in number.[112] This band of latter-day magi would exemplify the greater level of fulfilment open to those willing to grasp the full opportunities for spiritual enlightenment. Paracelsus was little interested in the path of elitist asceticism or esotericism, hitherto much associated with monasticism. Rather he emphasized that neither spiritual nor material rewards would be forthcoming without unremitting social activism and a strong work ethic. Such aspirations were open in principle to all believers. Those accepting the challenge of spiritual renewal were required to demonstrate conscientious application to their vocations and compliance with all the biblical commandments, with love of neighbour as a leading priority. For this purpose Paracelsus portrayed God as the master workman of the world. Humans were His labourers, who were charged to turn knowledge into works. To assist this effort, the Father had implanted His creative agent *vulcanus* in nature to catalyse the natural tendency to productiveness, but full fruitfulness was realizable only when assisted by conscientious application from the under-workers. Only by the sweat of their brow would their labours succeed.[113] In order to rehabilitate themselves, the learned classes needed to dispense with their academic gear, accommodate themselves to manual work, take on the begrimed appearance of the collier; then there was some hope that their medicine would work. Such characteristics of hard work were a true sign that they were treading in the footsteps of Christ and might aspire to a blissful existence.[114]

For such reformation of character, the learned classes, who were the equivalents of the *schriftgelehrten*, needed to dispense with their books and rely instead on their own efforts. As a path to knowledge, books were indeed inviting, accessible, but misleading. The established literature thrown up by the vocations represented the dead print that had exercised a stultifying effect in the religious sphere. The narrow but more profitable path required each person to be their own preacher and schoolmaster. Wisdom came from within, but it required constant inquisitiveness, consistent with the much-favoured injunction to seek and find of Matthew 7: 7. The Master rightly demanded from His workers consistent vigilance, since they were not born to sleep but to be wakeful, which was the only way to bring all works to their fruition. At this point Paracelsus drew attention to the parable of the wise virgins as an illustration of the need for preparedness.[115] Faithful to the intentions of the parable itself, the general emphasis on watchfulness, alertness and insightfulness in the writings of Paracelsus encouraged optimization of mental capacities and physical skills, and also it contained overtones about alertness to the imminence of the Second Coming.[116]

Like other mystics and radicals, he was greatly attracted by biblical sources relating to past states of paradise and the Garden of Eden. As already noted, he followed biblical precedent in using imagery relating to seasonality and various aspects of husbandry to illustrate favourite moral themes, such as extirpation of weeds in the context of retribution for sin, or fruitfulness as evidence for the reward of virtue.[117] Above all he favoured the metaphor of the fruit tree. Repeatedly he pointed out that the value of a tree was determined by the quality of its fruit.[118] The maturation of faith was likened to the ripening of a fruit. The believer needed to wait patiently until an inner feeling warned of impending ripeness, at which moment summer had arrived, symbolizing the time to act and the onset of a new age of fruitfulness.[119] Under the stewardship of believers the works of nature would prosper and be fruitful (*grünen und blühen*), a state of affairs that Paracelsus described as analogous to the condition of youthful chastity (*jungfraustand*), attainable only by the siblings of Christ and children of God.[120] Such unblemished fruitfulness marked a return to the condition of the primeval order of nature. As was consistent with the precedents described in Genesis, the highest fruitfulness was manifest in the older age. Paracelsus cited the hopeful contemporary signs of the resurgence of knowledge as a foretaste of the universal renewal that was held out as an expectation for final times.[121] As indicated by the passage at the head of this chapter, imagery relating to fertility was also selected to describe the regenerate household of God. Elsewhere, employing the imagery of growth, Paracelsus expressed his reservations about the attachment of excessive importance to the ritual of baptism. He warned that the outward sacrament should not be allowed to stunt growth and obstruct the full maturity, flowering and fruitfulness that were the rightful expectation of believers.[122]

Optimistic projections about the course of nature were characteristic of the general tenor of the writings of Paracelsus, which tended to place their emphasis on the generosity of the mercy of God. The systematic failings of mankind had produced no lessening of commitment on the part of the Creator. In common with the mystics, and applying their vocabulary, Paracelsus stressed that it was essential to the character of God to pour forth His grace. God made His material provision supera-bundantly (*überflussig und mannigfaltig*), sufficient to allow humans to subsist at the highest level of contentment.[123] Like the mystics, Paracelsus placed the emphasis on the Creator as the ground or spring from which the blessings of grace were derived without the use of any intermediary. Also, like them, he wrote about spiritual aspiration in terms of vegetative growth and fruitfulness.[124] Such metaphors were employed in the spiritual sense by the mystics, but in a broader context by Paracelsus, who duly accorded primacy to matters of faith, but also stressed the satisfaction taken by God (*wohlgefallen*) in making generous provision for every utilitarian need, not only of humans, but also of animals of all kinds.[125] Thus the virtues of herbs, the whole art of medicine, and indeed the whole of wisdom were seen as flowing directly from God without intermediary and they were available from no other agency. The basic requirement for intellectual renewal was recognition that the kingdom of God was the source of all wisdom. It was the duty of grateful recipients to prepare their inner spirit for reception of these various forms of knowledge. By this means they would act as the 'school of the ground of wisdom', in contradistinction to the rival high schools or academies, whose scholasticism represented folly and a labyrinth out of which it was part of God's purpose to lead His chosen followers.[126] The distinguished or heavenly school (*himmlischen schul*) delineated by Paracelsus was the recruiting ground for the apostles and prophets, who were later joined by all those eager to be instructed by God. The new generation of graduates from the heavenly school would demonstrate by the testimony of their fruitfulness and works that they were worthy of their elevated status.[127]

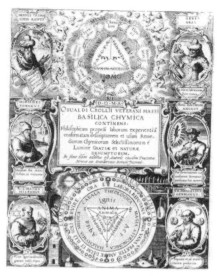

CHAPTER V

MATTER AND MAGIC

Die natur gleich ist in der zal und operation wie die trinitet ... alles nach der ordnung und monarchei götticher eigenschaft, zugleicherweis wie die bildnus des menschen von gott gehet.[1]

Integral to the process of renewal that Paracelsus believed was imminent was the expectation of return to the more perfect conditions that prevailed in former times. In Genesis and related texts, this earlier status was described as the exercise by humans of subjugation and dominion over all living things.[2] On the basis of scriptural assurances, it was certain that the anticipated transformation in the affairs of church and state would be accompanied by a restoration of human dominion over nature which, Paracelsus concluded, would involve the agency of the sciences, technical arts and medicine. Among the radicals Paracelsus was conspicuous for his advocacy of this concept of renewal. In light of such optimistic expectations, it seemed likely that in the short term the divine plan allowed for all manner of reforms and improvements, preparing the ground for the longer-term realization of such utopian objectives as a New Jerusalem. Paracelsus was convinced that progress towards such a blissful future would entail, as a matter of course, the triumph of his new philosophy.

Reflecting his preoccupation with medieval apocalyptic sources and their speculations about the periodization of history or procession of monarchies, in formulating his ideas about the new way forward Paracelsus presented himself as instigator of a new monarchy, set to outpace the best that all the preceding monarchies of medicine could offer.[3] He was convinced that the whole of the old order was bankrupt. As a consequence, despite the apparent invulnerability of his critics, they were destined to become discredited. In their place, Paracelsus was destined to establish a new monarchy of medicine. Under his leadership the Theophrastan sect would triumph, whereas his detractors would be reduced to the status of chimney sweeps. The unflattering portrait of the current decadent monarchy was embellished by images of abhorrent monsters, which assumed decisive significance through reference to the deformed creatures of the Book of Revelation.[4] Employment of apocalyptic imagery enabled Paracelsus to depict his mission as integral to the transcendental struggle between good and evil, with himself being allocated the role of divinely inspired arbiter, dispensing final judgement over his erstwhile persecutors.

Tria Prima

Paracelsus clearly faced the risk that he would be accused of operating with a false prospectus. He met this challenge head on by attempting to demonstrate a fresh perspective on leading questions of theory. While not able in practice to achieve complete consistency or eliminate every vestige of traditionalism from his outlook, his approach seemed to be both challenging and constructive, and also in line with his commitment to harmonization with his evangelical outlook.

His repeated and unceremonious attack on the ancients convincingly demonstrated his decisive rejection of the old. With respect to the more difficult task of reconstruction, by extensively drawing on ideas deriving from the Neoplatonists and by adopting a Trinitarian perspective on the theory of matter, his approach would have appeared innovative, credible and congenial, especially among the avant garde. Although Neoplatonism was not 'new' by universal standards, according to the values of the times the recent rediscovery of Neoplatonic sources injected a novel and controversial element into philosophical discourse. In his famous Oration, Giovanni Pico declared that he was embarking on an audacious plan for the reconstruction of knowledge, which he had no hesitation in calling a 'new philosophy'.[5] The Florentine Neoplatonists also made a point of underlining the medical applications of their novel philosophical perspective. In their individualistic ways, Agrippa von Nettesheim and Paracelsus highlighted the medical dimension of Neoplatonism. The appeal of recent medical Neoplatonism would have been all the greater to Paracelsus on account of its compatibility with the similarly Neoplatonically inclined medieval German mystics, who themselves were enjoying a new wave of influence after the advent of printing, as indicated by the Heinrich Seuse title-page (included as Illustration 6).[6]

On questions of basic explanation, no issue was more important than the theory of matter. This provided a key test of the ability of Paracelsus to compete with Aristotelian and Galenic authorities in their central areas of contention. Reference to this issue was inescapable. Paracelsus made no attempt to evade its importance, with the result that he allowed the theory of matter to become a focal point of his writings.

Given the religious framework in which he operated, it was inevitable that his initial perspective on the theory of matter was the conventional church teaching of *creatio ex nihilo*. Superficially, his position looks unexceptionable, but in practice, as Pagel has suggested, his theories were infiltrated by emanationist accounts of creation deriving from Stoic, Neoplatonic and Gnostic sources.[7] The intrinsic tension between the creationist and emanationist positions had long been appreciated, but a working reconciliation was achieved within medieval theology, permitting figures like Paracelsus the luxury of full exploitation of the Neoplatonic hierarchy of hypostatic entities, which were employed with great imaginative effect to confer dynamic vitality to every part of the macrocosm and microcosm.[8] The functioning of these hypostatic entities in the speculative and medical context has been sensitively outlined in the pioneering work of Walter Pagel.[9]

When it came to consideration of the important issue of the basic building blocks of nature, the standard classical model, embodying 'four' symbolism as a powerful unifying factor, remained too familiar and persuasive to be completely rejected.[10] However, the four elements, the four Aristotelian qualities, the four humours of Galen, tended to be assigned limited roles, consigned to the sidelines, or even lost in the mêlée comprised of such entities as the vulcanus, the iliaster, the aniadus, the ilech, and the archeus. Paracelsus recognized the need for substitutes for the elements of Aristotle that were more compatible with his hypostatic principles and capable of playing a more active and positive explanatory role.

In reaching towards his new conception Paracelsus drew on his familiarity with alchemy and applied chemistry. At the outset of his discussion on the limitations of the four-element theory, he cited an example from chemistry to illustrate the capacity of metals to generate a variety of strikingly different products, even by the use of quite simple manipulations. Often he illustrated his conclusion with reference to mercury, but in this instance he selected the equally appropriate example of lead, which took on entirely different physical and chemical characteristics according to its existence as minium, ceruse, or as a glass. The first form (lead oxide) was red, whereas the second (lead carbonate) was white. Both substances would have been familiar to his contemporaries owing to their use as artists' pigments. In all likelihood his glass was the glassy compound of lead salts and other substances, used in various formulations as cakes of 'glass', much valued for the fluxing of metals.[11] This example demonstrated the capacity of a metal to alter dramatically its properties by simple and controlled chemical manipulation. In explaining such chemical mutations, the traditional four elements seemed to be entirely irrelevant. In view of their chemical versatility, metals and salts recommended themselves as superior candidates for a basic place in the new theory of matter. Their links with the tradition of the seven planets meant that the seven metals represented a promising line of advance, also appealing because of employment of the number seven symbolism. On the other hand, this approach would have generated an impossibly complicated theory of matter. In any case the metals constituted a dead end, since Paracelsus became convinced that their number was not limited to seven. Because of the various pitfalls of larger base numbers, it was concluded that in laying down the essential principles of nature the Creator had opted for the simplest arrangements that were tenable, although Paracelsus acknowledged that the Creator might have selected the larger number if that had been His wish.[12]

When examining the possibility of a credible chemical basis for his theory of matter, Paracelsus was instinctively drawn towards a tripartite solution. He speculated that the Creator had intentionally granted precedence to the number three. As a consequence, this number unavoidably applied in the most fundamental ontological contexts and it lay behind all beings in creation. The Trinitarian principle was reflected in the essence of the deity, in the Word of God and therefore throughout the whole of creation.[13] An elaborate attempt by a leading exponent of Paracelsus to convey this shift to a Trinitarian conception in nature is shown in the central panels of Illustration 5.[14]

Since the number three was fundamental, it was decisive (*in grund*) in determining the adoption of three basic principles for the theory of matter evolved by Paracelsus. He warned that no other number should be contemplated and that any other approach would be false and inconsistent with nature. Accordingly, in all manner of contexts, he tended to fall back on tripartite alternatives. As noted, with respect to his anthropology he often opted for the trichotomous division into soul, spirit and body. This trichotomous anthropology possessed the advantage of a biblical source and a respectable lineage through Origen and Tauler, as well as being favoured by many radicals and spiritualists at the time of Paracelsus.[15] Such a preference was not only intellectually satisfying but also theologically significant since it diluted the impact of original sin and allowed greater latitude for the operation of free will and divine grace. In a quite different context, the proposals of Paracelsus for reforming the high schools adopted natural philosophy, astronomy and alchemy as his three 'pillars' or 'three things' (*drei dingen*), which he presented as his basis for the understanding of medicine, and from which he was determined not to diverge.[16] 'Three things' was precisely what he called the three chemical principles, which he presented as his new insight into the theory of matter. In outlining what he described as his new model for the art of healing, he instinctively described courses of treatment as comprising three stages. When explaining his approach to disease in general, his opening remarks invoked three fundamental dimensions of relevant knowledge: the heavens, the terrestrial sphere and the human microcosm.[17]

Paracelsus argued that three principles, analogous to the three members of the Trinity, were required to make up a perfect body in either the microcosm or the macrocosm. In view of their fundamental status, it was appropriate to recognize that these three entities were, just as much as the four elements, the product of divine fiat.[18] It was regarded as one of the greatest wonders of creation that God had separated all things into four spheres of existence, each reflecting the powers of an underlying material existence that was both unified and threefold in its character, just like the Trinity itself.[19] The three new principles were accordingly described in terms of both unity and trinity, *drei species in ein corpus*, and the progressive refinement that they supervised in nature was described as becoming 'transfigured, glorified' (*clarificirt*) – terminology usually encountered with respect to the Creator, the resurrection of Christ, or in the sacramental context, especially with regard to the Eucharist.[20]

This last example shows that the shift towards the tripartite emphasis in his theorizing drew together both theological and philosophical reasoning.[21] Paracelsus also pointed out that the unity within the Trinity was mirrored in the natural world, where all beings, whether sensitive or insensitive, were comprised of three entities.[22] Confirmation was provided by the Genesis pronouncement that humans were formed in the image of the Creator. The Trinity was as close to humans as they were to their own shadows on a wall, while all the wonders of nature were themselves like a shadow of the future paradise or New Jerusalem.[23] Furthermore, the Trinitarian principle and overall unity of being applied to every component in the created universe. Such conformity to simple numerical archetypes was taken as indicating that there was no superfluity (*überfluß*) in nature.[24]

From the prominence accorded to his announcement of the three principles and the comprehensive purposes to which this idea was applied, it is evident that Paracelsus attached the greatest importance to this aspect of his system. Subject to the strict definition of their function, he was content to preserve the general idea of the four Aristotelian elements, but this created the problem that confusion would arise if his new, more fundamental, entities were also called elements. He was obviously entirely uncertain about the label to apply; within a short passage he was liable to try out various names, among the commonest being *corpora, ersten, essentiis, species, stücke*, and *dinge*.[25] His terminology never became entirely settled, but *ding* became most favoured, which was awkward since this common word had many other applications. To avoid this difficulty, later commentators have tended to adopt 'principles', a practice which is followed in this study.

Just as important as the decision to adopt a tripartite basis for his theory of matter was his identification of mercury, sulphur and salt as his chosen primary principles. These three were in fact an obvious choice, since all of them occupied a significant place in the theory of medieval alchemy although, it should be stressed, it has so far not been possible to locate any source in the vast literature of medieval alchemy containing a considered statement approximating to the three-principle theory as it appears in the writings of Paracelsus. It is unclear what attention he paid to the mountainous complexities or nebulous and esoteric theorizing contained in the medieval alchemical corpus. By some procedure or other, on the basis of knowledge and intuition, he extracted the bold and simple conclusion that all created matter in the universe was derived from mercury, sulphur and salt and could be resolved back into these same three principles. This generalization was applied to the human body just as much as to metals or to the most remote celestial bodies. Once adopted as a basic tenet, this conclusion was reiterated throughout his writings and applied in every context as a major unifying theory. Inevitably, one of the main challenges for his new theory was its application in the field of rational pathology. The three principles were put to work in accounting for the normal operations of human physiology, in providing plausible explanations for disease, and, finally, to give insight into appropriate forms of therapy. These spheres of application involved drawing on analogies relating to many specific compounds and all the known forms of chemical action.

His radical objectives were pursued with consistency and rigour, with the result that his corpus of chemical writings looked very different in almost every respect from those of his medieval predecessors. He was sufficiently confident in his new theory to claim that any reasonable person would be persuaded to accept the existence of his principles on the basis of his experimental evidence. In this context he cited the simple experiment of burning a stick of wood. The burning process was the work of sulphur; the smoke was mercury; while the residual ash was salt.[26] Such 'proof' by fire assumed importance to Paracelsus and later to his followers, who were apt to call themselves philosophers by fire. Fire, like light, was a piece of symbolism that usefully linked religious experience with the sciences, especially alchemy. Sadrach, Mesach and Abed-Nego had proved their faith by fire.[27] One of the central ideas of the German mystics was the existence of a glimmer of fire (*seelenfunke, seelenfunklein*) in the soul, which was ignited by genuine religious experience. Vulcanus, the transcendent blacksmith, was accorded a prominent role as the model for any virtuous investigator. Just as blacksmiths or glassmakers acquired their art through fire, then fire should also be the vehicle for doctors to acquire their knowledge and their 'vulcanic art'. Fire provided the proof-stone for the doctor. As shown by his demonstration of the existence of the three principles, for Paracelsus fire provided the way by which the truths of science were made visible and confirmed by convincing experiments.[28]

Between them, the three principles were regarded as possessing the full range of properties needed to describe all chemical processes that occurred in nature. The attachment of equal weight to each of the principles contrasted with the usage of the alchemists, who predominantly saw their basic entities as part of a hierarchy. Even those who subscribed to the sulphur–mercury theory of metals tended to regard mercury as the metallic principle, while sulphur was relegated to the status of an impurity. Although the importance of salt was established through biblical authority and through its great utility, salt tended to be ascribed an even lower place in the alchemical chain of being. Alchemy was obsessed by the unique characteristics of mercury, which glistened like a precious metal but was liquid in form and easily mutable. Argument raged as to whether mercury should be regarded as the seventh metal. Owing to its special character, it was ascribed androgynous qualities, being part precious stone, part dragon, analogous to the sun and moon; mercury was even regarded as the analogue to Christ within the Trinity.

Paracelsus objected in general to the idea of ranking the works of creation in hierarchies. It was futile to argue that one tree was superior to another or that silver was less worthy than gold. The hierarchical approach may have been favoured, but such schemes were, in his view, contrary to the light and wisdom of nature.[29] The properties ascribed by him to mercury, sulphur and salt in their primal state were conventional chemical characterizations, stripped of esoteric terminology and meaning, or reference to hierarchy. According to his theory, the three principles closely approximated to the chemicals of the same names in their native form, of course allowing for the fact that salt was a generic term. Like the alchemists, Paracelsus recognized the biblical and practical basis for the adoption of salt as a principle, but the model for this primal substance was no longer confined to common salt (sodium chloride). No doubt reflecting his practical experience, his imagination was captured by a wide range of salts, especially nitre (potassium nitrate), but also the vitriols of copper, iron and magnesium, as well as the diverse and biologically active salts generated by metals such as mercury, arsenic, antimony and lead. The attractiveness of the mercury, sulphur and salt model for the explanation of physical change was facilitated by the capacity of each of these substances to exist in many physical forms, between them possessing a remarkable range of physical properties. Consequently these three principles between them readily seemed to explain complex phenomena such as change of colour in the organic or inanimate contexts.

The physical and chemical versatility of the three principles is reflected in the terminology adopted to describe their operations. It is usually stated with confidence that Paracelsus adopted mercury, sulphur and salt as his three principles, and this is correct. But he also freely drew on synonyms such as *ignis, feur, harz* and *resinam* for sulphur, and *liquor* for mercury, and even his self-invented *cataronium* for mercury.[30] Reflecting its preservative characteristics, the term *balsam* was used mainly for salt, but it was also applied to sulphur.[31] In his own definitions, Paracelsus allocated to mercury the quality of liquidity, to sulphur oleaginous qualities, and to salt alkalinity.[32] Alternatively, mercury was described as accounting for preservation, sulphur for combustibility, and salt for solidity.[33] In another source, mercury provided for liquidity, sulphur for combustion and salt for preservation.[34] In yet another case, mercury was credited with virtues, powers and arcana, sulphur with providing body, substance and structure, while salt was depicted as the source of all colour and was also attributed coagulative and balsamic properties.[35] In his mature account, Paracelsus attributed the burning property to sulphur, the capacity to produce smoke or to sublime was allocated to mercury, while the property of producing ash resided in salt. In order to burn, sulphur possessed the quality of oil; on account of its liquidity, mercury was responsible for all the humours; whereas salt possessed the capacity to generate all the colours.[36] When it came to diseases, whether in trees or human beings, they inevitably reflected the characteristics of the three principles. Syphilis, for instance, existed in three forms, each being determined by the impact of a poison derived from one of the three principles.[37]

The above characterizations of the three principles were not out of line with traditional thinking about the properties of the same substances, which indicates that Paracelsus was familiar with basic lore contained in the medieval alchemical literature. When it came to theory, any ideas imported from alchemy were filtered out to achieve conformity with his religious and cosmological convictions. Also, it is evident that, in working towards a formulation of the three-principle theory, Paracelsus was influenced by practical considerations. Medieval alchemical writings were of course very much products of their age and they reflected the priorities of their authors. They evolved into a distinctive literary tradition with its own elaborate system of arcane symbolism and particular preoccupations, such as the transmutation of base metals into gold, which Paracelsus scorned as a dangerous misapplication. His own approach reflected the priorities of a busy professional, concerned with the particular disease problems of his day and excited by the wealth of fresh and relevant information that was emerging from the industries and practical arts that were springing up around him. The importance of these technical considerations is suggested by the evidence concerning the evolution of his thinking about the three principles, which belongs to the early stages in his career.

Explosive Ideas

The first detailed exposition of the complete mercury, sulphur and salt theory featured in the *Opus paramirum*, which dates from about 1530; the three principles are almost universally employed in his writings from that date onwards. Such a chronology is consistent with a specific reference to the three principles in *De genealogia Christi*, which is thought also to date from about 1530.

It is evident that his theory had been taking shape for some time and was in all likelihood formulated before Theophrastus von Hohenheim had decided to translate himself into Paracelsus. Early writings such as the *Neun Bücher Archidoxis*, an alchemical tract that might be expected to be relevant, in fact retained the traditional four-element approach; indeed it departed little from medieval thinking in its remarks about mercury, sulphur and salt. The *Herbarius*, which may well date from about 1525, contains no reference to the idea of three principles, but a whole section is devoted to salt, which is described as a balsam necessary for the life of humans and other living beings, as well as for the preservation of food materials. In its dissolved form, in body fluids, salt actively supported life; in its precipitated form it strengthened the tissues of plants and animals. As an indication of its importance, Paracelsus argues, God provided reserves of salt in abundance.[38] A similar emphasis on salts is evident in his early writings on gout, which again contain no trace of the three principle idea.[39] The *Volumen paramirum*, a further early work, likewise contains no reference to the three principles, although in discussing poisons in the environment that were thought to account for much disease, Theophrastus suggested that more than fifty diseases were attributable to arsenic in its various forms, while many more were due to salts, mercury and sulphur. The same three substances were briefly mentioned in his account of the process of excretion.[40] These early comments, although not conclusive, suggest that at an early stage in his scientific writing Theophrastus was beginning to attach particular importance to salts, mercury and sulphur.

The *Elf tractat* provides another indication of his early thinking. In line with his assumptions about the macrocosm–microcosm theory, the aetiology of the eleven diseases was dominated by analogies drawn from meteorology. Much reference was made to the generation of storms, earthquakes, thunderstorms, etc. In this context, sulphur and salt, or specifically the salts nitre and vitriol, were often mentioned. In all probability Theophrastus was thinking of detonations of mixtures such as gunpowder. Although mercury was not much invoked, it is noteworthy that these short essays were interspersed with a few direct references to the three-principle theory. In Chapter 3, almost as an aside, it was stated that the human body comprised three entities, mercury, sulphur and salt. Colic could not be understood without attention to the solution and precipitation of salt. The latter acted internally in the stomach or epidermally in wounds; in both cases it exercised a caustic effect. In Chapter 8 he was even more explicit. Everything was said to comprise the *drei ersten*. The identity of these three things was not specified, although the subsequent text mentions arsenic, mercury, marcasite, salt and sulphur. Similar substances were invoked to explain the falling sickness, in the course of which, on one occasion, he highlighted three *stücke*, sulphur, nitre and mercury, which he speculated were responsible for the earthquake-like symptoms of this disease.[41] Such evidence suggests that in drifting towards the idea of three principles Theophrastus was influenced by the minimum number and type of ingredients he thought necessary to produce an explosive effect. His imagination seems to have been dominated by sulphur and nitre, with mercury added as something of an afterthought.

From this stage on it is quite likely that Theophrastus moved quickly to his final conclusion that all material bodies were composed from three principles and that these were sulphur, mercury and salt in their ideal forms. Support for this conclusion comes from *Von den natürlichen dingen*, which is an expansion of the *Herbarius* and, like the latter work, is attributed to an early date. Of the ten chapters of *Von den natürlichen dingen*, only three concerned plants; the remainder were allocated to chemical substances. Long chapters were devoted to salt and sulphur. The revised chapter on salt now stated without qualification that humans and all other bodies, sensitive and insensitive, were composed of three *stücke, corpora, species*, sulphur, mercury and salt. This seems to be the first occasion in the writings of Theophrastus that he made an unqualified assertion concerning the universal application of the three-principle theory.[42] In the section on salt, sulphur was allocated a burning property, mercury a liquefying property, salt a balsamic or preservative property. Similar conclusions were announced in the chapter on sulphur, although there the three principles were primarily described as the constituent parts of metals. This impression was modified at one point to suggest that sulphur was contained in all substances. With some care Theophrastus explained the operations of sulphur as a vital flame and potential source of powerful arcana. It was also indicated that sulphur as a principle was the equivalent of the Aristotelian element fire. The lack of prominence given to the most generalized statements about the three principles, as well as the absence of reference to the three-principle theory in the course of the other lengthy sections of *Von den natürlichen dingen*, are supportive of an early date of composition. The particular interest of this work for the theory of matter derives from the long and detailed sections on salts, sulphur and other substances such as arsenic and vitriol, which demonstrate the comprehensiveness of the chemical knowledge of Theophrastus at an early stage in his career.[43]

It is also striking that Theophrastus proposed, but seemingly failed to execute, a whole section on tartar, a salt to which he had already given some thought in the context of his speculations about such problems as gout and the diseases of miners. This humble substance assumed special importance in his pathology, since it was the basis for his ideas on the localization of disease processes.[44] Just as tartar seemed to appear from nowhere when it was deposited from fresh wine in wine casks, tartar-like deposits were laid down in places like the lungs, where they established themselves as the local seat for certain diseases.[45]

The macrocosm–microcosm theory facilitated this salt-orientated approach to disease, since it was assumed that all the minerals that occurred outside the body possessed rudiments on the inside. Paracelsus insisted that the deposition of distinct substances such as salts, rather than the balance of humours, accounted for diseases such as gout, and he speculated that there were as many forms of gout, as there were varieties of the relevant salt. With respect to such diseases the doctor needed to follow the example of the miner prospecting for ore by identifying the offending chemical substance and then tracing the relevant salt back to its original source.[46]

It was only a short step from *Von den natürlichen dingen* to the fully articulated three-principle theory stated in *Von den ersten dreien principiis*, the *De mineralibus* (both possibly from 1527) and certainly in the *Opus paramirum* (1530/31). The limited evidence available concerning the evolution of the thinking of Paracelsus on the three principles suggests that, although he was familiar with standard alchemical ideas about the constitution of metals, the three-principle idea seems to have been developed specifically in the context of his attempts to establish a unified approach to the aetiology of disease. In casting around for the most relevant analogies, he appears to have been most influenced by his knowledge of the chemistry of stock chemicals from the metallurgical industries, especially those used in explosive mixtures, as well as by parallels drawn from meteorology and geology.

Macrocosm and Microcosm

An important dimension of the three-principle theory was its application to account for natural phenomena at every level in the cosmos. This unified conception of the cosmos was essential to Paracelsus, since his theory of disease, as well as his other theories, assumed active commerce between the firmament and humans or other living organisms. This functional unity was not possible to the same extent under the Aristotelian cosmos, which assumed significant qualitative differences between the celestial and terrestrial spheres. In contrast, Neoplatonic cosmology and cosmogony entailed a more unified conception and continuous hierarchical gradation reaching down by a process of emanation from the cosmic mind, the point of contact with the Creator and source of celestial intelligences, eventually to the realms of nature and material existence. The entire system was linked by innumerable bonds of sympathy between higher and lower states of existence, facilitating the free interaction of spirit beings or demons and non-personalized spirits exercising seminal or energizing functions. Such agencies as the vulcanus or iliastrum of Paracelsus occupied an intentionally ambiguous status with respect to the hierarchy of being, allowing them to mediate between the higher and lower levels of the hierarchy. Although the main drift of influence was from the incorporeal centre to the material periphery, there was also a free flow in the opposite direction, enabling the circulation of influences and, among other things, permitting humans to make a stepwise spiritual ascent from the inferiority of material existence towards the goal of mystical union with God.

Paracelsus envisaged that the three principles exercised their influence throughout the whole firmament as well as occupying the terrestrial atmosphere. Throughout the cosmos the principles were responsible for the colours associated with each of the four elements. He rejected the commonly held Aristotelian opinion that the heavens, air and their related chaos were entirely transparent in their essential nature. According to the rival view of Paracelsus, their appearance of colour derived from the smoke or vapour emanating from the stars, which tended to be brown, blue or green according to the chemical source. Such pollutants were responsible for the blue or green appearance of the heavens.[47] Not content to leave any side of traditional cosmology unchallenged, Paracelsus poured scorn on the idea, favoured by the Neoplatonists, that the harmony of the heavens was responsible for the production of a heavenly symphony. To him, this was an idea for dreamers. In the light of the less romantic chemical and physical reductionism of Paracelsus, the heavenly symphony was something akin to the sound emanating from a water-mill or stony brook; heavenly sounds were merely the product of reverberations, the howling of wind, or the gushing of water.[48]

In outlining his ideas about the relationship of humans with their external environment, he drew freely on the ancient macrocosm–microcosm theory, which he emphasized to a striking extent.[49] In a manner somewhat reminiscent of Ficino, the two spheres of the macrocosm–microcosm were regarded as so closely analogous that they were like mirror images. 'Anatomy' was the science of the correspondences and sympathies between humans and the outer world. The macrocosm–microcosm relationship was also described in terms of pre-ordained harmony. The two spheres existed in partnership, or had 'received one another' (*einander annehmen*), which was precisely the language used in a celebrated New Testament passage describing the injunction to Christian unity following the model of Christ's unconditional acceptance of believers.[50]

The very first lesson of the macrocosm–microcosm theory was understanding that humans comprised the whole sphere of the cosmos and all of its constituent parts, something that was not feasible unless they were truly a small world (*klein welt*). When the macrocosm–microcosm relationship was described as being akin to the relationship between father and son, this was expected to invoke the biblical reference to humans being formed in the image of God.[51] It was assumed that everything in the parental macrocosm was replicated in the filial microcosm, with the important exception of matters relating to the human soul, partly to avoid the risk of astral determinism, and also to prevent the encroachment on free will. When it came to the basic material constituents of the humans at their point of creation, Paracelsus coined the term 'limbus' instead of the biblical dust, clay or mud (*limus*), to denote the special transcendent status of the type of ur-matter chosen for the purpose of conferring a unique status on humans.[52] On the positive side, the microcosm was strengthened by being able to draw on all the beneficial works of creation, but at the cost of being exposed to the manifold deleterious forces that also emanated from external sources.

The macrocosm–microcosm theory was also mobilized by Paracelsus to stress the analogy between the aspirations to salvation and health. Repelling the forces of evil, the legions of fallen angels that constantly afflicted humans from their point of origin in outer spheres, was analogous to employing the art of medicine to ward off external sources of disease. Both types of menace represented a fearful challenge, but God had granted the capacity to overcome the Devil through the religion of the heart and by drawing on the deepest powers of the soul (*ganzen herzen, gemüt*). Paracelsus was therefore confident that nature might be employed in an analogous manner to keep the forces of disease at bay.[53] This was a brave conjecture, but adoption of a theory of matter based on the three principles enabled him to articulate his theories in a credible manner, embodying reference to commonly understood chemical substances and employing descriptions of the disease process that would have seemed convincing to his intended readership. As indicated below, Paracelsus was not evasive about harnessing the macrocosm–microcosm concept to provide practical guidance concerning the treatment of disease.

The macrocosm–microcosm analogy was also applied by Paracelsus to emphasize his confidence in the generosity of the Creator's provisions in nature. The fundamental attributes of God implied that no human need was left unaccounted for and every benefit flowed without restriction from His creative power. Such munificence contributed to a plenitude in nature which were the other side of the coin from the unity and simplicity that were also fundamental to the character of the Creator. Paracelsus may well have been indebted to the medieval speculations associated with the concept of *principium*, which symbolized the reconciliation of the unitary and Trinitarian aspects of God - a perfect arrangement that expressed itself in an outflow of spontaneous creativity. The idea of *principium* may well have been congenial to Paracelsus on account of its central place in the thinking of Eckhart and his followers among the German mystics.[54] Such ideas were difficult to represent pictorially, but Illustrations 5 and 6 indicate two variant approaches stemming from representative mystic and spiritualist sources.

The concept of plenitude in both macrocosm and microcosm had further important consequences. Paracelsus portrayed nature as being in a continual state of flux, with species coming to their natural end and being replaced by substitutes occupying the same ecological niches. Consequently in every new season there was a renewal of life, including the emergence of a great variety of new metals and minerals.[55] In every direction, whatever the type of being, there was evidence of a multiplicity of species. Nature seemed to hold all creative possibilities in its hand, releasing them only at the most appropriate moment and allowing genera to proliferate their species according to the needs of the situation. Such huge variety in nature was all the more remarkable considering that everyone in this diversity of created beings was comprised of just three principles.[56] Like the mystics, Paracelsus emphasized the prodigious capacities of creation; but, whereas the divine dynamic was intrinsically harmonious, containing nothing superfluous, human intervention distorted the creative process, motivated by the various expressions of greed, which placed a premium on the superfluous (*überflussigen*). Such values were viewed by Paracelsus as unsustainable and would, he believed, in due course bring about the severest retribution.[57]

In view of his bias towards the principle of plentitude, it is not surprising that Paracelsus rejected conventional ideas about restrictions in the taxonomy of nature. Traditionally it had been accepted that metals were limited to seven on account of the appeal of symmetry with the seven planets. By contrast, Paracelsus suggested that metals existed in substantial numbers (*gute zal*). He was insistent that mercury should be counted among the metals and that the category should be extended to include substances such as arsenic, bismuth, cobalt and zinc, all of them either newly discovered or becoming much better understood. Following the recent discovery of new metals, he speculated that there might be no limit to the number of metals that might be discovered in the future.[58] Such a conclusion was consistent with his wider belief that imposition of any limit in numbers was likely to reflect limitations in human understanding rather than in the realities of nature. Just as the sculptor was able to shape his mental images into any number of concrete forms, so it was possible in nature to produce any number of diseases, remedies or arcana. Since the Creator, by the art of separation, had generated all the products of creation, it was within human capacity to develop this same art to locate all manner of substances useful in the treatment of disease.[59] Given this change of perspective, Paracelsus also disputed any meaningful connection between the seven metals and the seven planets as posited in astrology. He went so far as to state that there was no connection of any kind between metals and planets, a radical conclusion that was not reflected in all of his writings.[60]

Monarchy over Disease

Paracelsus viewed the problems of disease in the context of the universal contest between good and evil. Nature was pervaded by menaces to health analogous to the manifold threats to spiritual well-being. Both involved, equally, the challenge of regaining a decisive monarchy of good over evil. Such an approach stemmed from his melancholy reflections on the contemporary situation in state and church, which furnished abundant evidence concerning the dysfunctional character of the economic system.

His conflictual approach to pathology was put to work at an early stage in his career with respect to the diseases of miners. The first necessity was to understand that, within nature generally, as illustrated by the struggles in the animal kingdom, there existed a condition of enmity of all against all: *wie die natur wider die natur strebt, wie ie eins in der natur wider das ander ist.* Just as animals lived in fear of their competitors, humans were surrounded by every manner of threat to their well-being and existence.[61]

Alternatively, he suggested that illness was like civil discord. Any state relapsing into sinful behaviour and divided against itself was weakened and thereby open to being taken over by an unscrupulous neighbour. Once installed, the malefactor soon assumed complete control. Paracelsus likened disease to the eruption of civil war within the body. Concord between the three principles was thereby lost. Each was liable to rebel, exhibit arrogance and pride (*hoffart*) and then engage in acts of boisterousness, aggression and destruction, each principle according to its intrinsic chemical attributes. The result was fragmentation and the collapse of harmony between the three principles, making way for a foreign invader that ultimately inflicted death.[62] On the basis of these political analogies, Paracelsus conducted a precise technical review of the traumatic effects stemming from the adverse chemical changes known to be within the capacities of sulphur, mercury and salt.[63]

Hoffart among the three principles seemed like the key to explaining the source of many diseases, but the three principles were also effective in an alternative manner, by participating in 'spermatic' diseases, in which the principles acted like specific organisms, releasing poisons that gave rise to powerful morbid effects in particular organs. Spermatic diseases were significant in themselves, but they were also invoked to dispute the standard assumptions of medical astrology. On the basis of his macrocosm–microcosm theory, Paracelsus might well have favoured astral determinism. Indeed, on some occasions he fell back on such traditional ideas, but for the most part he rejected the standard astrological interpretation. Granted, humans were subject to the effects of the firmament, but such influences were not determined by the planetary dispositions to which astrologers attached importance. Since the Creator formed humans in His own image, it was an affront to His attributes to adopt any form of astrological determinism. Indeed, this was an error not far short of idolatry. Consequently it was essential to dispense with traditional ideas concerning the influence of the planets on human personality, and also with the humoral approach to disease that went along with such determinism. Paracelsus shifted the emphasis to chemical changes within the cosmos. Disease was occasioned when the three substances produced impressions or released spermatic bodies exercising specific and sudden physical effects, analogous to fire spreading through straw or saffron dye diffusing its colour through water.[64]

As already noted, nothing was more indicative of Paracelsus's antipathy to the ancients than his opposition to the Galenist proposition that disease arose from imbalance among the four humours and was addressed by correcting this disequilibrium, for instance by taking action to correct any excess.[65] Treatment was conducted according to the dictum, *contraria contrariis curantur*. Sometimes Paracelsus fell back on this approach, but for the most part he warned that diseases and cures needed to be viewed in a completely different light. He therefore rejected reference to qualities such as cold and hot, or identification of the sick according to their humoral disposition as choleric, melancholic, phlegmatic or sanguine. It was no help trying to heal the hot with cold or the cold with hot. If the treatment appeared to be successful, this was on account of some entirely different factor, the explanation for which resided in the three principles. The better alternative was to assume that like would be healed by like (*das ist aber wol geschehen, das seins gleichen das sein geheilt hat*) and thereby to confine therapy to suitably sympathetic expressions of the three principles.[66]

As with the three-principle theory, this new approach to therapy constituted a dramatic reorientation. In switching to the homoeopathic principle, Paracelsus was consistent with his Neoplatonic cosmology, particularly the idea that the macrocosm and the microcosm were bound together by a complex network of congruities, which constituted the hidden causes of all manner of phenomena, including health and disease. The challenge for the natural magician was to mobilize sympathetic powers that owed their origins to the heavens but were freely available in the terrestrial realm for appropriate uses. In his brief exposition on magic in his Oration, Pico identified sympathy, the mutual affinity between things, as the means of taking advantage of the deepest secrets of nature, which he extolled as the zenith of the art of natural magic.[67] Expressing the same idea, Agrippa von Nettesheim described magic as the location of sympathies in nature by exploiting the principle of attraction of like by like, or of bringing things together through their correspondences (*in attractu similium per similia et conveniendum per convenientia*).[68] Although it was repugnant to Paracelsus to accept that his homoeopathic principle was an ingenious extrapolation of a widely held Neoplatonic idea, his readership would have recognized that his innovation was consistent with notions expressed by a whole range of ancient and modern authors, from Pliny and Ovid to Ficino and Zorzi, with particularly clear and accessible statements emanating from Pico and Agrippa. Ironically, considering the strictures of Paracelsus about the pernicious influence of the poets, a good part of the Neoplatonic writing about sympathies took place in the context of odes exploring the power of love. Paracelsus may have been forgiving about this lapse since the theme of love was usually explored with some kind of reference to the religious context, thereby connecting with the concepts of similitude or equanimity (*gelicheit*) in the deliberations of the medieval mystics, who of course also operated within a Neoplatonic frame of reference.[69] As we are reminded by Illustration 6, the writings of Heinrich Seuse were characteristic of this mystic genre. In poetic, philosophical and theological contexts, magnetism was repeatedly invoked as providing experimental demonstration of the power of sympathy.

It is possible to detect a trend towards the homoeopathic bias in the early writings of Paracelsus. Literary influences may well have played a background role, but once again his practical experience of mining and metallurgy seems to be relevant. In reflecting on the diseases of miners, he was struck by the existence of beneficial and harmful substances in close proximity. It seemed as if they were related to each other rather than comprising polar opposites, an approach that was reminiscent of the Dionysian idea of the Good, which looked on disease and disorder not as a contrary evil, but as a lesser form of the good.[70] Good and bad seemed almost part of one another; accordingly, it was necessary to reach an understanding of the good that lurked in the bad *(zu wissen das gut in dem bösen)*, for which purpose chemistry was specifically ordained *(in den Vulcanum verordnet)*.[71] This conclusion was illustrated by reference to the coexistence *(dan in eim ston sie beide)* of poisonous and less poisonous compounds of substances like arsenic. Since all chemicals were formed from the three principles, any poison was reducible to these three. Similarly, all medicines were reducible to mercury, sulphur and salt.[72] The three principles made it easier to understand that chemically the poison and its remedy might be so closely related that they could be described as neighbours. Alternatively expressed, the good that was designed to heal the bad was likely to be its neighbour. Hence, whatever the source of jaundice, it could generate an arcanum for the same condition.[73] Once this conclusion was reached, it was often repeated. It became a standard part of the rational pathology of Paracelsus that the disease must be traced to its roots, which would then indicate a source from which the cure might be derived.[74]

The rooting out of disease by derivatives of known poisons inevitably led Paracelsus to be accused of poisoning his patients, to which he replied that he was merely elevating into a principle a practice that was already widespread, for instance in the treatment of syphilis, where compounds of mercury were in established use. He insisted that expertise in the arts of correction and separation could lead to widespread conversion of poisons into non-poisons, and he provided many instances to illustrate this practice.

Under the three-principle theory, just as in the case of medicines, all metals were seen as products of mercury, sulphur and salt and were regarded as being reducible to these same principles. Paracelsus speculated that, when participating in the formation of a metal, the three principles reached a higher level of refinement. As was consistent with this conclusion, when metals were subjected to separation it was possible to extract their root chemical in a particularly pure form, in which it exhibited its ideal virtues. For instance, processed sulphur was thought to possess greater purity and potency than the initial native sulphur. The benefits of purity extended to the therapeutic context, since a much smaller dose exercised a great effect. There were thought to be similar advantages to apply when sulphur was obtained in a sublimated form from its various native sources. Through such chemical manipulations, the higher the degree of purity attained, the greater the therapeutic effect. This important generalization was pertinent to his homoeopathic approach, since it suggested not only that it was possible to treat like with like, but also that compounds that were harmful in large doses might exert a positive effect in modest doses. Such radical benefits from small doses might have seemed improbable, but Paracelsus invoked the examples of magnetism and static electricity, where a small magnet or piece of amber demonstrated a capacity to attract surprisingly large amounts of other materials. Also relevant was the basilisk or other mythical beasts, whose slightest glance generated fearsome effects. In view of such analogies, it was reasonable to believe that a drug taken in minute amounts was in principle capable of extracting severely malignant influences from the human body by some kind of sympathetic action.[75]

The importance attached to dosage resulted in the ultimately famous dictum of Paracelsus that all things are poison and nothing is without poison; it is the dose alone that frees a thing from its poisonous nature.[76] This statement said what it meant, as indicated by the clarification that all nutriments are poisonous if taken in the wrong amounts. However, the context of this dictum indicates that Paracelsus's main objective was to insist on the modification of poisons by their chemical correction and not primarily by their dose. Consequently, it could be argued that Paracelsus was only to a limited extent the anticipator of the modern dose-response relationship, or of the homoeopathic principle of serial dilution.[77]

Demonstrations of unexpected powers by simple substances suggested that the vulcanic arts were capable of revealing remarkable capacities inherent in nature. It was therefore evident that the Creator had provided a plentiful supply of drugs in nature, but it was necessary to learn the arts of preparation, especially the separation of the active from inactive substances. This stress on the importance of isolating active ingredients was contrasted by Paracelsus with the prevalent practice of apothecaries, on the instruction of ignorant physicians, of making up their prescriptions from indiscriminate mixtures of mainly useless substances. Such high regard for simplicity and purity in his own approach to medication led Paracelsus to castigate his competitors for their habitual dispensing of complicated and unrefined products that were no better than pig swill or slops (*sudler, sudeln*, etc.).[78]

Magnetism was invoked on many other occasions by Paracelsus to illustrate the existence of hidden sympathetic powers in nature capable of exerting remarkable effects. The magnet provided experimental proof that minute amounts of a substance possessed the capacity to exert substantial influence, often at a considerable distance. In the long-running philosophical dispute, the magnet persuaded Paracelsus to come down in favour of action at a distance rather than action by contact. In view of its wider salience, it is not surprising that the magnet was allocated one of the six chapters of his *Herbarius*, and one of the ten chapters of its revision.[79] Arcana derived from herbs were thought to operate by a power akin to magnetism, with the precise purposes to which their sympathetic powers should be applied being suggested by signatures, outward physical signs that correlated with some striking characteristic of the target disease. Signatures were of course not an invention of Paracelsus, but they were provided with a new level of rational authority by his system.[80]

Magnetism was also invoked to explain the operations of mumia, defined by Paracelsus as the life-giving force conferring resistance to decay in all living beings.[81] Mumia owed its vital activity to the element air, from which it was fed, in a manner analogous to the maintenance of a flame. Additional virtues were absorbed from the firmament, with the greatest exaltation of mumia deriving from the sun and moon. The potent influence of mumia was manifest as a kind of magnetism, the effects of which were illustrated by the remarkable powers exercised by peasants and hunters over all the types of animals that came under their bidding. Among other things, this great magnetic capacity allowed the presence of a small trace of mumia within the human body to exercise dramatic effects in the relief of pain and cure of many diseases. Such effects were called magnetic cures, and the mumia was in effect a magical magnet. Its powers were supposed to excel those of all other arcana known in medicine.[82] The status of mumia was high, but it was not as elevated as balsam. The former gave resilience to the body, but the latter reached over to the world of the immortal spirit.[83] As a link between the material and spiritual realms balsam was intrinsic to physical bodies while at the same time belonging to the spiritual realm through possession of virtues associated with the kingdom of God and the Trinity. On account of these associations, it is not surprising that the seemingly inauspicious turpentine was accorded a special place of prominence in the pharmacopoeia of Paracelsus, since it was regarded as a particularly potent source of balsam.[84]

Mumia proved that the human body had unusual powers of resilience. Paracelsus warned the doctor to remember that the body itself possessed more powers to drive out disease than were ever available to the doctors with all their medicines. Each human organism had the capacity to act as its own doctor. Individuals had the duty and capacity to understand and control their health by encouraging the balsamic powers of their mumia, which constituted the true 'curative' medicine. The medical specialist's first responsibility was to reinforce or 'defend' these autonomous healing powers of nature, compared with which outside medical interventions were at best a poor substitute.[85]

Magnetism and electricity were also invoked by Paracelsus to explain the powers exercised by the imagination. Since, like the magnet or amber, the imagination could exercise its effect over a distance, it could give rise to many diseases and misfortunes.[86] This model was widely applied. Plague was explained by reference to an internal sympathetic power in humans which, in susceptible persons, had the effect of attracting poisons from the atmosphere. Such poisons were then passed from person to person by virtue of the same magnetic power. In that case the infection might be repelled by the wearing of an amulet that had the effect of calming the magnetic powers of the body. The same kind of magnetic power was thought to reside in particular organs, such as the reproductive organs, which were apt to attract materials capable of instigating morbid effects. Magnetism was thus used to explain the sympathetic powers attributed to the uterus, thought to cause the falling sickness in women, or the attraction of semen to effect fertilization.[87]

Paracelsus adopted an alternative approach to infectious disease, and described the plague as an infection from Mars. To explain its instantaneous impact, Paracelsus invoked the basilisk, which possessed the power to harm or kill by its glance. A poisonous look from Mars was equivalent to the glance of the basilisk and enough to spark off an epidemic of plague.[88] The basilisk was used almost as often as the magnet to account for diseases of sudden occurrence.[89] Other beasts were called upon for similar purposes. Diseases of miners were explained by exhalations, which were sudden events with widespread and dramatic effect. They were analogous to the breath of the crocodile which, like the glance of the basilisk, possessed the immediate power to kill humans.[90] Notwithstanding its evil effects, the basilisk taught positive lessons about the nature of the disease process, including the suggestion that just as the slightest glance could destroy, the smallest drop of medicine might generate a cure.[91]

The human condition was a delicate balance. The threats to health and well-being were potent and numerous. It seemed almost impossible to repel these legions of adverse forces. Yet the worldview of Paracelsus identified equally potent reserves of resistance, some of them intrinsic to the human frame, whereas others might be summoned from the visible or invisible realms by the diligent practitioner to deal with any problem confronting the sufferer. Reflecting this positive outlook, most of his little monographs on disease not only contained a rational pathology drawn up according to his own particular system, but were also replete with ample guidance on therapeutics, strongly practical in emphasis and widely accessible in terms of cost and availability. In modern terms the value of these medical recommendations seems hard to fathom, but they must have been compelling to his contemporaries, for whom they must have seemed like a welcome and realistic manifestation of therapeutic optimism.

The Light of Nature

On the basis of some presentations by Paracelsus, his Light of Nature is often regarded as roughly equivalent to the medieval conception of the Book of Nature, or even as an incipient expression of Baconian empiricism.[92] As already indicated, Paracelsus was influenced by medieval sources, for instance Konrad von Megenberg's *Das Buch der Natur*, which itself drew on the encyclopaedic digests of Thomas of Cantimpré and related sources. Paracelsus not only made active use of the range of ideas about the Book of Nature as expressed by the medieval mystics and Neoplatonists, but extended its use and made it central to his outlook through his conception of the Light of Nature.[93] The Light of Nature was accordingly not seen in limited terms as an imposed taxonomy of nature, or even as an inbuilt system of law-like regularities designed to testify to the power and will of the Creator, as suggested by advocates of natural theology such as Raimond Sebond. Paracelsus subscribed to the above ideas to some extent, but he opted for a more ambitious conception in which the Light of Nature was regarded as more of a hypostatic presence, sometimes diffuse and impersonal, on other occasions an elevated astral body or even a demonic agency.

Paracelsus was of course not original in his attraction to light symbolism, the prevalence of which in Old Testament, New Testament, patristic and Neoplatonic sources prepared the ground for its extensive employment among the medieval German mystics and the spiritualists of the sixteenth century.[94] Even against this background, Paracelsus remains quite exceptional in the prominence he accorded to the Light of Nature, which he employed for the widest spectrum of purposes in his writings.

Besides the manifold and obvious points of attractiveness of light as a metaphor for the Creator and for the Trinity, this symbolism was applied also to the prophets, apostles and saints, and it was used for denoting faith, love, or other religious aspirations. Paracelsus would have found light imagery particularly appealing on account of its positive connotations in the cycles of nature and in relation to sustaining life. Light metaphors provided a ready way of describing religious aspirations and indicating positive incentives towards health and fertility more generally. Such a unified conception was supported by the association of light and life both in the opening chapter of Genesis and in the opening verses of the gospel of John. As is indicative of the importance attached to this conception, Paracelsus elevated the Light of Nature to a status akin to that of the Holy Spirit in the religious sphere.[95] The Light of Nature was therefore not understood as a neutral agency, but as a teleological influence drawing human intellectual capacities and the creative processes in nature into more perfect congruity.

Already, from occasional comments in earlier parts of this study, it is apparent that Paracelsus regarded the Light of Nature as the definitive court to which he referred his ideas and from which he expected to receive justification in his contest with rival authorities. He declared that the Creator had made two lights available for the direction of humankind, the Light of Nature and the Light of the Father. The two operated alongside one another, each keeping to its separate territory. The Light of the Father, or Holy Spirit, communicated with the soul. According to the will of God at the first point of creation, the Light of Nature was allocated to the material world for the purpose of regulating the forces operative in nature.[96] Alternatively, he described the Holy Spirit as a single entity with two virtues. The first was the Light of Nature, which revealed everything about the created world, while the second operated through faith and only reached its full potential in the context of the sacrifices made by Christ.[97]

On account of its broader theological relevance, the Light of Nature always possessed a range of connotations for Paracelsus. On the negative side, insensitivity to the Light of Nature was identified as the recipe for ignorance, which, Paracelsus believed, was manifest among his professional competitors. In its most elementary aspects, the Light of Nature generated acquaintance with obvious truisms about nature or familiarity with the empirical basis of the practical arts and sciences. However, the Light of Nature was not conceived as the equivalent of Baconian experimentation, which Paracelsus regarded as being of no more worth than the superficial and fragmentary knowledge of the laity. As a consequence, *experimentator* was generally used by him as a term of abuse.[98] Since the Light of Nature involved an element of deeper understanding than was possible under any form of empiricism, this means of intellectual illumination was frequently tied up with the uses of magic and kabbalah. Hence, Paracelsus insisted that the interpretation of prophetic images created with the inspiration of the Light of Nature necessitated the application of magic, while the particularly intractable problem of understanding the apocalyptic time frame required reference to the kabbalistic arts (*die gabalistica*), which at this point he described as the mother and origin of astronomy.[99]

At the level of the individual, within the microcosm, the Light of Nature was equated by Paracelsus with the human faculties of reason, circumspection and wisdom. This asset was granted by God to enable humans to optimize their rational abilities, at least sufficiently for them to determine their future and prevent themselves lapsing into error.[100] One of the main uses of the Light of Nature was to facilitate the discovery of practical arts. For this purpose the Light, although unified, operated at two different levels, first in the microcosm, where it sharpened the awareness of the intellect, and secondly in nature, where it was responsible for generating each of the applied arts. Since the two modes of the Light of Nature existed in harmony, practitioners were drawn towards a requisite goal by some kind of sympathetic action, analogous to the experience of gold prospectors, who were drawn towards the precious ore hidden in their mines.[101]

The conception of the Light of Nature adopted by Paracelsus also possessed transcendent qualities. Since it was not bound by the flesh or by mortality, the Light of Nature had a status akin to that of angels. Indeed it could be described as our personal protector (*gönner*), or domestic god or angel.[102] As such, the Light of Nature was the key to the expression of remarkable capacities such as the ability to acquire insight into the practical arts, understand the significance of past events, or foresee the future. Such understanding came about particularly during sleep. Such an elevated form of knowledge was described as the 'great kabbalah'. Since this type of wisdom had been freely available throughout Old Testament times, as shown by the examples of Adam and Moses, this provided an additional reason for applying the term kabbalah. It was conceded that Satan and the evil spirits in his thrall were also great kabbalists. For prophylactic purposes, examples were supplied of characteristic temptations offered by these malign beings. Only by deriving their own kabbalistic powers exclusively from the uncorrupted Light of Nature was it possible for vigilant believers to avoid such pitfalls. Untainted commerce with the Light of Nature was presented as a real possibility because the human spirit was able to transcend the limitations imposed by the flesh. The Light of Nature was therefore free to reside in the spirit and act like an effective schoolmaster unhindered by corporeal influence. On the basis of Old Testament and New Testament authority,

Paracelsus was satisfied that the prophetic powers manifest in dreams derived ultimately from spirits serving an augural function. In such cases of application of kabbalistic or magical arts the practitioner was rightly called a magus.[103]

At the prophetic threshold, the Light of Nature reached its boundary; further penetration into the supernatural was reliant on a yet higher light, unique to humans and only accessible by virtue of their capacity to free communication with good and evil demonic agencies. This higher light was often given no particular name, but was sometimes called the *leicht des menschen*, indicating powers analogous to those deriving from the Holy Spirit. On account of their special nature, humans had the ability to transcend the Light of Nature, and might even attain the capacity to travel freely within the wider demonic universe and make use of this experience to extend their powers into the highest realms of magic.[104]

The rich variety of operations supervised by the Light of Nature represented a major source of belief in the possibility of maximizing human capacities and gaining relief from every kind of problem and debility. Typically, in relation to the diseases of miners and associated artisans, Paracelsus insisted that workers were never forsaken by God, whose Light of Nature provided the means to overcome the poisons that afflicted their lives, thereby granting them monarchy over the diseases that were such a threat to their lives and well-being.

Paracelsus was confident that his new approach to pathology and therapeutics would confirm that God had created a ready cure for every disease. Success was assured, but only if all practices were subject to the guidance of the Light of Nature and the Holy Spirit, thereby also conforming to the ethical norms laid down by the hierarchy of divinely inspired agencies such as vulcanus. These were rigorous demands, unlikely to be met by the botchers who dominated medicine, yet the sacrifice was worthwhile on account of the high level of effectiveness of the new arts that would be revealed. Such full appropriation of the Light of Nature was self-evidently not to be attained by any short cut, by illicit arts such as sorcery, or even by straightforward scientific procedures. The fullest blessings of nature would only be dispensed to those who developed those very special qualities of acumen and foresight that were needed for the fullest consummation of the arts of magic and the kabbalah.[105]

Magic and Kabbalah

In view of the wider spiritual, ethical and technical ramifications of the Light of Nature, it is evident that the engagement of Paracelsus with nature was not subject to the limitations of science as it is now understood. Nor was he addressing anything as narrow as natural philosophy or any of the rough equivalents of science in older terminologies. Given the broader remit of his commitments and the more ambitious pretensions of his programme, at every stage of his career and in writings of every kind, the term magic was favoured as the label for both the speculative and utilitarian aspects of his engagements with nature.[106] He also had a distinct preference for linking magic and kabbalah as conjoined, if not synonymous, operations.

Any doubts about the wisdom of making magic central to his avocations would have been dispelled by the scriptures, which provided ample testimony to confirm his instinctive preference for the magical worldview. As indicated by the episode of Moses and the magical serpent featured in Illustration 4, Paracelsus's audience would have shared his familiarity with the magic of the Old Testament. It was therefore not unreasonable for Paracelsus to present himself as the reviver of an honourable tradition, evident already among the patriarchs and prophets of the Old Testament and further exemplified by the activities of the Magi and apostles of the New Testament.

By emphasizing the consistency of his magic with the evangelical faith, by conspicuously distancing himself from popular practitioners who were commonly suspected of engaging in sorcery and by rejecting the heathen sources venerated by the Neoplatonists, Paracelsus hoped to endow his own magic with superior credentials and establish the magical arts as a legitimate basis for the betterment of the arts and sciences with which he was engaged. As is already evident, oblivious of the warning signals, from an early stage in his career Paracelsus became a committed advocate of magic and the kabbalah and he took every opportunity to advertise his engagement with these disciplines. With characteristic abandon, he made himself more vulnerable to criticism by canvassing his ideas about magic and the kabbalah without troubling about restraint or precision of meaning.

Throughout his writings, in most contexts magic denoted what other authors described as natural magic, although it is striking that this latter term was little used by Paracelsus. Thereby he failed to apply terminology that was of obvious utility for defensive purposes, since it avoided the connotation of demonic involvement.[107] Perhaps he was just being candid since in many contexts he adopted an extremely relaxed attitude to the possibilities of demonic intrusion in nature. Despite using terminology liable to stress the demonic angle of his theories, in most contexts his magic involved no more than the location of useful properties of natural bodies or isolation of active chemical compounds, often for the purposes of medical intervention.[108] Like most natural magicians, Paracelsus explained this mobilization of hidden powers with reference to such entities as quintessences, occult properties or celestial influences. At one level, ability to control such powers required no more than professional competence, but also such operations entailed a degree of engagement with cosmic forces that went well beyond the capacities of the uninitiated technician. Natural magic was important, but it represented only one side of the magical operations to which our reformer was committed. As with other contemporary enthusiasts for magic, in the thinking of Paracelsus there was no clear line of division between the spheres of natural and demonic magic.[109] Demonic magic was adopted as an integral and indispensable part of his system and it was considered essential to the realization of the ambitious objectives to which he was committed.

Confirming the impact made by Giovanni Pico della Mirandola, Reuchlin and their allies among the advanced thinkers, Paracelsus habitually mentioned magic and the kabbalah as conjoined operations, essential for the revival of knowledge and spiritual understanding. Such an association echoes Pico's Oration, which culminated in an apologia for magic and the kabbalah. Although ancient in their origins, the two disciplines were recognized as possessing enormous innovatory potential.[110] Even more than in the case of magic, the Christian kabbalists acknowledged that they were espousing an unpopular cause. They needed to overcome the prejudice and misrepresentation that habitually closed minds to the supreme command of 'mysteries' that were known to the ancient Hebrews. Since it stood to reinforce the fundamental truths of the Christian religion, there was no reason to fear the kabbalah. By neglecting the kabbalah, the critics had rejected a source of divine revelation. From the perspective of Pico, Reuchlin and Colet, the kabbalah comprised those mysteries or secrets of divinity handed down by God to Moses that were perceived as unfit to be disclosed to the multitude. Such precious truths were consolidated into a tradition, handed down over the generations and preserved as the property of a select circle of the wise. They were the subject of the injunction by Christ not to cast pearls before swine (Matthew 7: 6).[111] John Donne likened this tradition to alchemy. The kabbalists were 'the Anatomists of words, and have a theologicall Alchimy to draw soveraigne tinctures and spirits from plain and grosse literall matter, and observe in every variety some great mystick signification'.[112] According to Pico, such speculative understanding of the kabbalah took precedence over any of the more practical magical associations, although he was also adamant that the kabbalah would equip operative magic with fresh insights and incentives.[113] Indeed, Pico believed not only that the Orphic hymns required kabbalistic insights for their interpretation, but that all magical operations were enhanced by reference to the kabbalah.[114] This view was taken up by Reuchlin, who described the kabbalist as a figure steeped in the mysteries of the macrocosm and microcosm, possessing kinship with angels and able to manipulate the lower powers of nature to perform miracles. Although open to the accusation of sorcery, like the Old Testament patriarchs, the kabbalists performed their wonders in a spirit of godliness.[115] Paracelsus evidently shared these perspectives on the magical associations of the kabbalah, which accounts for the frequency with which the two disciplines were mentioned conjointly in his writings.

Each of the kabbalists adopted his own rendition of this discipline. As was his habit, Paracelsus adopted an idiosyncratic approach, for the most part displaying no interest in the sefirot, numerology, or manipulations of the names of God or the Hebrew alphabet. Indeed he ignored the whole content of the specific medieval kabbalistic literature. He bypassed most of the speculative fields about which other recent Christian kabbalists displayed such passionate concern. His usage of the term kabbalah, a word that was subject to amazing spelling variations in his writings, fell within the range of meaning of magic as it was applied in his writings. Either the two were used as synonyms, or kabbalah was assigned as a subdivision of magic. Since it fulfilled no settled purpose and was for the most part synonymous with magic, retention of the term kabbalah might therefore seem perverse. It was nevertheless indispensable, since it was an essential component in his rhetoric, more than any other word decisively conveying the idea of Mosaic authority for the most elevated conception of magic to which Paracelsus aspired.

He was neither apologetic nor evasive about his advocacy of magic. As far as he was concerned, magic possessed the firm sanction of biblical authority. To him, the modern magician operated entirely within the honourable tradition of the magi and others who had earned this status by their spiritual insight, hard work and altruism. On the basis of such discipline and enlightenment the magus might expect to be rewarded with special wisdom and a command over nature superior to that of the generality of scholars and professions. Although jealous of his reputation as a magus, Paracelsus was vigilant in distancing himself from sorcery and idolatry, which he regarded as dangerous and illicit activities that were rampant at all levels in society.

Not infrequently he directed harsh words at village conjurors.[116]

This numerous and bizarre fraternity was perceived by Paracelsus as a menace, since it risked discrediting the whole magical operation. It was therefore essential to distance his conception of magic from the antics of these notorious competitors. Otherwise there was a risk that the new brand of magic that he was attempting to launch and the new elite cadre of responsible magical practitioners might be strangled at birth. He was extremely sceptical about the elaborate magical rituals that were in common use in connection with the deployment of medicinal herbs. Such misguided practices not only failed to add anything positive to the treatment, but in the process the herbs lost their freshness and even sometimes rotted away, thus eliminating their health-giving properties. The manner of using herbs should be determined entirely by scientific considerations, while sorcery should be shunned. He pointed out that the action of herbs was no different from the operation of a magnet. Just as a magnet drew upon its kind such as the needle of a compass, the herb was capable, through its sympathetic powers, of drawing out poisons from wounded flesh. In the case of herbs, these powers were released when the plant was collected and they lasted for the precise time required to deal with the problem being addressed. Such powers were exposed through the offices of the Light of Nature. Since they were demonstrations by God of his wonderful works, they were rightly called mysteries, secrets and magnalia of nature.[117]

The village sorcerers may have been remiss in their handling of herbs, but Paracelsus regarded the church as a more culpable proponent of discreditable magical practices. Through assiduously cultivating the veneration of saints, pilgrimages and the sacramental system, the church had built up its own misapplications of magic into a massive and lucrative institution.[118] Coincidentally, Einsiedeln, the place of his birth, was also one of the main pilgrimage sites in Europe. There, he must have personally witnessed this ecclesiastical magical system at the height of its development. It is even possible that the prevalence of healing functions at the shrine at Einsiedeln had adverse implications for his father's medical practice. His own prospects in Salzburg may also have been adversely affected by the dominance in this area of the pilgrimage site associated with St Wolfgang that was at the peak of its popularity at precisely this date. Major artistic embellishments such as the Michael Pacher retable at the pilgrimage church of St Wolfgang, Abersee were indicative of the entrepreneurial spirit pervading the headquarters of the Wolfgang cult.[119]

In view of the continuing ascendancy of saints in the sphere of healing, doctors stood to gain when the religious reformers made the veneration of saints one of their main targets of attack. Indeed the assault on the healing employments of images and relics of the saints was one of the few issues upon which, at least for a short time, a broad spectrum of reformers could agree. Johann Eberlin von Günzburg suitably expressed this consensus when he attacked the prevalence of the use of saints for extorting money on pretence that this would improve protection from hazards and provide relief from misfortune. His strongest strictures were reserved for claims about the healing powers of saints such as St Quirin, St Anthony and St Wendelin, who were supposed between them to bestow protection from gout, plague, St Anthony's fire and diseases affecting sheep, although these benefits were only available on compliance with demands for exorbitant payments in money or kind.[120] In criticizing such excesses and associated fraudulent practices, Paracelsus found himself in the company of Erasmus, Franck, Luther, Karlstadt and many others among the reformers. In the columns of the *Flugschriften*, the reformers hotly contested the claims by the church to a monopoly on magical healing.[121] The abuse of magic by the church even alarmed artists and prompted leaders of opinion such as Albrecht Dürer to revise their thinking about religious artworks.[122]

In view of its evident self-interest, for once the humanistic medical establishment might well have been quietly supportive of this aspect of Paracelsus's critique. The opportunism of the medical profession was frankly admitted by Henrich Stromer of Leipzig, one of the known enemies of Paracelsus: 'For all the arts the Reformation was a setback, except for medical practitioners. It is the case that all painters, sculptors and goldsmiths were apt to lament that they were driven to hunger; on the other hand the medical practitioners cashed in because when the saints ceased to care for the sick, the people were again forced to seek the refuge of the doctors.'[123]

Although Paracelsus lined up with the reformers on this issue, as was often the case, he displayed an independence of outlook that indicated carelessness about his own interests. Even in this context, where there was an opportunity for reconciliation with reformers and the medical elite, he proved perverse and unreliable. Contrary to the growing scepticism of the times, to which he had himself powerfully contributed, Paracelsus conceded that magical powers were genuinely exercised and cures were indeed performed at sites of pilgrimage. Such events, he believed, could be explained naturalistically, particularly by powers akin to magnetism exercised by the bodies of the dead. Wonders that took place during pilgrimages seemed to support his theories concerning powers latent in images, regarded as being akin to vibrations from bells or other musical instruments. At this point he momentarily fell into line with the standard teaching of the church, conceding that the ceremonial of the mass, including church music and images, possessed some of the virtues that were traditionally claimed for them. They presented dramatic and visible symbols that reinforced the influence of preaching. For the sake of simple people it was legitimate to use oral and visual media to communicate the Christian teaching, provided that there was an adequate defence from idolatry. As a consequence, Paracelsus resisted the pressure to subscribe unconditionally to the wave of iconoclasm to which he was a witness. Instead he called for an act of discrimination, recognizing that simple, unadorned figures and symbols retained some value since they involved no element of deception about their inner (*inwendig*) nature. On the other hand, powerful dangers resided in the more prevalent church imagery, which was highly pretentious and ornamented, hence dependent on outward (*auswendig*) appearance, the sign of a deep-seated, corrupting nature.[124]

Because of such dangers, Paracelsus decided that it was better to aim at communicating the message of Christ without the help of such physical symbols and magical practices.[125] In the end he concluded that the use of the saints' images for healing purposes inevitably involved the intrusion of evil influences. It was conceded that in past ages the Father had granted impressive powers to his saints, including authority over all kinds of wild animals, but any such feats in modern times were signs of the intrusion of Satan. In order to avoid such spiritual risks, God had facilitated a supply of medical practitioners and through the gifts of magic and the kabbalah they were furnished with every manner of treatment requisite for their professional work.[126]

There was in fact no real convergence of opinion between Paracelsus and his professional rivals on the issue of magic. His bold conflation of medicine and magic was an embarrassment to them, since it drew unwelcome attention to the intrinsic tension between the church and their profession concerning activities over which they were in contention. The posture adopted by Paracelsus also made it more difficult for the medical establishment to maintain their ambiguity. Formally they preferred to maintain an aloof attitude to suspect arts, while quietly practising magic in some form or other. Since basic to their confrontations with Paracelsus was disparagement of his magical outlook, it was awkward for the critics to engage in the covert practice of the same arts. Accordingly, the overt emphasis of Paracelsus reduced the liberty of action of his competitors and strengthened the polarization of attitudes.

According to Paracelsus, in order to gain access to the great powers latent in nature and made available by God for the treatment of all diseases, it was necessary for medical practitioners to make a complete commitment to magic, as if they were born again. They needed to undertake a complete intellectual reorientation. This required abandoning the whole of their current infrastructure of beliefs; instead they were told to adopt the three arts, philosophy, alchemy and astronomy, strictly in the form understood by Paracelsus, as the three pillars of their outlook. From this foundation they would then naturally extend themselves into magic and the kabbalah, studies they were known to reject, but which constituted a necessary basis for their rehabilitation. As far as he was concerned, unless medical practitioners embraced magic and the kabbalah, the medications applied in their professional work would be no more effective than pig swill.[127] Habitually he censured his competitors for their neglect of magic and the kabbalah, pointing out that both were essential guides to discovering the arts. Indicative of the diverse applications of the magical disciplines, he had found that his chiromancy had benefited from being handled kabbalistically, while magic had proved essential for his physiognomy and anatomy.[128] Such asides, while not particularly meaningful in themselves, confirmed that magic and the kabbalah were not confined to the margins of the new system that Paracelsus was developing.

The magical arts were invoked in many different contexts, including with reference to diseases such as epilepsy that counted among his most serious preoccupations.[129] In this case the macrocosm–microcosm analogy was a helpful starting point. The falling sickness seemed to occur when the mental faculties were overcome by a subtle poisonous vapour of foreign origin. Such agents might arise from sudden chemical ignition, after which they seemed to invade the cells of the brain, where they overwhelmed reason. Such explosive events were among his favourite explanatory devices and suggested the susceptibility of the human constitution to traumas akin to mine accidents. Poisonous fumes generated by this means were easily explained by the three-principle theory. For example, sulphur might readily, by the effect of heat, be converted into a corrosive vapour. However, ordinary chemical processes seemed insufficiently rapid or dramatic to provide a complete explanation. Further understanding required a reference point beyond the usual confines of natural philosophy. Epilepsy seemed to involve the wider cosmos, as it was understood through magic and the kabbalah, rather than sorcery, which frequently intruded on the explanation of epilepsy and contributed to the tendency to regard this condition as a dangerous form of deviancy.[130] By invoking the operation of magic and the kabbalistic kabbalah (*gabballia gabalistica*), Paracelsus ruled out the participation of demonic spirits of the kind invoked in sorcery. Magic and the kabbalah suggested a more naturalistic point of origin, reflecting interference from the realm of the most subtle substances. He was emphatic that the macrocosm–microcosm analogy, magic and the kabbalah, and the chemistry of sulphur, between them constituted a comprehensive understanding of the falling sickness. Any additional speculations about humours invoked by the Galenists were dismissed as completely superfluous.[131] Although his dissertation on the falling sickness was brief, magic and the kabbalah were central to its argument. It is also evident that they were seen as vehicles to demystify understandings of this condition and to undermine rival approaches that fell back on sorcery and demonic spirits.

One of his main dissertations on plague provides a further case of the application of magical theory to a further specific and serious disease. As usual, he insisted that plague was not amenable to humoral interpretation. Instead, it seemed analogous to the infliction of wounds, which in this case were located at three specific sites. His explanation called for a factor that could exercise specific effects at these separate locations. Various explanations based on poisons emanating from the atmosphere were considered but rejected.[132] Consistent with his localized approach to aetiology, plague needed particular attention to specific locations or sites (*stat*).[133] Some force seemed to be implicated, which possessed no obvious natural origin but nevertheless had the power to cause a crippling disease that was resistant to all usual methods of treatment. By a process of elimination, he turned to the power of the imagination, which was described as the root of all magical operations, responsible for even more potent effects than the powers exercised by magical characters. Physicians were warned not to forget the magical and kabbalistic arts. Despite having been used to great effect by Apollo, the magical arts were neglected by all the standard medical authorities. Owing to their ignorance of the kabbalah and magic, Paracelsus believed that his competitors, the 'alleged doctors', had no hope of understanding diseases such as plague. Since it was a disease with supernatural associations, it required the application of magic for its interpretation.[134]

At this stage, Paracelsus invoked the harmful effects stemming from enmity between father and son. Either could adversely affect the other. The trauma of such tensions was so profound that great harm could be inflicted without the stroke of a sword. For once he agreed with another authority, no less than the famous Johannes Müller of Königsberg (Regiomontanus), who had concluded that the French pox originated on earth but then was transmitted to the firmament, from where it rebounded to the earth. Likewise, Paracelsus concluded that plague also originated in the earthly environment. For instance, displays of personal enmity might prompt malign imaginations to spark off an ignition on the planet Mars, which acted like a fire-iron on sulphur. Sulphurous fumes then shot to earth and incited an outbreak of plague that took effect at one of three relevant bodily sites, according to the specific form of the sulphur implicated. Sulphur was the cause of the fever, but if a worse condition developed, this was the direct effect of Mars which, as already noted, was capable of acting like a basilisk if conditions were appropriate.[135]

It was accepted that customary ideas about the aetiology of plague were not entirely wrong. Since it was a visitation from the stars, this disease was indeed an act of God. However, such traumas were also susceptible to chemical explanation, which was duly provided by Paracelsus. It was conceded that chemistry constituted only a partial explanation since, in line with the Neoplatonic theory of reciprocal action between the macrocosm and the microcosm, the original inducement for the infection was the action of the malign imagination. The best preservative against future occurrences of plague was the avoidance of reprobate behaviour, since this had the effect of inciting the heavens into fearful responses. God had so framed the macrocosm that it constituted a mechanism for punishment of the wicked, as demonstrated by instances such as Noah's Flood, the destruction of Sodom, or the crippling epidemics that were currently afflicting western Europe. Accordingly, only by avoiding inciting the heavens would there be any relief from the ongoing suffering from supernatural retribution.[136]

The tendency of Paracelsus to revert to the power of the imagination in the explanation of disease is a reminder of the significance of the spiritual dimension of the human constitution in his medical theory. The seriousness of this theoretical commitment was indicated by the first synthesis of his medical theories, which was divided into two parts: the *Opus paramirum* concentrated on corporeal aspects of disease, while *De causis morborum invisibilium* dealt with the spiritual dimension of health, which he regarded as equally weighty in its importance. His *geist* terminology facilitated transactions between the mental attributes of the human constitution and the world of personalized or demonic spirits. In his view, the demonic universe completed the picture of plenitude and was no less significant than the material part of creation represented by physical beings. In this respect Paracelsus was consistent with other writers on magic, especially those such as Agrippa von Nettesheim, who represented the Dionysian bias in the Neoplatonic tradition. However, unlike the Dionysians, Paracelsus ignored the complicated taxonomies and nomenclatures traditionally employed to describe the hierarchies of angelic and evil spirits, as for instance those popularized in Agrippa's *De occulta philosophia*. Instead he opted for a simpler and naturalistic alternative. The body/spirit distinction was stated in the customary manner, emphasizing dichotomies such as between visible and invisible or mortal and immortal. On this basis the body belonged to the earth, while the spirit derived from the heavens and hence related to God. Our reformer's vital forces were also fitted into this scheme: mumia belonged to the body, whereas balsam was associated with the spirit. He attempted to give greater clarity to these distinctions by expressing them in physical terms. Corporeal objects possessed the qualities of turbidity and darkness. Since the spirit, by its nature, was clear and transparent, it had the capacity to clarify dark objects so that they were rendered transparent, just as if they were made of crystal.

As in standard Renaissance theories of *spiritus*, the characteristics attributed to the human spirit were allowed to shade over into the kinds of powers that were exercised by demonic beings.[137] Following conventional practice, such demons were divided into conflicting factions representing good and evil. Paracelsus conceded that malign demons represented a formidable menace; their wiles could be circumvented, but only by determined effort and the strictest regard for the dictates of faith. He took consolation from the aid that was available from beneficent spirit beings, which not only provided moral comfort but also gave access to material benefits, even to the extent of helping to detect precious substances deposited in the deepest recesses of a mountain. For such beneficent purposes Paracelsus invoked spirits that inhabited every part of the universe. Each of the elements, air, earth, fire and water, contained its characteristic rich assembly of spiritual residents. On the evidence of myth and common experience, it was demonstrable that humans possessed the capacity to enter into free concourse with representatives of all of these groups of spirit beings, from whom mankind was eligible to derive many special benefits.

Paracelsus gave careful consideration to the basis for such remarkable interventions emanating from the universe of spirit beings, concluding that their prowess derived from their superior virtue. As was consistent with the distinctions already considered in the previous chapter, spirit beings, like children and the handicapped, were endowed with uncorrupted souls. Hence, when they turned their hands to the arts, they succeeded with less effort and achieved more conspicuous success. All of these spirit beings needed to be treated with special reverence, since they were specifically recognized by Christ and were as important as humans in His estimation.[138] Owing to their unexceptionable conduct, such spirit beings had valuable lessons to teach. Their secrets had been freely communicated to magicians of old but subsequently this knowledge had been squandered and largely lost. Spirit beings were not only the stuff of legends; they had lived on, and their wisdom was still accessible. It was speculated that such arcane wisdom was most likely to be transmitted during sleep. The magician, astronomer and alchemist all stood to learn from these spirits. The operational relevance of such spirits to divination and the prophetic activities of Paracelsus will be discussed more fully in the final chapter. Access to their secrets opened up utopian vistas for the living; as for the dead among the spiritual virtuosi, Paracelsus speculated about the translation of their saintly spirits to the heavens, following the famous precedents of Enoch and Elijah.[139]

At such points of contemplation about the higher realms of magic, Paracelsus tended to revert to admiration at the wonder and mystery of the workmanship of the Creator. He was ambitious in his aspirations, but humble concerning immediate expectations. He compared his own work to that of the painter. Artists were capable of representing the diversity of nature efficiently of and producing impressive simulations of life, but even their best efforts, when compared with the works of God, were no better than the merest shadows (*schattending*). The finest colours were generated not in art but in nature. It was therefore necessary to accept that there were grave limitations to even the most informed and spirited attempts to explain such visual splendours as the colours produced by plants in terms of plant pigments derived from salts to which the plant had access. The properties of the rich variety of chemical derivatives of the three principles went some way to explaining the diversity of appearances in nature. But such explanations, at best, provided only a limited understanding of the fundamental mysteries that were implanted by nature into its creations. With God's continuing help, Paracelsus believed that humans would be granted further insight into such mysteries. As with spiritual enlightenment in general, the first prerequisite for such understanding was humility about the mysteries of nature. Wonderment was the only right initial response to such phenomena as morphogenic transitions of plants. He cited the case of the little grey or black seed which turned into a tree combining beautiful shades of green in its leaves with the contrasting bright hues of its fruits and flowers. Such things were indeed a great mystery that would always evoke amazement and would never be completely fathomed. God was wonderful in His works, which He performed day and night without intermission, inspired by the hope that humans would conscientiously apply their labours to achieve a humble and proper appreciation. The mission to come to terms with the works of creation, envisaged by Paracelsus as part science and part magic, was seen by him as one of the surest paths leading believers to reconciliation with their God.[140]

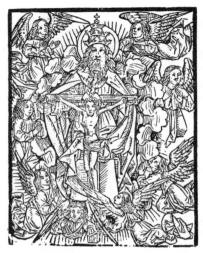

CHAPTER VI

RADICAL REFORM

Der weg zur seligkeit will still sein, will nit mit geschrei gehn, sonder von innen aus dem herzen heraus und nit von außen an kleibt.[1]

Paracelsus was raised in a Catholic environment and his body was interred according to the rites of the same tradition.[2] Little else was conventional in the religious affairs of the inveterate reformer. The Catholic church was subjected to unrelenting criticism, which is liberally distributed throughout his writings. Just in case his attacks on the old church were interpreted as a sign of sympathy for the incipient Protestant movement, he distanced himself from the magisterial reformers, who were condemned individually, as were the 'parties' or 'sects' they inspired. Luther was first on the list of offenders, with Zwingli running a close second. Dissenting groups were less frequently mentioned, but none was entirely spared. The Anabaptists (*Täufer, Wiedertäufer*), the most identifiable element within the radical movement, were identified as misguided zealots.[3] Paracelsus was particularly apt to lump together the Catholic, Lutheran and Zwinglian priesthoods. All of them were judged to be equally corrupt, concentrating on gratifying their religious instincts on stinking carrion to the neglect of the proper work of Christ. None of them would, at the Last Judgement, be regarded as eligible for the ranks of the apostles or prophets.[4]

Even in his early maturity Paracelsus had no doubts about the superiority of his own religious credentials. He was determined to make an assertive contribution over a wide front, with every confidence that his reform objectives carried the stamp of divine approval. In his work as spiritual reformer he exhibited the exalted ambitions that were evident in his revolutionary medical programme. He was sure that the moment had come for the embattled community of believers to seize the initiative and bring about the universal betterment of both church and state.

Radical Reputation

In the course of time the main confessions have claimed Paracelsus as their ally. This positive estimate contrasts with the judgement of his own century. As a strident critic and outsider, he became an object of suspicion during his lifetime, while after his death his reputation for religious unorthodoxy was unscrupulously exploited by his jealous enemies. Their campaign of character assassination was based on the related propositions that Paracelsus was both sorcerer and heretic. There was ample material in the unpublished writings to indicate that he was guilty of doctrinal unreliability, but these incriminating sources escaped the notice of his critics. His published works contained many pointers in the same direction, but the critics also made inept use of this evidence. The suspicions of the critics contained a grain of truth, but they conspicuously failed to substantiate their accusations.

The community of brilliant humanist physicians stumbled towards their conclusions on the basis of intuition rather than meaningful evidence. In Konrad Gessner's correspondence with the distinguished Johannes Crato von Kraftheim, and in a preface composed by the latter in 1562, Paracelsus was maligned as a leader of the fanatics or enthusiasts.[5] The reputation of Paracelsus as a dangerous radical continued to be peddled. His famous disciple Valentin Weigel came under criticism for adopting Paracelsus as his model. Johann Schelhammer accused Weigel of being the prime mover of a cell of enthusiasts, where 'Bombastic' figs were cooked and consumed, the resultant unripe concoction being derived word for word from the writings of Paracelsus. As definitive proof of the iniquity of Paracelsus, he was linked by Schelhammer with the revolutionary Thomas Müntzer, who was identified as a further source for Weigel's outlandish opinions.[6] Regardless of the lack of supporting evidence, such adverse representations of Paracelsus retained currency among his critics for more than a century.[7]

The usual starting point for modern estimates of the religious orientation of Paracelsus is the evidence concerning his slight personal acquaintance with Sebastian Franck and the distinct similarities of his outlook with that of other leading spiritualist writers of the sixteenth century.[8] In recent years, specialists such as Goldammer, Biegger and Gause have also noted some specific points of doctrinal affinity with other radical thinkers, although few have followed George Hunston Williams in identifying Paracelsus as a significant figure in his spiritualist division of the Radical Reformation.[9] Since the exposition by Williams, there has been much reflection on the characterization of the Radical Reformation, which now tends to be defined with respect to specific social situations and local realities in church politics rather than exclusively with regard to abstract theological positions.[10] Recent reformulations have produced some major shifts in perspective. If anything, this modern research strengthens the grounds for including Paracelsus among the radicals deriving their inspiration from the medieval mystics, whose writings became much more widely accessible owing to the impact of printing. Illustration 6 provides a reminder of this trend to make some of the leading mystic classics more freely available.

Like many of the other independent and enigmatic figures, Paracelsus fails to identify with any of the main sectarian groups.[11] On some issues he subscribed to a broad consensus, while on others he occupied a virtually unique position. As a critic of abuses within the Catholic church, he was in the company of Erasmus, Berthold of Chiemsee, or Johann von Staupitz on the Catholic side, magisterial reformers such as Luther and Zwingli, well-born rebels such as Hutten, or the motley spectrum of Heinold Fast's 'left wing' of the Reformation. In common with these latter rebellious elements he developed distaste both for the clerical hierarchy and for the existing system of secular authority. Like Grebel and Karlstadt, Paracelsus was not satisfied that Luther's version of justification by faith represented a real improvement on the 'ceremonial works' righteousness of the Catholic church. Each of these three radicals demanded immediate and decisive action to address the lengthy agenda of anticlerical grievances and eliminate all vestiges of idolatry, objectives that were unachievable without largely dissolving the clerical estate. By this means they aimed to root out all externalities, excesses and abuses preventing the realization of the inner and deep personal faith to which they subscribed. Such a sweeping reorientation was defensible since it seemed consistent with the gospels and was necessary to capture the spiritual purity of the early church.

Creating conditions for inner renewal through the agency of the Holy Spirit was the first priority, but it was not sufficient in itself to bring about the universal betterment to which radicals like Paracelsus aspired. Reform was seen both as a personal and as a communal endeavour. Also, the meaningful expression of collective action involved not only the congregation but also the wider community. Integral to the conception of justification adopted by figures like Paracelsus was the full practical realization of Christ's injunction concerning the primacy of love of one's neighbour in the context of family and community. Paracelsus was witness to the potency of this idea with respect to his particular calling. If a humble medical practitioner like Paracelsus was able to realize anything like the programme to which he was committed, then, through collective effort, it was reasonable to expect a revolutionary transformation of society. Given the apocalyptic framework that predominated among the radicals, such a remarkable prospect seemed entirely practicable in the light of the great spiritual awakening that appeared to be taking place.

Understandably, Paracelsus elected to demonstrate his Christian witness through the calling for which he possessed such conspicuous aptitude. Adoption of this specialist role gave him the opportunity to make a decisive contribution to the end-time mission as it was understood among the radical congregations. The whole ethos of his professional work was determined by this sense of a broader ethical and religious mission. Although he resisted the temptation to work specifically as an apostle, the missionary ideal was never far from his thought. Indeed, as a magus, he claimed special insights relating to the interpretation of such sources as images and dreams, which added to his confidence as an interpreter of the scriptures and other sources of prophetic wisdom. In view of such special aptitudes, it was impossible to resist the urge to participate in spreading the Word. He felt equipped to contribute from a position of strength to any informal gatherings of serious believers and students of the scriptures. It is therefore understandable that from time to time Paracelsus found himself being stigmatized as a *winkelprediger*. This preaching mission would undoubtedly have become more overt, had conditions been more favourable to the unrestricted expression of opinion.

Winkelprediger

Even before the full impact of Anabaptism, the spread of preaching by unauthorized personnel, attacked at the time as *schwärmer* (fanatics or enthusiasts), was a cause for alarm.[12] Writing from Nuremberg in March 1524, Andreas Osiander expressed concern about the collapse of congregational discipline. In his view, Lutherans had been justified in discrediting their neglectful Catholic predecessors, but instead of allowing the new reforming authorities the opportunity to consolidate their influence, zealots tempted poor people to listen to dangerous talk by preaching in all kinds of secret locations and holes in the corner (*heimlichen orten und winckeln*). Lutherans, in most places where they were newly ascendant, complained that they were being overwhelmed by these *winkelprediger*. Osiander, like Luther, accused these agitators of spreading rebellion and anarchy throughout Germany. In principle the Lutherans accepted the priesthood of all believers; in practice they issued a blanket condemnation of unauthorized preachers, all of whom were liable to be represented as dangerous fanatics in the mould of Thomas Müntzer.[13]

Similar fears were evident in Catholic areas such as Salzburg. There the first trouble arose from Lutherans, but soon centre stage was occupied by more diverse groups, some of them linked to militant Anabaptism.[14] Almost from the date of taking office as archbishop in 1519, Matthäus Lang von Wellenberg wrestled with the problems of improving discipline among his priests and stifling the growth of nonconformity.[15] The mining centre of Schwaz in the Tyrol, which may have been a port of call for Paracelsus before his arrival in Salzburg, was a leading centre of social and religious unrest. Jakob Strauß began his preaching career at Schwaz and then Hall, in each place being met with opposition from the Catholic establishment, including one 'Bruder Michael', who seems to have been a counterpart to Remigius and Valentius, the opponents of Theophrastus during his stay in Salzburg. When Strauß was expelled from Hall in 1522 he was succeeded by Urbanus Rhegius, who in turn was forced out of this living in 1524 because of his own expressions of dissent. Both Strauß and Rhegius anticipated Theophrastus in their indignant attack on endemic malpractice in the church.[16] Also like Theophrastus, Strauß campaigned to eliminate spiritual orders and lay fraternities, while proposing to turn their more acceptable practices to the advantage of the whole community.[17]

Mounting discontent stirred the Catholic authorities into action. Following high-level deliberations in Regensburg, in July 1524 a mandate on religious discipline was issued in Salzburg. This programme constituted the first major response to Lutheranism. Although the measure was intended to remove many of the causes of discontent, its effectiveness was undermined by unpopular constitutional and taxation measures that were introduced at the same time.[18] As a consequence of these policing measures, when Theophrastus arrived in Salzburg he was met by a prohibition on the publishing and distribution of books of the Lutheran type, as well as by harsh punishments for those found guilty of infringing the rules or otherwise propagating Lutheran or other heretical ideas. By April 1525 it was evident that the situation was drifting out of control, which prompted Lang and other church leaders to express despair about the relentless growth of damaging Lutheran teachings and even worse forms of heresy. Blame for social unrest was laid at the door of this nonconformist activism.[19] At the beginning of May a trial of strength against religious dissidents was attempted; a subversive preacher from Unterinntal was apprehended, but this episode only served further to inflame popular anger.[20]

The arrival of Theophrastus in Salzburg coincided with a plunge into civil strife. The Catholic authorities displayed an unyielding determination to enforce their traditional mandate, while a widely based reform party detected the chance to obtain redress for its grievances and shift the constitutional balance to its own advantage. In view of the evident buoyancy of the reform movement, it is understandable that Theophrastus was carried along by its tide. By education, training and early career, he followed in his father's footsteps and earned his living as a medical practitioner, acting as both surgeon and physician. Yet the very first statement made by Paracelsus himself about his vocational activity, which dates from his stay in Salzburg, relates to his activities as a preacher, to which he admitted, while objecting to being labelled a *winkelprediger*. In the prevailing tempestuous atmosphere, such an accusation was no light matter. A degree of notoriety was a positive recommendation among the rebellious townspeople and their peasant allies. On the other hand, the church and provincial authorities regarded any *winkelprediger* as a dangerous agitator. As is indicative of the perceived influence of these unauthorized preachers, Georg Kirchmair, the chronicler, in 1524 reported to the Innsbruck provincial authorities that in the Tyrol lay people, both men and women, who were preaching openly and in secret *in den winckeln*, to the detriment of the simple and unlearned.[21]

Already in 1525 the authorities were rounding up prime suspects. Only the temporary collapse of social discipline prevented them from reaching down to figures like Theophrastus. As indicated in Chapter III, his actions certainly merited intervention from the policing authorities. Instead of evasion or denial, he drafted his *Septem punctis*, clearly intended for publication on the *Flugschriften* market. This blistering critique of alleged abuses within the Catholic church was more than enough to make his position in Salzburg untenable when conditions returned to normal. Understandably, he conducted a timely retreat. Over the next few months, owing to a collapse of momentum within the radical movement, he must have appreciated the vulnerability of the position of any alleged *winkelprediger*. In this situation it seemed preferable to make enemies on one front rather than two. The instruments of attack sharpened for use against the church in *Septem punctis* were adroitly honed once again for application in his confrontations with the Galenist medical orthodoxy, which in some respects served as a proxy for the various clerical establishments.

The sound sense of his decision to leave Salzburg was confirmed by subsequent events. The Catholic establishment deferred action against the social elite who had Lutheran sympathies in order to concentrate on persecuting the less well placed independent lay preachers and their sympathizers, who were indiscriminately labelled as Anabaptists. Notwithstanding the overt pacifism of their victims, the authorities pursued a policy of complete extinction. As a consequence, Anabaptists continued to be treated indiscriminately as dangerous militants. By the time Theophrastus arrived in Basel, the Salzburg archdiocese and the lands controlled by Ferdinand I had instituted a regime of brutal persecution, and this approach persisted for the rest our subject's lifetime.[22] Since much of the rest of his career was spent in the provinces of Ferdinand, the fate of the Anabaptists was very evident and must have contributed to reinforcing our reformer's policy of prudence in outward expression on matters of faith. Some of his places of stay, such as St Gallen, were centres of relative tolerance, but even here the *winkelprediger* were subject to harassment.[23] More commonly there existed a policy of more active persecution. Ferdinand's local authorities were instructed to look out for *winkelprediger*.[24] These preachers were known to be operating from hostelries and the shops of artisans. At one of these pub gatherings in Sterzing in April 1526, Hans Vischer expressed sentiments about the failings of the priesthood that were entirely consistent with the line adopted in *Septem punctis*.[25] Sterzing was a centre of nonconformity and the home of Michael Gaismair. Jakob Hutter came from the nearby Puster Valley. By the date of Paracelsus's arrival in Sterzing in 1534, Gaismair had been hunted down by Ferdinand's assassins and a determined attempt had been made to clear out Anabaptism from this episcopal seat. Suppression was not entirely successful: Hutter was able to return to Sterzing in 1535, although he was soon captured and executed after frightful torture.[26] No doubt Paracelsus was alert to the dangers of even covert religious activity, and he must have been aware of the Sterzing authorities' vigilance against Anabaptist cells. Just before Paracelsus's transfer to nearby Meran, the authorities there arrested and executed one Wölfl, a goose tender and notorious preacher, and they broke up the circle of his followers.[27]

Septem punctis dates from before this cranking up of the regime of oppression. In 1525 Theophrastus had the luxury of unimpeded use of hostelries for spreading the word. He insisted that such meeting places should not be regarded as *spelunken*, dens of thieves. By default, the hostelry rather than the church had become the focus for spreading the gospel and for attacking the vices of the idle and negligent priests who, with their titles and degrees, had turned their churches into dens of thieves.[28]

By turning the tables on his critics, Paracelsus applied the *spelunken* imagery to remind his readers where the true gospel resided. Those looking for the house of God were warned to avoid churches, since these had become the home of murderers or a den of thieves, from which ravening wolves preyed on the faithful.[29] Naturally Paracelsus invoked the precedent of Christ clearing the Temple of money-changers. The pursuit of riches caused churchmen to neglect their proper duties. They had turned into dealers and money-changers, and hence made their temples into dens of murderers. What use had Christ for all the ceremonials, sacramentals, various tithes, mass offerings, or other levies? The churches conferred benefits neither on their priests nor on their flocks. Priests were slaves to materialism and the people were robbed of their assets.[30] If there was doubt about the extent of this corruption, not only the old church, but also the followers of Luther and Zwingli were condemned for turning their churches into dens of thieves.[31]

The above comments indicate that, although Paracelsus learned the art of discretion with respect to his public utterances, his later writings showed no divergence from the radical stance adopted in *Septem punctis*. The flow of his religious, social and ethical works showed no sign of interruption. Many of his most ambitious pieces of writing, including some of his most notable expressions of radicalism, were generated in inhospitable circumstances, where the authorities were tireless in their efforts to locate and exterminate the remnants of the radical leadership. Despite their overall success, the policing authorities failed to notice that the flow of seditious writings from the pen of Paracelsus was continuing without interruption, demonstrating that his appetite for radical reform remained unextinguished.

Architect of Reform

Given the extreme dissatisfaction of Paracelsus with the church in both its Catholic and reformed manifestations, it is tempting to conclude that there was no collectivist arrangement that could command his confidence. His scepticism has tempted even Paracelsus experts to regard him as an impartial outsider who adopted a disengaged, philosophical approach to religious issues, necessitating dissociation from all sectarian groupings and from the religious and social controversies that absorbed the lesser mortals among his contemporaries.[32]

Such a conclusion is scarcely consistent with the evidence. While his writings possess a distinctive flavour owing to substantial cross-fertilization between all parts of his interests, his approach to theological or doctrinal disputes reflected standard lines of argument and his conclusions indicated alignment with identifiable positions in the contemporary debate. His expositions related to the main issues of the day were intentionally accessible and designed to influence opinion. They were specifically aimed at a wide readership, who would have recognized them as a product of the radical camp. Such was his passion about issues of social and religious controversy that his views on these subjects found their way into his prognostications and even intruded as frequent digressions into his scientific writings. Paracelsus was capable of caution, but there is little to support the idea of his disengagement with current affairs, and very little sign that he was inclined to retreat into Ginsburg's Nicodemism.

With respect to his rejection of the dominant confessional parties, Paracelsus was by no means unusual. Many leaders of opinion also found themselves stateless persons with respect to the emerging confessional system. Such figures as Johannes Bunderlin, Hans Denck, Christian Entfelder, Sebastian Franck, Ludwig Hätzer, Andreas Bodenstein von Karlstadt, Valentin Krautwald or Caspar von Schwenckfeld either avoided alignment or shifted their positions, sometimes on various occasions in their careers. The same absence of decisive confessional commitment is evident with respect to lesser figures such as Martin Borrhaus, Otto Brunfels, Hans Greiffenberger, Simon Haferitz, Jörg Haugk von Jüchsen, Jakob Strauß, Gerhard Westerburg and Clemens Ziegler. Paracelsus arguably belongs to a broad segment of opinion that subscribed to the propositions that the old church was profoundly corrupt, that a drastic measure of reform was urgently required, and that the new order needed to capture the spirit of the primitive church. Having opted for the path of critical evaluation, it is understandable that this same group was cautious about making premature commitments or offering unconditional support for any of the hastily contrived panaceas of the sectarian market place. Events largely justified their caution. Hence, even avid partisans of reform were apt in the final instance to reject separation from the old church. Through disillusionment, caution, inertia or the expectation of regeneration from within, many found themselves in the position of Paracelsus and either reverted to the old church at some stage before their death or allowed themselves to be buried according to traditional rites.[33]

The attitude of Paracelsus to reform is reminiscent of many other radicals whose attitudes were formed before the confessional system took shape and when there was still an expectation that a powerful expression of discontent from below would inspire concessions from above, including a sincere attempt to address their collective grievances. In the light of experience, radical voices like Paracelsus must have appreciated that there was no realistic prospect that their demands would be met. The purification of church practices to which they aspired required reversal of the ongoing bureaucratic centralization, dismantling of the clerical estate and strengthening of lay influence to an extent that was entirely unacceptable, not only to the Catholics, but also to the magisterial reformers. Faced with this reality, separation was accepted with various degrees of reluctance. Once cast adrift into separatist congregations, many groups, by inertia, ended up by being categorized as Anabaptists.[34] Rather than follow this tide, figures such as Paracelsus placed their confidence in the capacity of non-aligned congregations to drive forward the reform programme on an opportunistic basis. As exemplified by the Castelberger study group in Zürich and similar distinguished meetings headed by Johannes Kessler in St Gallen, the informal gatherings inspired by Paracelsus himself, or more humble examples such as those associated with Hans Vischer or with Wölfl, the goose tender from the Puster Valley, associations of lay people were springing up and evolving into autonomous congregations or study and debating groups potentially capable of sustaining the demand for reform.[35] Such groups were indicative of a major sentiment in favour of more active lay participation, even a growing autarchy of lay gatherings of believers, with opportunities for greater equality among those sharing in spiritual experience, including both brothers and sisters in Christ.[36]

Symbolic of this shift in orientation was the distancing of Karlstadt from his former academic colleagues, his abandonment of his title of doctor and designation of himself as a 'new layman' (*neuer laie*), in which capacity he took up the life of a peasant farmer. At Orlamünde, he abandoned his old ways as a priest and introduced a more communal approach to worship.[37] Transformation of attitudes of this kind converged with the approach to religion and communal life expresssed by Paracelsus, or indeed many of the others listed above.

Paracelsus's conception of the church as some kind of loose confederation of spiritually inclined believers was akin to congregationalism as it took shape over the next century. This conception also fitted well with his eschatological expectations, which anticipated that the established churches would continue to be agents of Antichrist, while believers would remain subject to dispersion and oppression. Paracelsus placed a high degree of confidence in the spiritual capacities of all individuals, but he was entirely collectivist in his expectation that believers would advance to their eschatological goal in congregations that had a firm unity of purpose. In view of all the grounds for reservations about the existing sectarian options, in the end Paracelsus followed the route of Schwenckfeld and observed the rule of *Christichen freyheit*, which entailed leaving to divine dispensation the final resolution of the church order to be adopted by the community of saints. Since a positive outcome for such a body of believers was seen as the inevitable product of the divine plan for latter times that was rapidly unfolding, Paracelsus was content to leave the warring sectarian groups to sort out ecclesiological issues and concentrate his own energies on broader issues of principle.

His frequent reference to the gospel commission showed his confidence in the success of the great missionary effort that he believed would characterize the final stages of history. By whatever means, he was sure about the prospects for a definitive sorting out of the 'dead' church from the 'living' body of believers. The former would go to their graves, but believers would be rewarded by being constituted into some kind of united church. Both in his scientific and spiritual capacities Paracelsus believed that he was the agent of a collective endeavour that was destined to triumph.[38] His non-scientific writings demonstrate that he was continually elaborating plans for the 'contented' community which, he was confident, would take root in later days.

In *Septem punctis* Theophrastus had already warned that, if the churches were unwilling to forsake their arrogance and pride and recapture the simplicity of children of the street, they would never participate in the promised great rebirth.[39] Hopes for the future rested on the return of witness to the Holy Spirit within the church, so allowing the degenerate *gemauerten kirchen* or *menschenkirchen* to be converted back into a community of saints (*gemeinschafte der heiligen*), or truly *christenlichen kirchen* or *catholischen kirchen*.[40] Such renewal could only spring from the living faith.[41] He was confident that the power of love springing from the truly catholic heart could effect such changes and eventually reverse the tide of commodification that was responsible for so many evils. However, he appreciated that there was little sign that this positive transformation was being accomplished. With respect to the current wave of reform, Lutheran, Zwinglian, Anabaptist and like sects had turned out to be false prophets of the kind predicted for the final times. The Holy Spirit resided with the much narrower circle of the *stillen im lande*, comprising those who remained aloof from the dominant confessions.[42] Papists, Lutherans, Zwinglians, Anabaptists, Hussites and Bohemian Brethren were all ruined by their corruption and intolerance. Most of them imposed their will through the use of bloodshed rather than through the message of Christ. Only those expelled from all the other sects were likely to be recruited into the eternal congregations (*ewigen kirchen*), which offered the one hope of secure salvation.[43]

Part of the problem was the church as an institution, which possessed an inbuilt tendency to growth. Since it was preoccupied by greed for resources to support its own inflated weight, the church headed the ranks of the exploiters, which was quite contrary to the intentions of Christ, who promised his followers that they would carry a light yoke and a slight burden. The teaching of Christ required elimination of all who idle parasites (*müßiganger*), bloodhounds and poisonous snakes who constituted the current regime of exploitation (*schinderei*). As it was intolerable to countenance continuing suffering under the pope, bishop, monks, priests and other godless types, their removal was the only way to free the people from oppressive laws, ordinances, tithes, offerings and other ingenious devices for stripping them of their possessions.[44] It was entirely consistent with New Testament teaching to terminate the tenure of priests and remove such trappings as benefices and tithes. Believers would then be free to realize their aspirations according to the gospel commission. They might then wander the world and preach without restriction, calling their message from the windows and rooftops, and engage freely in the Lord's Supper. Priesthood was a symbol of misguidance; all believers should regard themselves as brethren, since all were equal in the sight of Christ.[45] The New Testament gave little authority to priests, so removal of the priesthood would help to restore the apostolic ethos. As a consequence, believers should only be served by preachers of the Word of God and not be subject to the current regime of wizardry exercised by *kreuzmacher, segensprecher*, etc.[46]

Paracelsus contested the claims of the priesthood to a monopoly in the administration of the sacraments. With respect to the Lord's Supper he drew a distinction between practice under the Holy Spirit and under ordained priests. Only direct experience of the Holy Spirit could lead to true spiritual renovation; when the Eucharist was administered by priests it was hardly right to use the term sacrament. Such rites and ceremonies, like theological hair-splitting, were futile since they were not helpful to the work of the Holy Spirit. Christians should therefore not expect any benefit to derive from priests. It was impossible to avoid the conclusion that the ordained priest was an obstacle in the way of salvation.[47]

Like many other radicals, Paracelsus rejected existing hierarchical church arrangements. In fact he was more radical in his rejection of hierarchy than Anabaptists such as Melchior Hoffman.[48] For Paracelsus there were only two types of Christian: apostles and laity. The former would fulfil the gospel commission and wander the world preaching the gospel in a condition of complete poverty. The laity were described as their own apostles, which implied that congregations should operate on a self-help basis. Paracelsus warned that any clerical order was likely to be arrogant, lazy and debauched; also, they would invent institutions like the mass to aggrandize themselves.[49] One of the objectives of the Lord's Supper, which he wanted to be substituted for the Catholic mass, was that all believers be seated at the same table, giving the chance for the upper echelons of the church hierarchy to translate themselves into humble preachers operating as equals with other members of their congregation.[50]

Owing to their arrogance, false apostles, otherwise known as epicurean *winkelprediger*, meaning the Lutherans and other magisterial sects - had thrown away their advantages and had replicated the vices of the papists. As a consequence the sheep-stall of Christ was even more filled up with wolves, toads and foxes. Since they had failed to emancipate themselves from the vices of the old church, the magisterial reformers had already sacrificed the credibility of their new confessional systems.

The guidelines for the new congregational order favoured by Paracelsus were stringent but not unreasonable, as shown by the prevalence of such terminology as *einfältiger bauern weise* (in the manner of the simple peasant), or the idealization of the child or fool, respecting the normative values within the new congregation. Simplicity was an essential protection against the intrusion of the various forms of idolatry that were still prevalent owing to the continuing preoccupation with ceremonial and supervision by the priesthood. Repelling the wily forces of Satan required strict compliance with Christ's command for his followers to be consistently simple (*einfältig*) in their expression of faith. With direct reference to the proverb *je gelehrter desto verkehrter*, Paracelsus warned that the faithful should not yearn after the wisdom of the learned; the only way forward in faith was straightforward and uncompromising simplicity (*nur einfalt ... straks onverrukt*). The criterion of simplicity suggested that traditional forms of learning were detrimental to the teaching of Christ and bound to lead to the intrusion of Satan. The same approach also demanded that in celebrating the Lord's Supper it was necessary to eliminate all superficial symbols of beauty and finery, which were merely the manifestations of sorcery, witchcraft and augury. The only way to join the table of Christ was to reject all superficially attractive human ordinances and observe the rule of simplicity in faith.[51]

For Paracelsus, the way forward lay with what he variously described as the *ewigen kirchen, christlichen kirchen, catholischen kirchen, kirchen Christi, kirchen der heiligen,* or order of the cross. As already indicated, he envisaged some kind of congregational arrangement that would be separatist in its nature. Notwithstanding hints about universality, he clearly envisaged a believers' church based on the voluntary subscription of a small group of the spiritually enlightened or 'chosen' believers, with baptism playing a crucial part at the point of entry and the Lord's Supper occupying a symbolically important role in the process of individual and collective renewal. His comments about these congregations make it evident that they would face rejection and persecution by church and state as well as by the majority of the population, all of whom were set on the path of eternal damnation.

Given that there were only twelve apostles, Paracelsus concluded that the community of true believers was likely to remain small. Only a small minority was likely to accept the rigours of the associated regimes of the apostolic mission, poverty and a wandering existence. Paracelsus insisted that the rest of the community should expect to adhere strictly to the teaching of the scriptures and resist all pressures to depart from the Word of God. Inevitably the sheep would be subject to temptations from false priests, but they should be determined not to be deflected from the single, narrow way, door and light, all epitomized by Christ.[52] The moment had come for the weeding out of good from bad. Comfort was taken from the biblical passages stating that the last shall be first and the first last, or that many shall be called but few chosen.[53] Since the way to life was narrow, few would gain entry.[54] Also relevant was the forecast that the harvest would be plenteous but the labourers few.[55] The accumulated evidence suggested that the new congregational order would be small, but, on the model of the early church, extremely potent in its influence. Many of the ascetic standards outlined by Paracelsus for the congregations of believers are reminiscent of the codes adopted during the medieval reforms of the monastic orders and mirrored in lay devotional groups. However, despite such borrowings, Paracelsus had no doubts about opposing monasticism, which was consistent with his high valuation of marriage and acceptance that the discipline of the new congregational order should be open to all. As is evident from both his scientific and social ethical works, there was no sense that the new congregations would be inward looking. Rather it was their mission to minister to all the needs of the poor, with the goal of bringing about an almost utopian social order in the local community, along the lines of the secular framework designed by Michael Gaismair for the province of the Tyrol.

The new congregations were poised to take on great challenges and were expected to achieve major objectives. Although affiliation was founded on voluntary association, the congregations of Paracelsus were clearly seen as inheriting the mantle of the Catholic church and not as merely an addition to the ranks of the sects. Just as there was only one correct order for the Lord's Supper, there was only one legitimate organizational vehicle for the community of believers. Multiplication of sects was inimical to the unity of purpose that was essential for the success of the saints.[56] Paracelsus insisted on a precise equivalence between true believers and the church. Using the bridegroom imagery much favoured among the radicals, his church of Christ or community of saints would be glorified in the sight of God and its members would be eligible to regard Christ as their bridegroom, as well as being rewarded with many other wondrous signs.[57]

Given this exalted status, it was possible for the community of saints to approach the future with a sense of optimism. As further outlined in the next chapter, the future order was expected to exhibit an indivisibility of religious and secular aspirations. In strict regard for the teachings of Christ, the saints would renounce the use of force and commit themselves to peace, humility and patience. Fulfilment of the eschatological scheme depended entirely on the providence of God. On this account Paracelsus envisaged strict renunciation of revolutionary activity to force the pace of change. Only by complete reorientation of values was it possible to locate the path to heaven, which was the way of Christ and the cross and meant acceptance of repentance, poverty, suffering and martyrdom. It also involved simplicity, stillness and love, including commitment to love of neighbour, upon which social regeneration depended. In this transformation, those in a position of authority would assume more burdens than their vassals; preachers would work harder than any of their flock. The way of the cross not only promised spiritual realization, but also wider satisfaction and the achievement of a 'blissful existence' (*selige leben*), which represented the full fruits of spiritual and social regeneration.

Working out the full implications of the *selige leben* was recognized by Paracelsus as one of his major commitments. Although this remained one of his great incomplete projects, the surviving drafts are sufficient to demonstrate the seriousness of the undertaking. Indeed they provide confirmation of his determination to produce a comprehensive plan for future betterment. This plan was sketched out with regard to the eschatological frame of reference. Only those capable of renouncing sin and achieving complete rehabilitation could expect to reach the *selige leben* and then be spared at the Day of Judgement.[58] The seriousness of this expectation concerning the *selige leben* is confirmed by the quotation at the head of the next chapter and by the subsequent discussion of the contribution of Paracelsus to the apocalyptic debate.

Anabaptist Relations

With respect to formative influences on the theological outlook of Paracelsus, most attention has been attracted by Luther and Zwingli, and Erasmus to a lesser degree. Among the reform-minded in Paracelsus's generation, these influences were inescapable. Notwithstanding his inevitable debt to the writings of these seminal figures, Paracelsus decisively rejected both the Catholic church in its current state and the alternatives implemented by the magisterial reformers. Thereby he inevitably became aligned with more radical voices. This shift in the separatist direction raises the question of his attitude towards the Anabaptists, who were at the height of their influence when Paracelsus was formulating his religious position. Anabaptism was of course a diverse phenomenon at this stage, comprising a multiplicity of congregations, the characteristics of which were greatly influenced by certain remarkable and charismatic figures who, for brief periods, dominated their affairs. Anabaptism is relevant for the many minor figures it helped to give a voice to, also for the democratic impulse that allowed congregations to exercise decisive influence in all religious affairs. When these factors are taken into account, it is evident that Anabaptism exercised an influence well beyond its numbers. Friesen has skilfully argued that in some important respects even an Olympian figure like Erasmus was inclined to the perspective adopted by the Anabaptists.[59] Zambelli conducted a spirited enquiry into the radical links of Agrippa von Nettesheim, and she underlined the relevance of Anabaptism in this context.[60] In view of his more obvious radical standpoint, the same enquiry ought to be conducted with respect to Paracelsus.

One of the challenges facing the modern Anabaptist industry has been the sorting out of the unruly cohorts into more natural taxonomic categories. There is now agreement on the identification of some broad divisions within the Anabaptist movement. Such groups displayed a reasonable degree of doctrinal homogeneity and exerted their influence in different regions. Especially pertinent to Paracelsus was the south German type of Anabaptism flourishing in the areas with which he was most associated. This form of Anabaptism happened to exhibit apocalyptic and spiritualist tendencies, both of which constituted obvious points of contact with his outlook.[61]

The wanderings of Paracelsus coincided closely with areas that witnessed a high level of Anabaptist activism. It is quite likely that he was familiar with Anabaptism in its embryonic form during his first stay in Salzburg. Thereafter, his visits to Strasbourg, Nuremberg and St Gallen coincided with phases of preoccupation with the perceived Anabaptist menace. It would indeed have been difficult for him to remain ignorant of Anabaptism. In view of the risk of his own exposure to accusations of dissent and his occupation of a similar ideological niche, this group must have attracted his special curiosity.

Particular tracts by the Anabaptists might have been difficult to locate, but it is evident that their ideas enjoyed wide circulation, as demonstrated for instance by the large common denominator of content in the vast corpus of proceedings against Anabaptists or in the writings of various south German Anabaptist leaders. Many avenues existed whereby Paracelsus might have gained access to intelligence about the Anabaptists and their opinions.

Since he made a fair number of direct references to the Anabaptists and expressed his opinions with confidence, it is evident that he regarded himself as well informed. As ever, he expressed himself in categorical terms. Since almost all of his direct references to the Anabaptists were uncomplimentary, it is tempting to conclude that he absorbed the standard establishment view of this movement. Anabaptists were indeed included in his blanket denunciation of the modern 'sects', although they were much less evident as a target than either the Lutherans or the Zwinglians. As a pacifist, Paracelsus would have regarded militant Anabaptism with abhorrence, but in fact this side of the Anabaptist movement scarcely entered his considerations. Of more concern was the bizarre behaviour and gratuitous craving for martyrdom within some aberrant Anabaptist cells, about which he would have received ample testimony at St Gallen, which was the source of some of the most disturbing stories. On this basis he concluded that Anabaptists suffered from fanatical self-delusion (*kibs*) or mental derangement.[62] On a couple of occasions he even seems to have rebuked the Anabaptists for their undue obsession with the baptismal sacrament.[63]

Considering the evidence as a whole, Paracelsus seems for the most part to have avoided the obvious invitation to make Anabaptists a target for criticism. *De causis morbis invisibilium* constitutes the one obvious exception, where, somewhat gratuitously, Anabaptists were hauled over the coals; this may be explained by special circumstances applying in St Gallen, where the tract was written.[64] It is even possible that Paracelsus scalded the Anabaptists for the benefit of Joachim Vadian who, as a conservative humanist, needed delicate handling and was known to be preoccupied by the Anabaptist issue. Rebukes directed against the Anabaptists were an easy means to purchasing a modicum of credit. There was very little else about Paracelsus that was likely to create a favourable impression on Vadian. Indeed it was not even clear that our reformer was totally out of sympathy with the Anabaptists.

Although recent commentators occasionally remark on points of similarity, sometimes on issues of importance, links between Paracelsus and Anabaptist writers have not been explored systematically.[65] The above survey of the religious leanings of Paracelsus has already exposed his general compatibility with the radical movement and his particular drift towards a congregationalist perspective. It is consequently worth considering whether, beneath the façade of outright rejection, there is any further evidence of his convergence with the Anabaptists, especially those with spiritualist and apocalyptic leanings.

Already in *Septem punctis* Theophrastus had adopted a strong New Testament bias in his theology. He therefore cited gospel authority against his oppressors representing the old church. The same line of defence was applied by dissenters against their establishment persecutors. At the climax of the debates between the radicals and the magisterial reformers in St Gallen in 1532, the dissenters made capital out of the habitual tendency of their critics to fall back on the Old Testament, which was contrasted with their own constant regard for the gospel message.[66] As Hans Marquart of Wißenhorn warned his critics: 'just take note, we are now children of the New Testament'.[67]

During his stay in the St Gallen area between 1530 and 1533, Paracelsus must have been familiar with these exchanges, and also with the anxiety experienced by Vadian and his allies concerning continuing Anabaptist activism.[68] Vadian carried the scars of his feud with Conrad Grebel, his own brother-in-law, over the direction and speed of reform. As a doctor, Vadian was irritated by the refusal of local Anabaptists to flee to places of safety at times of epidemic disease. In the past he had subscribed without hesitation to the common view that flight was the first policy of choice. During the 1529–30 outbreak of sweating sickness, the stubborn Anabaptist resistance to flight prompted Vadian to defend his line in an immense diatribe, which remained incomplete and is still unpublished.[69] Notwithstanding his distaste for the Anabaptists' argument, Vadian abandoned his old practice and remained in St Gallen during the 1529–30 epidemic. Paracelsus disliked some aspects of the fatalism of the Anabaptists, but always insisted that the doctor's duty was to combat diseases at their place of occurrence.[70]

Paracelsus was alarmed by stories about the excesses of local Anabaptist zealots, but the culprits had been punished and disowned by the sect. At St Gallen, bizarre and sinister charades were things of the past. On the main issues of contention between the authorities and the Anabaptists, it was far from clear that the sympathies of Paracelsus rested with Vadian rather than the dissenters.

On the basis of the competent summary by Bonorand, Vadian characterized local Anabaptists as subscribing to twelve dominant tenets.[71] With respect to Bonorand's listing, the first four Anabaptist beliefs were shared by Paracelsus to a limited extent; the second set of five was accepted by him without reservation; he was unsympathetic concerning the final three, but these were also alien to the Anabaptist mainstream.[72] Paracelsus had few difficulties in accepting: (5) the community of goods,[73] (6) rejection of unjust taxation,[74] (7) objection to use of the death sentence,[75] (8) scruples about civil oaths,[76] and (9) the adoption of non-violence and opposition to wars or the right of resistance.[77] On most of these five issues of agreement he expressed himself as vehemently as the Anabaptists in many different writings and in some cases at considerable length.[78]

With respect to Bonorand's first four points, Paracelsus was sympathetic towards (1) Anabaptist reservations concerning the abuse of office by magistrates and other civil authorities, but would not have agreed with the minority of rigorists who adopted a policy of total non-compliance with social controls exercised by outsiders. With regard to Vadian's charge of perfectionism (2), Anabaptists would have denied the charge and claimed that they were being penalized for demanding fidelity to evangelical aspirations that ought to command universal acquiescence. Paracelsus would have approved of their stern judgement concerning the laxity of existing standards without approving of their literalism, legalism or introduction of institutions such as the ban, which he would have regarded as the equivalent of excommunication. He was perhaps also open to the charge of perfectionism, particularly on account of his advanced ideas about divinization of believers, which connected especially with the Docetic tendency of his Christology and sacramental theology. With respect to their exclusiveness and claim to be the only true church (3), the Anabaptists would have denied the charge as stated, but Paracelsus would have sympathized with Vadian's suspicions. However, Vadian would also have regarded the congregations outlined by Paracelsus with just as much abhorrence as the Anabaptist congregations. With reference to (4), the rejection of infant baptism and the substitution of baptism of believers, as further discussed below, Paracelsus paid lip-service to infant baptism, but his considered viewpoint can only be interpreted as acceptance of the baptism of believers.

Given the substantial area of agreement between Paracelsus and the Anabaptists according to the criteria applied by the long-suffering Vadian, it is not surprising that in their general ethos the writings of Paracelsus betray striking similarities with various of the declarations of belief emanating from Anabaptist sources. The parallels are most pronounced with Anabaptists representing the spiritualist and apocalyptic perspective.

The author of the *Septem punctis* would therefore have discovered little with which to disagree in the concise *Sieben Artickel* produced by Jakob Kautz, who carried the baton for Denck after the latter's expulsion from Strasbourg.[79] Paracelsus was in a position to witness the confrontation between Denck's team and the Strasbourg authorities in the late autumn of 1526, which ended with the expulsion of the radical leaders in early 1527. This celebrated test-case provided a practical demonstration of the problems raised by the evolving social ethic of the Anabaptists. Reflecting the spiritualism of Denck, Kautz emphasized the free accessibility of the 'light' of the Holy Spirit, which had been purposely obscured and made inaccessible by both the old church and its Lutheran successors. Following Müntzer and Denck, and also reflecting the usage of Paracelsus, Kautz relied heavily on the outer/inner distinction in outlining the escape from sterile externalities to the living Word or Voice of God.

Such reorientation involved a radical rejection of ceremonial, which he regarded as incompatible with the qualities manifested in Christ himself. Kautz cited the gospel commission of Matthew 28: 19 and Mark 16: 15–16 as laying down the criteria for the sacraments, on which basis he rejected infant baptism and called for a spiritual understanding of the Lord's Supper. He also implicitly rejected predestination and placed the emphasis on free will. In line with this universalism, he stressed the role of Jesus Christ as the new Adam, whose redeeming role was exercised, not by his single act of sacrifice as understood by Luther, but by his general example, the consistent following of which constituted an essential means to salvation. Individual commitment to a life of suffering, faithful to the way of Christ, was contrasted with the Lutherans and their *schriftgelehrten* advocates, who corrupted the gospel and made Christ into an idol (*abgott*).

The articles drafted by Kautz contained much that was congenial to Paracelsus, and indeed they exercised distinct appeal among the church leadership in Strasbourg. On aspects of faith such as free will, predestination, the universality of grace, and also more generally on questions of anthropology, Christology and soteriology, Paracelsus was more in agreement with Denck and Kautz than with the Lutherans. He may also have noticed with approval that Denck's Anabaptists in Strasbourg favoured dispensing with the office of priest, which was contrary to the position adopted by the Swiss Anabaptists in their Schleitheim Articles.

Ten years after Kautz, Calvin conducted discussions with Anabaptists in Strasbourg; indeed he married the widow of an Anabaptist. The main literary product of these discussions was a two-part tract, the first part of which was a critique of what he perceived to be the Anabaptists' most typical points of delinquency. The first chapters concentrated on the Schleitheim Articles relating to baptism, the ban, civil authority and oaths. The final chapter attacked the Anabaptist interpretation of the incarnation on the basis of alleged Valentinian and Docetic tendencies. The second part was devoted entirely to the question of sleep of the soul, an idea which was obviously widely shared among Anabaptists at this date. Calvin would have discovered that virtually the whole of his critique could be applied to Paracelsus, who not only subscribed to most of the Schleitheim principles to which Calvin took exception, but was also a prominent exponent of heterodox opinions on the question of incarnation, and even made use of the idea of sleep of the soul.[80]

In light of the above evidence it is not surprising to find that, both in incidental detail and general outlook, expositions by Paracelsus readily find their counterparts in classic tracts emanating from the wider Anabaptist movement. It has already been pointed out that both Paracelsus and Jörg Haugk von Jüchsen were attracted by number symbolism and both used seven as an organizing principle, Paracelsus in *Septem punctis*, and Haugk in his *Ain christlich ordenung* (c. 1524).[81] Where Haugk differed from Kautz, he tended to agree with Paracelsus. Like Kautz, Haugk attacked the prevailing worldliness and preoccupation with externalities; he drew more than Kautz on mystic terminology and concepts in his account of the ascetic quest for salvation. Like Kautz, Haugk prominently invoked the fear of God and the need for suffering, in accordance with the example of Christ.

The outlook of Paracelsus was also consistent with the extensive preamble to Hans Hut's *Von dem geheimnus der tauf*.[82] Hut insisted that poor people had been badly let down by their priesthood, which was corrupted by its misguided, worldly, avaricious and soft way of life. Nobody would learn the secrets of godly wisdom through these Pharisees, who had made their churches into dens of thieves (*spelunken oder mörder-grueben*).[83] The only way forward was to eliminate the system of benefices and thoroughly reform the existing priesthood, thereby paving the way for a new evangelical regime of Christian love in which all brothers and sisters would be united in righteousness under the cross of Christ. This new discipline demanded a decisive return to the simplicity of faith, with believers recapturing the purity of childhood or even reverting to the ways of simple people (*narren*). For Hut there was no better way of symbolizing this decisive break with the past than by the institution of baptism of believers.

Like Paracelsus, Hut developed his programme for reform in a strongly apocalyptic context. The apocalyptic motif was also dominant in the writings of Melchior Hoffman, and it was evident in Haugk. For a short period, at the popular level, south German Anabaptism was predominantly apocalyptic. As we shall see in the next chapter, Paracelsus developed his own distinctive approach to apocalyptic analysis and prophecy. He was more cautious about commitment to rigid timetables than some leading Anabaptists, but in other respects his outlook was similar, and this also applied to his approach to such various themes as the sleep of the soul, the Sabbath rest, and the perceived Ottoman Turkish menace, each of which was relevant to his eschatology.[84]

The Gospel of Creatures

A further point of confluence in outlook between the Anabaptists and Paracelsus related to their common attachment to the injunction to preach the gospel as authorized in the gospels of Matthew and Mark. The importance of this injunction to Paracelsus has already been established and it was equally essential to the Anabaptists.[85] Among the last instructions of Christ to his disciples was the order to go into the world and preach the gospel to every creature. Believers were instructed to accept baptism as a mark of their salvation, after which they were promised many gifts, including the power to heal the sick.[86] Evangelization of the world was seen by Anabaptists as part of the new dispensation initiated by the Resurrection, which thereby fulfilled the prophecy of Daniel and granted Christ dominion over the whole world until the end of time.[87] Believers were told to turn this eschatological expectation into a reality. The combined functions of preaching, baptizing and healing therefore assumed a special level of significance in the final days. These dramatic challenges added to the dynamism of the Anabaptist mission, which of course was not restricted to ordained priests, but was open to the entire baptized community of their saints. The force of impact of the gospel commission was amply confirmed by the evidence of personal testimonies when Anabaptist activists were subjected to criminal inquisitions.[88] Although Paracelsus adapted the gospel commission to his own aptitudes and circumstances, he saw himself as contributing to this collective missionary endeavour to which the Anabaptists were equally strongly called and in which they were the main players. He was confident about making a conspicuous contribution in his capacities as preacher and healer, and his affairs were conducted with a view to maximizing his impact on both fronts. On this account he avoided any gratuitous confrontation with secular and religious authorities that might prejudice his liberty and survival. Marginalization, disapprobation and a persistent harassment were willingly accepted as integral to the experience of martyrdom, which both Paracelsus and the Anabaptists regarded as a necessary consequence of their apostolic vocation.[89]

Both Paracelsus and the Anabaptists were committed to the instruction, generally interpreted as a duty, to preach the gospel to the whole creation (*prediget das evangelium aller creatur*).[90] If acquainted with Haugk's tract, Paracelsus would have been struck by his liberal use of analogies from nature, including the idea that human decadence had involved reversion to a base animal type. Haugk interpreted the gospel commission as an instruction to preach the gospel according to its manifestation in the created order. For a short time this construction became general among the Anabaptists. The most influential proponent of this interpretation of the gospel commission was Hans Hut. Anabaptists tended to refer to this teaching as 'the gospel of all creatures' (*das evangelium aller creatur*) and to justify it with reference to other New Testament passages.[91]

The gospel of creatures was the means by which believers, even the simplest people, could abstract essential Christian teachings from the natural world. The main sources related to the behaviour of imagined beasts or domesticated animals, from which it was possible to learn about the necessity of suffering and understand better the message of the crucifixion. At the same time the gospel of creatures warned of the need to root out materialism and avoid the temptations represented by the creaturely level of existence. It was a forceful reminder of the universality of the power of God, which had to be observed in a spirit of fear and earnest endeavour with a view to maintaining, and where necessary restoring, the order in nature that was implanted at the time of the creation. Through the gospel of creatures the whole world assumed figurative importance as an object lesson in the search for redemption through suffering.[92]

Although the gospel of creatures as developed by the Anabaptists was idiosyncratic, it possessed some obvious points of reference to the natural theology that occupied a contested, but distinctive niche in medieval theology.[93] It also connected with the idea, cultivated by mystics such as Seuse, that Christ was sent to earth so that the attributes of the Creator, obscured since the creation, would be revealed by physical example and would then be understood throughout creation. In particular, as is indicated by the strong overlap of the images of the crucified Christ and the Creator as represented in Illustration 6, the might and divinity of God was most perfectly revealed through the humanity that Christ assumed.[94]

The injunction by Christ for his followers to preach the gospel, baptize and perform acts of healing was of course treated with great seriousness by Paracelsus.[95] With respect to the preaching obligation, he tended to quote the fuller relevant text, referring to preaching the gospel to all creatures (*das evangelium allen creaturen*), thereby adopting the more conventional vernacular translation rather than the alternative favoured by Hut.[96] However, in common with Hut and other Anabaptists, the creatures text was taken to indicate that nature, especially the animal kingdom, provided a source of object lessons for human edification. In their liberal use of analogies drawn from nature or mythologies relating to nature, both Paracelsus and the Anabaptists recognized the value of standard reference points in popular culture for the communication of their message.[97]

From his naturalistic perspective, Paracelsus concluded, like Haugk, that on account of their propensity for sin humans habitually tended to plummet down the scale of nature. As already pointed out, central to his macrocosm–microcosm theory was the idea that humans encapsulated the characteristics of the animal kingdom, their inferiors in creation. Animals were regarded as a mirror in which human nature might be better understood.[98] As a corollary of this animal ingredient of personality, exacerbated by the fall of Adam, humans were endowed with degenerate creaturely instincts (*wir alle von Adam tierisch geborn seindt*).[99] This inheritance rendered humans vulnerable to replicating various types of base behaviour prevalent within the animal kingdom. The negative creaturely (*vihisch*) aspect of human personality was explored in great detail, drawing on an impressive range of animal types to provide a lurid portrayal of this form of moral danger.[100] Since moral degeneracy was occasioned by succumbing to base animal instincts, Paracelsus concluded that the task of preaching and rehabilitation was a mission akin to ministering to animals, with the goal of persuading the reprobate to shed their 'old creature' and take on the characteristics of the 'new creature'. Such a complete transformation was the only way to attain the blessed existence. By means of this argument he arrived at his own characteristic understanding of the *evangelium allen creaturen*.[101] It was assumed that John the Baptist and Christ himself were reflecting the same point of view when the former called the Pharisees a generation of vipers or when Christ explored images about ravening wolves, pearls before swine and so on.[102]

Humans were endowed with the capacity to attract both positive and negative sidereal influences. Through their exclusive affinity with favourable virtues, the regenerate could assume the identity of lambs or turtle doves.[103] The more usual human propensity was signified by the assumption of the identity of wolves, basilisks, serpents or vipers. Degeneration to the level of a pig and assumption of a '*säuisch*' personality placed a person beyond redemption. Such persons were incapable of being born again to the new life.[104] In some respects humans could be regarded as a sum of the personalities of various animals, replicating both their positive and negative characteristics. The gibberish of scholars reflected the dominance of instincts derived from the parrot; and the posturing of graduates was no more significant than the noises emanating from parrots with their bent beaks and clumsy feet. Aggression and competitiveness were derived from the fox or wolf.[105] Some animal characteristics provided valuable survival instincts, but it was essential to rise above this inferior aspect of personality, among other reasons because animals were subject to the control of planetary forces. Only by engaging with higher spiritual powers was it possible to transcend the level of the creature and escape from the influences emanating from the stars. Notable among those who failed to achieve this emancipation were the secular princes, as was evident in their habit of provoking wars in order to build up their empires. These were *viehischen menschen*, who were in thrall to the stars and their base animal instincts. As a consequence, they would eventually be hunted down as easily as the hunters secured their game. By contrast, believers subdued their animal instincts and lived in the wisdom of God; from this higher moral vantage-point, they coexisted in peace and refrained from the letting of blood.[106] Believers thereby evaded the dangers of the ubiquitous dens of iniquity and were able to prepare themselves for the future golden age.[107]

Consistently with their ideas about the gospel of creatures, the Anabaptists and Paracelsus adopted a common approach to preserving the *rechtschaffener ordnung* or *gottliche ordnung der tiefe* in the natural and moral world. Here the most relevant dichotomies were higher/lower and outer/inner. Believers faced the challenge of maintaining this order, free of all impediments stemming from falsehood in its various guises. They were caught up in a cosmic contest between the Holy Spirit and the legions of Satan. Acceptance of the enlightening spirit from above served to uphold the order of things (*ordo rerum*) imposed by the Creator.[108] Succumbing to infernal forces entailed reverting to the level of the creature and subverting the order of nature. Only the inner working of the Holy Spirit led to new birth and to the enjoyment of the fruits that resulted from the seed that God sowed in the innermost parts of nature. The inferior way led to outer and superficial knowledge, symbolized by husks and sterility. Plato and Aristotle and their followers were censured for throwing away the opportunity to transcend their animal nature. Their seed was planted among thorns and was destined to come to nothing. They represented the dominance of evil spirits and the path to certain ruin. The only hope for rebirth rested with those who followed the gospel injunctions to knock and seek. In response to earnest praying and fasting, God would see to it that they were born again; their seed would flourish and their wisdom would flow freely as a reward for their strict regard for the gospel message. They would emancipate themselves from the level of the creature to such a degree that, in the end, their spirit would be without stain or any imprint of animal nature. Their goal should be to base everything on gospel precedent and allow everything to flow from this source (*alles im evangelio gegrünt und aus im fließ*). Every action needed to be consistent with this source and there should be no departure from its requirements. Anyone contemplating aggression should consider whether there was any basis in the gospel for their actions; similarly, since their professional decisions were matters of life and death, jurists or doctors should apply these same criteria. Only those observing the gospel imperative and contributing to the preservation of God's order would be counted among the regenerate. Delinquents undermining this order, for instance through rapacious greed, would be ruthlessly punished by destruction and none would be spared.[109]

The gospel and order of nature were invoked for important and similar purposes by Paracelsus and the Anabaptists. In this context the approach adopted by Paracelsus was consistent with Grebel, Kautz and the Schleitheim Articles. Compliance with the stringent discipline of the gospel message promised all the liberal benefits associated with the new birth that flowed from God's copious grace. On the other hand, failure to heed the gospel message would entail continuing entrapment by base creaturely instincts and the values of the material world. Owing to the misuse of nature and transgression against the moral order ordained by God, both Paracelsus and the Anabaptists held out the prospect of severe retribution for every kind of delinquent under the apocalyptic timetable that, they were certain, was already unfolding.

The Sacraments and the Way to Heaven

Paracelsus was a critic of the Catholic mass, the sacrament of penance and most other aspects of the sacramental system of the old church. He decisively rejected the standard Catholic teaching that the seven sacraments represented seven necessary remedies for the soul, all contributing to the build-up of credit on the path to rebirth.[110] Paracelsus adopted the usual reformist position that only those sacraments justified on a scriptural basis should be retained. It was generally accepted that the sacraments of baptism and the Lord's Supper were acceptable. Beyond this point the spurious unity broke down and the whole sacramental question became the subject of bitter and prolonged controversy.

Paracelsus gave every sign of acquaintanceship with the sacramental disputes that were raging around him.[111] But rather than fit into any of the obvious confessional niches, he tended to his habitual independence of outlook, indeed not hesitating to strike out towards idiosyncratic and unexpected conclusions, especially when these seemed called for by their consistency with his general dispositions. The result was often a distinctive but not entirely remote point of view, arguably closer to certain of his Anabaptist counterparts than to any of the mainstream positions. Even though most of the relevant primary sources remain unpublished, the active interest of Paracelsus in the sacramental issue has long been appreciated and this subject is now attracting the attention that it merits.[112] In view of the existence of much promising ongoing work, the following remarks will concentrate on questions relating to points of convergence between Paracelsus and the spiritualist Anabaptists.

The centrality of the issues surrounding the sacraments was not lost on Paracelsus. The crucial role of both baptism and the Lord's Supper is indicated by his unqualified claim that these sacraments constituted the way to heaven.[113] They were seen as integral to shaking off the traditional, corrupt, '*Hagarisch*', inheritance associated with the old flesh. Only by accepting this essential core of the sacramental system was it possible to attain total rebirth and renewal as children of the Holy Spirit, which in turn conferred eligibility for membership of reformed congregations and participation in the wider community of the kingdom of heaven.[114] Alternatively expressed, the two sacraments offered the means for believers to shake themselves free of the corrupt, old flesh of Adam, in order to participate in the heavenly blood and flesh of Christ. Thereby they assumed the status of '*neu mensch*', qualified to be regarded as brethren to Christ and God.[115] The sacraments were therefore the sole means of accessing the greatest mysteries. Consequently, although they were reduced in number, the sacraments were not at all diminished in significance. If anything, their status was enhanced, since the most profound mysteries were placed within reach of the most humble believers entirely on their basis of their own independent action, without reliance on the mediation of any form of priesthood.

Since baptism was portrayed as the first and decisive step in the process of rebirth, it was likely to feature in any of the writings of Paracelsus, as was the figure of John the Baptist, who assumed a striking exemplary role.[116] The powerful voice of John crying in the wilderness (*schreien stimm*) seemed to foreshadow the situation of Paracelsus himself.[117] Through his hard life and suffering, John made himself receptive to the Holy Spirit.[118] He knew that exposure to trials of the desert (*die rechte wüeste*) represented the only way to God. This wasteland was, in the view of Paracelsus, the only place for believers to live.[119]

From an early stage in his career, Paracelsus accepted that baptism was a fundamental institution of the church. This was an unremarkable conclusion, and one of his didactic expositions on baptism suggests an entirely conventional outlook. Infant baptism was accepted without demur, and resorting to a second baptism of believers was rejected. He insisted on simplification of the baptismal ceremony on the grounds of removing idolatrous features, but this objective also was widely supported. For once he seemed to be entirely at peace with the general evangelical outlook, also obviously avoiding partisanship with respect to the ongoing dispute between Luther and Zwingli.[120]

Other comments about baptism suggest a less conventional approach. As befitting its association with John the Baptist, baptism seemed to belong to the province of believers rather than infants. In all of his expositions Paracelsus underlined that the crucial aspect of baptism was not the water ceremony, but the acceptance of the Holy Spirit. The latter was appreciated only by true believers. The Holy Spirit washed away all sins and suitably initiated a new life and spiritual rebirth that was able to transcend the wasteland of mortal existence and bring about identification with the suffering and satisfaction offered by Christ.[121] Baptism was described as a great transformation, the discarding of the old, decadent flesh and tainted blood of Adam and elevation into a new body infused with the blood of truth inherited from Christ, that would bring release from the experience of death. The new situation was also described as a state of virginity. Baptism was seen as a fresh incarnation mediated by the Holy Spirit, marking the end of a form of life restricted by natural laws and the limitations of animal nature. Understandably, without baptism there would be no ascent to a state of purity. The baptized community operated under a new dispensation or office that conferred an ability to make the transition to a higher level of spiritual wisdom, through which they could reach the highest, angelic level of enlightenment, *englische weisheit* or *höchste erleuchtung*.[122]

With respect to the earliest comments of Paracelsus on baptism, Gause points to possible parallels with the thinking of the early Anabaptist activist Balthasar Hubmaier,[123] who was the main target of attack from Zwingli on this issue.[124] Gause also points out that it is difficult to think of some of the Paracelsus expositions on baptism as applying to anything other than the baptism of mature believers.[125]

Although Paracelsus avoided explicit discussion of the relative merits of infant and adult baptism, comments in many of his mature writings on this subject reinforce the impression that, for most circumstances, he envisaged adult baptism as the norm. Amplifications by Paracelsus suggest that he regarded baptism as a matter of choice, and consequently a challenge suitable only for mature persons and for believers. All were faced with the choice between Adam and Christ, the two figures who epitomized the dichotomy between matter and spirit. Adam stood for all the limitations of the creature and material existence, while faith in Christ entailed a life of sacrifice, but also the promise of new flesh and blood. Baptism was the beginning of a process that ended with resurrection at the Day of Judgement, after which baptized believers would join Christ in the kingdom of heaven.[126]

This transition to the new flesh and blood was announced as a direct gift, spontaneously flowing into humans (*eingeflossen*) from the Father, without any other mediator (*ohne alle mittel*), and infused from above (*von oben herab*) exclusively by the Holy Spirit.[127] Baptism was therefore a way to unlock transcendent powers (*kraft, macht*) not obtainable by any other means. Such spiritual transformation was possible only through faith, without which the Holy Spirit would be impotent.[128] Only those possessing an active faith and who had reached a state of enlightenment could benefit from baptism and be receptive to the Holy Spirit. It was therefore advised that baptism should take place immediately after coming to the new faith, since this would expose believers to the optimal powers of the Holy Spirit. This order of events was correct because it recapitulated the baptism of Christ by John the Baptist. As in the work of John the Baptist in the Jordan, the baptismal sacrament was designed for willing believers who, of course, were persons of maturity, but could be described as being new born.[129]

When viewed in context, baptism emerged as a high priority, but only on the understanding that those who participated in this sacrament were acting in the spirit of faith.[130] Also suggesting the design of baptism for mature persons, Paracelsus warned that those taking the conscious decision to reject the way of faith and baptism were destined for eternal damnation.[131] Baptism was associated with a crucial spiritual decision. Rejection of baptism irredeemably tied people to their mortal body and confined them to the blind alley of their terrestrial existence. Faith and baptism were passports to the province of heavenly wisdom or 'astronomy', and eventually eternal life. Baptized believers would prosper in their capacities as theologian, prophet, apostle or martyr. In each of these spheres they would display a capacity for 'fruits and works'.[132]

Sometimes, references by Paracelsus to the involvement of adults in the baptismal ceremony seem to mean nothing more than the taking of pledges on behalf of infants. But this is not always the case, as for example the reference to David, who took up his pledge on his own behalf in front of his people. This ceremonial action was described as the analogue to baptism. Hence David separated himself from the behaviour of the Pharisees by his actions. In the same way baptism acted to pledge the person baptized to the fear of God and thereby to a life of poverty and honesty in all of their dealings. The collectivity of those fulfilling the baptismal obligation would comprise the community of saints who would join in Christian unity ultimately to achieve a state of affairs that could be described as a new Jerusalem.[133]

For the scriptural justification of baptism, Paracelsus relied heavily on the gospel commission of Mark 16: 15–16. According to this hard-worked passage, Paracelsus proclaimed, the faith was to be preached throughout the world to all-comers; thereby the chosen people would be drawn to the faith and would offer themselves for baptism.[134] This same scriptural passage was also taken by the Anabaptists as evidence that the gospels firmly restricted baptism to mature believers, an interpretation that was of course contested by Zwingli.[135] Paracelsus used Mark 16: 15–16 to emphasize the shortcomings of the existing priesthood, who restricted themselves to their parishes and therefore made no contact with complete unbelievers. Preaching the gospel to all creatures was here taken as an instruction to take the Word to all unbelievers, even Turks and Tartars, who would then be baptized as a sign of their faith. Among the Anabaptists, the above gospel text was taken as an instruction to preach to all unbelievers with a view to achieving their conversion, after which baptism was viewed as a necessary consequence.[136]

Given the above instances, it is arguable that Paracelsus regarded baptism as a practice that might apply in many circumstances to mature persons in response to their conversion. Such practice seemed an entirely correct understanding of the gospel commission, which itself was in keeping with the precedent set by John the Baptist. When he wrote approvingly of the mission of John the Baptist in preaching the true faith and overthrowing the practices of false apostles concerning baptism, Paracelsus was not, as was supposed by Goldammer, inveighing against the Anabaptists, but more likely against the Catholics and perhaps also the magisterial reformers, all of whom persisted in the unscriptural practice of confining baptism to infants.[137] This radical perspective is more consistent with the context, which is an attack on the general wantonness of the clergy and also on their magical pretensions. He appealed to believers to follow the example of more enlightened teachers, his *gesandten*, who operated according to the dictates of the gospel commission.[138] The position of Paracelsus on baptism coincides more closely with that of the Anabaptists than is generally appreciated. Given the sensitivity of this issue, prudential considerations would have led him to leave his expositions to speak for themselves rather than to engage in direct controversy. In view of his other expositions which were more accepting of infant baptism, he may well have sided with those Anabaptists who adopted a lenient attitude to this old tradition, especially because infant baptism was not specifically prohibited in the gospels. He also appreciated that infant baptism was a source of consolation in cases of deaths in infancy, or for persons with mental a handicap.[139] It is even arguable that the insertion of remarks that could be taken as tolerant of infant baptism was an intentional defensive device, since dogmatic subscription to adult baptism was one of the surest paths to the executioner's blade. It is also possible that expressions of lenience about infant baptism were designed to signify reservations about the mainstream Anabaptist movement, which had employed adult baptism as the basis for a form of intolerant and rigid sectarianism that was just as offensive to Paracelsus as the other manifestations of sectarianism he criticized.

The proximity of the thinking of Paracelsus to that of the Anabaptists seems not to have been lost on his immediate followers. In one of his many references to Mark 16: 16, Paracelsus concluded that those who believed and were baptized were also deeply blessed. Alert to the sequence of belief and baptism, an early adherent inserted 'W.' in the margin, which may well have been taken by his contemporaries as signalling '*Wiedertäufer*', an interpretation that has been accepted as likely by the modern editor.[140]

For both Paracelsus and the Anabaptists, baptism was not a single, isolated event but the beginning of a developmental process of discipleship, modelled on the life and suffering of Christ. The water baptism of John was a prelude to spiritual baptism in Christ, in the course of which the new life was sustained, reinforced and rendered fruitful by the Holy Spirit. Essential to this stepwise undertaking was participation in the Lord's Supper. This sacrament was not expected to be intrusive in the life of the ordinary lay person, but it was symbolically important, and consequently the subject of intense literary attention from Paracelsus, who was keen to place on record his own distinctive analysis.

In line with the attitudes of Paracelsus expressed in *Septem punctis*, more than any other sacrament or liturgy, the Catholic mass seemed to encapsulate the shortcomings of the church. Once again, Paracelsus was expressing a widespread grievance when calling for the dismantling of this elaborate practice and for the elimination of its many associated financial penalties.[141] The elaborate liturgy of the mass was described as pure idolatry, totally inappropriate for remembering the suffering and death of Christ, which should be the sole concern of believers. This remembrance ceremony needed to reflect the spirit of the poor.[142] As with the baptismal ceremony, he went further than most reformers in his demands for simplification of the Lord's Supper. He called for the total rejection of input from mealy-mouthed clerics (*murmeler*). In the interests of the congregation, he advocated the use of ordinary bread and wine, both accessible to all participants, who would accompany their Lord's Supper with the reading of relevant verses from the sixth chapter of the fourth gospel.[143] In this conception, the Lord's Supper represented such a potent force that it was not needed daily; for the laity, having it once a year would be sufficient for full communication of its virtues.[144]

Paracelsus dissociated himself from all the main streams of interpretation of the Eucharist, rejecting the idea of the sacrifice of the mass, Catholic transubstantiation, Luther's consubstantiation, and Zwingli's symbolism, which was shared by many Anabaptists.[145] In the view of Paracelsus, the Lord's Supper entailed a great mystery, to which he applied his own unorthodox understanding. For this purpose he drew on insights from his Marian writings, his evolving Christology and his cosmological theories and their metaphysical presuppositions. It was accepted that this sacrament served the purpose of achieving union between the believer and Christ, but Paracelsus rejected the idea of a 'magical' conversion of the elements assumed in Catholic or Lutheran practice. Instead, the communicant experienced engagement with the spiritual being or heavenly flesh that comprised the essential nature of Christ. Thereby, unwittingly or not, Paracelsus stumbled towards various ancient heresies that had been the subject of protracted controversy before they were finally rejected, in some cases a thousand years before his birth. In the late medieval period the relevant heresies were known mainly through the denunciations contained in classic ante-Nicene works such as Tertullian's *De carne Christi*.[146] The attacks by Calvin on the alleged Valentinian heresies of the Anabaptists were founded on his reading of Tertullian.[147] If Paracelsus was familiar with such a source, he was clearly more attracted by the targets of Tertullian's attacks than by the powerful patristic invective against the heretics.

As in the case of baptism, Paracelsus avoided systematic exposition or direct confrontation with the awkward issues raised by his speculations. It is nevertheless striking that, on some occasions, his interpretation of the Lord's Supper can only be taken as implying that the human appearance of Christ was an illusion. He therefore drifted towards denial of the two natures of Christ, with substitution of the proposition that Christ had only one nature and that this was a divine existence. The roots of this diffuse heresy are traditionally traced back to the Docetic position, the development of which was blamed by Tertullian on groups such as the Gnostics and on individuals such as Valentinus. It has rightly been pointed out that Docetic (and indeed monophysite) tendencies were already evident in the early Marian writings of Paracelsus.[148] If anything, such an idea became even more prevalent in his later thinking.[149] He insisted that the corporality of Christ was more apparent than real.

After his birth and baptism, Christ retained the appearance of all the usual human qualities, but without possessing any normal kind of corporality (*die empfindlicheit in Christo ohn ein corporalitet*), since his blood and flesh were completely taken away. Christ then bore his body like a piece of angelic or heavenly clothing. As a consequence he was able to shed this apparent physicality at the moment of his resurrection and give full expression to his eternal or heavenly corporality. This same exalted change was held out as a realistic expectation for all those who subscribed to the order of Christ (*die ordnung Christi*) through their new birth.[150] Paracelsus believed that the Lord's Supper enabled communicants to engage personally and directly with the 'heavenly flesh' or 'spiritual limbus' of Christ and thereby glimpse the full possibilities of eternal life.[151] Participation in the Lord's Supper provided the chance to claim just reward for the life of sacrifice that stemmed from observance of the gospel commission and spreading the word to unbelievers throughout the whole world.[152] The Lord's Supper therefore offered a source of inspiration to the community of saints that they expected to draw upon until the end of the world.[153]

As already noted, recent commentators on Paracelsus have highlighted his teachings on the sacraments. They draw particular attention to his concept of the heavenly flesh, which is pertinent to his theological, philosophical and scientific outlook. As in the case of his ideas about baptism, his interpretation of the Lord's Supper was not without its contemporary counterparts; again, the closest parallels were with the Anabaptists and the spiritualists. Similar ideas were at least considered in the Eucharistic speculations of Melchior Hoffman and Clemens Ziegler, as well as in the Caspar von Schwenckfeld/Valentin Krautwald partnership, all of whom were linked with Strasbourg.[154] All of them came round to the idea of heavenly flesh in the context of their Christology and Eucharistic thinking. Their aberrant approach to the sacraments and drift towards a Docetic or monophysite position stimulated controversy and added to their notoriety. Calvin's alarm at the prevalence of such ideas among Anabaptists in Strasbourg had prompted him to compose a fierce denunciation of these views on the incarnation of Christ. Had the ideas of Paracelsus been known, he also would no doubt have been drawn into this critique. In light of the distant connections of Paracelsus with Vadian, it is worth noting that the latter was one of the most notable combatants on the side of the Zwinglian establishment in the Eucharistic controversy. Although Strasbourg provided a possible source of direct contact between Paracelsus and this wider Docetic group, it seems unlikely that the mature views of the other discussants had evolved by the date of his visit. On balance it seems likely that the Docetic position was reached entirely independently by Paracelsus, although in this case, as on other tenets of faith, the whole group may well have been drawing on common sources of influence from late medieval theology.

Spiritual Reform

Attention to his understanding of the sacraments of baptism and the Lord's Supper provides further confirmation of the affinity between Paracelsus and the radical movement of his time. On the basis of many points of agreement on essentials of their faith as well as additional similarities on non-essentials, it is tempting to categorize Paracelsus as an Anabaptist. However, because of distinct reservations on his part about certain tenets of the Anabaptists, or his distrust of zealots exhibiting sectarian aspirations, for present purposes it is sufficient to emphasize that Paracelsus had more in common with the Anabaptists than some of his adverse comments might suggest. His closest affinity lies with other individualistic opinion formers, who had Anabaptist links but ultimately favoured a more independent stance. Like Paracelsus, they were attracted by certain aspects of Anabaptism but disappointed by its practice, which exposed all the classic manifestations of sectarian intolerance and demagogy. Paracelsus would not have been beset by a sense of isolation. The literary exploits of a host of minor figures such as Hans Greiffenberger, Hans Hergot, Jörg Haugk von Jüchsen or Clemens Ziegler suggest striking compatibilities of approach on both spiritual and secular issues. With respect to more weighty authorities, the mature religious thinking of Paracelsus approximates to that of such near contemporaries as Brunfels, Denck, Franck, Bunderlin and Entfelder, all of whom shared his links with Strasbourg. On key matters of faith their expositions are almost interchangeable with respect to language and concept. All of them were committed to the II Corinthians 3: 6-inspired objective of discrediting the authority of the *schriftgelehrten* in the name of freedom of the spirit.

Although publications such as the *Paradoxa* of Sebastian Franck seemed a perfect complement to his own literary output, Paracelsus would have been alert to definite differences of emphasis among the radicals. For his taste, Franck, like the Florentine Neoplatonists, was too immersed in the classical tradition. While Paracelsus, in line with the Anabaptists, habitually deferred to the apostolic imperative of Mark 16: 15, in the *Paradoxa* this verse was studiously ignored by the more reticent Franck.[155] On the other hand Paracelsus would have welcomed the eschatological framework adopted in Franck's great *Chronica*. The primacy of eschatological considerations was also shared by Hans Hut and other leading militant Anabaptists. However, Franck and Paracelsus disapproved of the dogmatism of the militant Anabaptists in their apocalyptic forecasts. They were offended by the mature ideas of Hoffman on the same grounds, as well as finding alien his outlook on hierarchy within the church or on the sinfulness of the Virgin Mary. On these latter issues, among the indigenous Strasbourg radicals, Paracelsus had more in common with Ziegler.

Similarities of outlook are of course to some extent indicative of the operation of common influences from the past. As a corrective to the dominant preoccupation with old dissenters as progenitors of modern Anglo-Saxon sects, recent research on individual radicals, as well as the broader Anabaptist movement, has established their greater reliance on late medieval traditions of piety than was hitherto suspected. A similar debt is evident in the case of Paracelsus, who seems to have been attracted by precisely the same sources. The final chapter of this study underlines this conclusion with respect to the Franciscan apocalyptic tradition associated with Joachim of Fiore. Indeed virtually the whole apocalyptic exercise of the Reformation rested on medieval foundations. Paracelsus was also by no means alone among the radicals in preserving the idea of an elevated status for the Virgin Mary, which reflected a strongly developed theme in piety on the eve of the Reformation.[156] In common with the broader evangelical movement, Paracelsus was alarmed by idolatrous aspects of the cult of veneration of the saints, and he shared the movement's opposition to monasticism or lay orders and confraternities, as they functioned on the eve of the Reformation. Yet it is evident that many aspects of the ascetic and communal ideals of the radicals were derived from such medieval models, which were silently transposed to meet the requirements of the later age and thereby incorporated into the sectarian social ethic.[157] Although the Anabaptists rejected the Catholic tradition of sacramental and sacerdotal mediation by the priesthood, they absorbed much of the regenerationist and ascetic tradition of late medieval piety.[158]

Most of the older expressions of piety assimilated by the radicals would have emanated from intangible currents of religious practice. Such congenial precedents were reinforced by expositions such as the *Imitatio Christi*, the *Theologia Deutsch*, and even the *Horologium sapientiae*, which were already launched on their path to becoming spiritual classics.[159] Although it is impossible to establish the precise basis for Paracelsus's literary inspiration, recent researches have drawn attention to the general influence exercised by the sermons of Johannes Tauler which, from 1508 onwards, were widely available in their original German-language form. This collection provided a readily accessible and comprehensive insight into late medieval mysticism that was actively exploited by reformers of all colours.[160] Paracelsus shows every sign of indebtedness to the same source for a great deal of his most favoured language as well as for some of his most actively used concepts.

The association of Paracelsus with mysticism is of course a familiar notion. C.G. Jung laid the foundation for identifying Paracelsus with a generalized form of transcendental mysticism, but this connection is difficult to sustain if consideration is limited to works of unquestionably authentic origin. Of more tangible importance is the evidence suggestive of indebtedness to late medieval German mysticism. The latter movement produced a prodigious literary legacy, the appeal of which remained undiminished in the sixteenth century. The influence of this indigenous expression of mysticism penetrated many sections of the radical movement. In his first overview of Paracelsus, Goldammer acknowledged that his subject belonged broadly to the mystical religious type. In particular, he recognized that key elements in the language of Paracelsus, as well as many basic ideas, were likely to have been derived from the German mystics.[161] This source was for instance invoked to explain his habitual reference to the dichotomy between interiority and exteriority, a deep-seated idea in Christian spirituality that was explored exhaustively by the German mystics. Goldammer stood by this conclusion; also his team sometimes cited examples of links with the mystics in their editorial comments. However, this conclusion was not actively developed by Goldammer, and possible sources of direct influence such as the sermons of Johannes Tauler rarely entered his deliberations.

In considering the impact of Tauler on the early thinking of Luther, Ozment naturally focused on the key concepts *gelassenheit, gemuete* and *grunt*.[162] None of this terminology or related speculation originated with Tauler, but it is evident that his writings were the main conduit through which these notions reached Luther and his contemporaries.[163] These same expressions and their derivatives are also pervasive in the writings of Paracelsus. But his debt to Tauler was more extensive and persistent than in the case of Luther. Much of the spiritualist belief and terminology alluded to in Ozment's study is typical of the late medieval mystics. A good instance is provided by the quotation at the head of this chapter, which employs the outer/inner dichotomy and calls for believers to defer to the inner recesses of the heart and dissociate themselves from outer preoccupations. Communion with the Holy Spirit was held up as a goal attainable through the stillness of introspection rather than through the shrillness of liturgical practices.[164] This Paracelsus quotation is characteristic of German mystic piety and could have been derived from many different sources of either male or female authorship.

The aspiration to reconciliation and unification with the Trinitarian deity, as expressed by Paracelsus, reflected his sensitivity to the virtues of the mystic path. He understood the requirement for complete emancipation from worldly influences, a process of emptying out of extrinsic factors, removing all gratuitous interference in order to open the innermost soul to the wellspring of spiritual enlightenment emanating from God.[165] To an even greater degree than the mystics, and in common with other radicals, Paracelsus adopted the most liberal view on access, which he believed was directly available to all who were willing to submit to the disciplines and sacrifices of the new life that was freely on offer. Paracelsus and his counterparts preserved the idea of stepwise spiritual progress, but this was more loosely conceived and freed from the formalistic requirements common in medieval piety.

Also in line with the mystics, Paracelsus and other radicals insisted on demanding sacrifices, complete humility and emancipation from human pride and avarice, before the universally available gift of grace was able to flow spontaneously according to the earnest intentions of the Trinitarian deity. Thereby the direct reconciliation of sinful humans with their

Creator would finally be achieved; believers would be freed from their lengthy bondage, and the way opened to great spiritual and intellectual rewards. For this reason, the mystic plea 'without any intermediary' (*ohne alel mittel*) was adopted as something of a motto by Paracelsus and was accorded prominence, as for instance in the introduction to *Astronomia magna*, which stressed the need to reject transient, material values and to defer to eternal sources, which it promised were available '*ohne mittel*' from either the light of the Holy Spirit or the Light of Nature, each 'school' or 'schoolmaster' in its province offering a faultless source of insight. These sentiments of Paracelsus replicated Parodoxa, Nos 161–3, of Sebastian Frank, who himself acknowledged Johannes Tauler as his main source of guidance.

The Light of Nature represented knowledge that derived from below, since it came from the material world (*von unten hinauf*), whereas the Holy Spirit conveyed a higher level of enlightenment since it emanated from the most elevated source (*von oben herab*).[166] Both forms of knowledge were legitimate and complementary, but, following sound scriptural and mystic precedent, Paracelsus frequently emphasized the aspiration to ensure as much as possible that the foundations of wisdom, arts and knowledge derived *von oben herab*, since only this source was endowed with the authority of the 'fiery tongue'.[167] The sacraments of baptism and the Lord's Supper, as conceived by Paracelsus, were particularly appealing because they were means of accessing the outpouring of grace *von oben herab*, without intermediary.[168]

Many sections of the writings of Paracelsus exhibit intensive reliance on mystic terminology and metaphor. For instance, with respect to the above discussion of the order in nature, closer inspection of a few adjacent paragraphs from the commentary on Psalm 91 (92) indicate that the whole discussion was compounded from sentiments favoured among the mystics and readily accessible through Tauler.[169] Illustrating an obsession with pursuing things to their ultimate source, the commentary calls for engagement with the secrets of nature, called the *ordnung der tiefe* or *grosse tiefe ding*, only to be attained by various *tief* means: *übergehbar tief, tiefen gedanken, tief herzen, tiefen grund*, or *in den grund*.[170] Such knowledge of nature was quiet or hidden (*still und geheim*); the way forward required saturation (*ersättigen*), reaching the deepest level of the soul (*gemuete*), a depth of penetration initially accomplished through use of the outer senses but also requiring participation of the heart.[171]

Utilizing metaphors associated with productive organic growth, of a kind much favoured by the mystics, it was promised that enquirers reaching the requisite depths of wisdom would experience such fruitfulness, growth and flowering (*grünen, blühen*) that they would overcome their sinful existence and regain a general dominion over nature.[172] The various organic growth and inflorescence metaphors widely employed by Paracelsus provided him among other things with the opportunity to employ *fliessen* and its compounds, which again reflected a usage favoured by the mystics.[173]

In the course of a few lines Paracelsus was likely to employ much of the above mystic vocabulary. For instance, when characterizing the shortcomings of the monastic orders, their regimes and aspirations were condemned for being *eusserlich* rather than *innerlich*, thereby neglecting the opportunities of the religion of the heart, which enabled the Holy Spirit to exercise its powers and silently flow (*fleust*) into the innermost ground of the soul (*innerlich gemute*).[174] Elsewhere social hierarchies and inequalities of wealth were regarded as suspect because they were contrary to the order of nature and inconsistent with the teaching of Christ. They exemplified the futility of resisting the order that flowed from both God and the Holy Spirit.[175]

The *grünen* metaphor, employed by Paracelsus to describe his own prospects for success, was contrasted with the sterility and dismal expectations of his competitors.[176] The *wüeste* metaphor was employed with respect to John the Baptist and the challenge for later generations to participate in his way of life. This same image also held a fascination for Eckhart, being employed by him and his followers to invoke the terror of the unknown expanse, but also the challenge of hidden aspects of divinity.[177] When, in his early writings, Paracelsus was looking for a term to describe the identification of the believer with Christ, he instinctively turned to the favoured mystic metaphor *versmelzung*. Such usage turned out to be ideal for application in the Docetic perspective adopted by Paracelsus, since it suggested the completeness of the identification of the human spirit with Christ through the medium of the heavenly flesh.[178]

A recent account of the debt of Thomas Müntzer to Tauler could equally well apply to Paracelsus. Tauler is credited with contributing to Müntzer's emphasis on the experience of conversion through the power of the Holy Spirit, which was seen as the only way to cast off the influence of the material world and become a 'friend of God'. Intimacy of this kind was denied to those who relied on the written word, especially the *schriftgelehrten* and the Pharisees of the church. Reception of the Holy Spirit in the abyss of the soul enabled believers to plumb the depths of God's wisdom. By this means, such aspirant friends of God would see their labours blessed by fruits and the performance of miraculous deeds. The regenerate would soon reap the benefits of their enlightenment and be rewarded for their courage in breaking away from the corrupt church. Such compensations were part of the witness of the separation of the wheat from the tares, destined for the end of time.[179]

Metaphors were appropriated from the mystics by Paracelsus and others, not merely for the sake of adding local colour, but by virtue of appropriateness to their theology and worldview. Even apparently neutral pieces of usage were likely to possess some deeper meaning and to have both philosophical and theological ramifications. This conclusion has recently been exhaustively demonstrated with respect to Eckhart's employment of the term *grunt*.[180] *Grunt* is described as an example of a 'master metaphor' possessing remarkable 'complexity, creativity and power'.[181] As McGinn indicates, Eckhart's concept of *grunt* was relevant to many religious and philosophical issues that were also of concern to Paracelsus. Eckhart's treatment of these questions was distinctly Neoplatonic in its bias. Indeed, Eckhart played a significant part in the transmission of ideas derived from Plotinus, Proclus, Pseudo-Dionysius, Origen and Augustine, as well as drawing on Neoplatonically influenced summaries such as the *Liber de causis*.[182] The same Neoplatonic influences were incorporated into the work of Tauler and hence were available to the spiritualists of the sixteenth century.[183] Thereby, Tauler became an accessible and congenial source from which Paracelsus and other radical thinkers could absorb such important Neoplatonic or Gnostic ideas as dualistic light metaphysics[184] or trichotomous anthropology.[185]

Tauler is also relevant as a source on less weighty matters that nevertheless attracted keen interest, such as exploiting magnetism as an analogy,[186] or number symbolism. With respect to the number seven symbolism, following the injunctions of Isaiah, Tauler laid down the seven stages whereby the Father led his disciples to the full gifts of the Holy Spirit. Such a stepwise, ladder-like process towards spiritual realization was of course a central theme of the mystics. The incremental stages outlined by Tauler were described as a key to the mysteries of the scriptures. This mystic discipline or 'school of greatness' provided insight into 'simple naked truths' of a kind that was obscured and rendered inaccessible in the scholastic system. In conformity with the seven liberal arts that these gifts replaced, and also consonant with the seven sacraments, the gifts of the Holy Spirit were sevenfold. On the basis of the distinction between the Light of God and the Light of Nature, the fifth of these gifts was the capacity to observe and judge the products of creation.[187] Such sentiments were consistent with the interpretation of the Psalms by Paracelsus and would have convinced him that Tauler was inspired by the same spirit as the prophets, perhaps even to the extent of sharing their ideas about a messianic future. Whether or not they were directly indebted to Tauler, radicals shared his ideas about the special importance of the seven gifts of the Holy Spirit. Indeed this theme was adopted as the organizing principle for Haugk's *Ain christlich ordenung*.[188] Completion of the ascending scale of the seven stages of divine wisdom was to Haugk a duty demanded by God, the fulfilment of which brought believers into conformity with Christ. The chosen people would face the opposition of the whole world, but there was every confidence that they were destined to succeed, at which stage they would be within reach of their final Sabbath state of rest.[189] Such progression towards the Sabbath state of rest was of equal concern to Paracelsus.

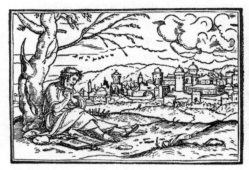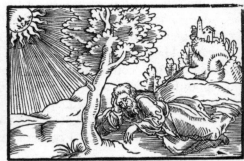

CHAPTER VII

ENDZEIT

... die zeit der philosophia ist zum ende gangen. der schnee meines ellends ist aus. die zeit des sommers ist hie ... so ist auch hie die zeit, zue schreiben, vom seligen leben und vom ewigen.[1]

The above quotation is a reminder of the pronounced eschatological and apocalyptic thrust in the mission of Paracelsus.[2] Predictably, he shared the conventional Christian teleological view of history, which embraced the idea of some future age when all the imperfections of material life would dissolve away. Such events would occur during a final dispensation marked by the second coming of Christ. The Reformation age was particularly alert to the apocalyptic interpretation of the confrontation between the forces of good and evil. It is therefore not surprising that Paracelsus became preoccupied with the interpretation of the end stages of the historical drama. Naturally, he enquired into the final trials and tribulations of the saints, but he also displayed particular curiosity about the prospects for some kind of golden age, or New Jerusalem, perhaps in the period of Sabbath rest before the Last Judgement. The granting of tangible relief to the scattered communities of saints was seen as an appropriate reward for their protracted and intense suffering. Any indications that their commitment and sacrifice would be rewarded by some positive outcome before the Day of Judgement would have constituted a particularly welcome boost to morale.

Paracelsus protected his credibility by refusing to be drawn into precise commitments about the chronology of future events. Reticence about affiliating with any of the specific apocalyptic dogmas that were gaining the support of his radical contemporaries was no indication of his lesser commitment to the general idea. As far as he was concerned, Christian civilization had reached a turning point. Since the providentially determined stages of history had largely run their course, the age of mundane secular affairs was over. The summer season and time of harvest had been reached. Having duly served their time of suffering, God's chosen people would at last enjoy the fruits of their labours and bear full witness to their state of salvation. Quite when this conclusion would be reached was a mystery not revealed in advance, but Paracelsus was convinced that it was safe to conclude that all the evidence pointed to the imminent dissolution of earthly monarchies. His generation was not yet witnessing the end of time, but it was safe to call their situation the beginning of the end.[3] Since false prophets had succeeded in turning the western world into a den of pestilence,[4] the end of the existing order was inevitable and would come so quickly that the false prophets and their churches would be taken by surprise and discover that there was no escape from punishment for their blasphemies against the Holy Spirit.[5] Just as much as Hans Hut, Paracelsus believed that he was operating in the spirit of the prophets of the biblical age. Both of them believed that they were superior to the luminaries of the established churches as guides to the last and most dangerous age of human existence.[6]

The Calling of Time

It is evident that the perspective of Paracelsus on every aspect of his work was pervaded by the sense of living at a momentous point in time. Central to his important macrocosm–microcosm conception was not only the understanding that that the pattern of the cosmos was stamped into the essence of the human constitution, but also, by natural extension, that the whole course of history, as determined by the Creator, was similarly imprinted on the human consciousness. It was therefore possible to draw on this reservoir of clues to achieve a better understanding of past, present and future. Time was a silent witness implanted in the human personality, awaiting the opportunity to reveal the full body of its secrets.

Unveiling his new theory of disease, Paracelsus was satisfied that it was consistent and well grounded. But he appreciated that he had still not fully taken the question of time into account with respect to matters of life and death. All entities within creation, without exception, were granted an appointed period of life, which constituted their own 'year'.[7] After their term of life, a new world began in the form of a next generation. Whether a living being or a process like building a house or healing a disease, all possessed an assigned duration.[8] It was wrong to attribute these periods to the influence of the stars; they were intrinsic to the processes themselves, determined by their particular seed. Ultimately, of course, all durations were appointed by God. Despite our feelings of control, all events, including our own actions, took place within the context of a decisive providential plan.[9] This applied whether the individuals concerned were good or bad. Limitations were imposed on all human lives, even on those of the saints.

God set such limits regardless of the level of virtue displayed by the human subject. Death was constantly at our shoulder, waiting for its appointed moment to act, which was never revealed to the person concerned. The amassing of treasures, great power or affluence were no protection against death. The mighty king, with all his capacities to surround himself with earthworks and with reserves of every kind of military personnel, was certain to be killed, if only by an apparently stray bullet.

Rather than try to evade such inevitabilities, it was better, with John the Baptist, the prophets and apostles, to accept that the Day of Judgement was imminent. At that point all would be brought before God to face their summons, including the dead, who would be resurrected for the same purpose. For the living it was best to regard life on earth as no more than a prison in which we languish. At death our body reverted to the earth, while the spirit was released to await the Day of Judgement. Both body and spirit would then come together again in order for the three chemical principles to achieve their final flowering and express their definitive character. The subsequent course of events would not be revealed in advance to humans, although it was evident that there would be no further disease, no need for medication or for doctors, since there would be no sickness. Indeed there would be an end to all the limitations of the previous state of existence. While waiting for this conclusion, the only right path was to continue with the advancement of knowledge so that humans would be able to claim that they had pursued their calling in a full spirit of righteousness.[10]

Time embodied its own imperative for change in all spheres of existence. This was something that physicians seemed not to understand. New clouds were constantly appearing on the horizon, as indicated by the French pox, which was unprecedented and had taken doctors entirely by surprise.[11] Physicians had chosen to bury themselves in the past and had not appreciated that the universe was caught up in a cycle of change analogous to the stages of human existence. Current society tended to be just as ignorant of its debased condition as the citizens of Nineveh, the site of the prophetic warnings contemplated by Jonah, as indicated in Illustration 7(a). On account of their complacency, the moderns would be subject to the same judgements as their biblical predecessors. It was of course necessary to take account of changed physical conditions. Granted, the modern environment was nothing like the past. The world was a more crowded place than ever before and it was more corrupt. It was accordingly no surprise that society faced entirely different disease problems, many of them of greater severity than ever before, that called for new names and a different understanding.[12]

As is already evident, the crisis of health that afflicted Paracelsus's generation was not seen as an accidental occurrence. New afflictions like the plague or syphilis were at least in part the result of endemic vice, which stirred up the wrath of the firmament. The macrocosm–microcosm theory, as developed by Paracelsus, facilitated the attribution of misfortune to human misconduct, which seemed capable of causing trauma in the stars. In all cases the ultimate command over events resided with God, so that it was correct to describe such epidemics as a punishment for arousing the scorn of God. Such misfortunes were God's way of punishing those who stepped out of line with the divine order; they represented the divine equivalent of the maintenance of order by civil authorities.[13] For punishment, God employed the various intermediaries known to communicate poisons and infections. The basilisk was the medium for inflicting poisons from Saturn; rabid dogs were a similar vehicle. Many monstrous beings were also used for this punitive purpose. Among the latter was the office of pope (*papa*), which was the clerical equivalent of a serpent or a basilisk. Hence, as long as the papal office was in existence, epidemics were held out to be a regular expectation.[14]

On some occasions Paracelsus underlined the distinction between two kinds of misfortune stemming from the heavens, which he called natural and supernatural. These terms coincided approximately with the medieval theological distinction between the *potentia ordinata* and *potentia absoluta* of God. These two modes of action represented two aspects of the operation of God's scorn. Occurrences of plague typified the natural category, in which humans brought down deleterious effects on themselves by means of naturally occurring reciprocal interactions between the macrocosm and microcosm. Although the pattern of causation was complicated, in principle it was possible to detect naturally occurring omens of such imminent disasters. Success in such matters constituted a potent test of the depth of the astronomer's initiation in the Light of Nature.[15]

The more serious menaces fell into the supernatural category, where God intervened directly in nature for the purpose of punishing the evils of humankind and occasionally of rewarding upright conduct. Classic instances of this direct intervention were Noah's Flood and the destruction of Sodom and Gomorrah. In such cases it was not possible to predict these events by natural means. Accordingly, both of these Old Testament instances came as a complete surprise to the culprits. In general it was the habit of God to provide signs in the heavens, and this intention was confirmed by the statements of Christ and the prophets. Such signs were not natural occurrences and were not susceptible to being interpreted astronomically.[16]

On the question of time, Paracelsus agreed with Hippocrates, whose respect for astronomy he applauded. Astronomy was duly incorporated as one of the main pillars of the new medical system, its role being to provide an understanding of the influence of everything in the macrocosm that was liable to impinge adversely on the microcosm. Such outer influences impacted in time and were delivered over the course of time. Attention to time was acutely sensitive, because time determined the seriousness of all diseases or adverse experiences. In order to attain a complete understanding of such phenomena, it was necessary to pay attention not just to the present, but to all points in time, past and future, indeed every step up to the end of time. It was also necessary to pay full regard to the seasonality of all phenomena, including diseases.[17] The seasons would give an idea of what was realistically possible in medicine. Paracelsus placed emphasis on the acuity or sharpness of time (*ist die zeit scharpf*), which was proved by its ability to generate new things perpetually, so that every hour was different and unpredictable in its effects. As a consequence nobody was in a position completely to fathom the secrets and intentions of time. Certainly this was not within the capacities of medical practitioners, who should remember that time exercised command over them. In fact time could be said to play with the practitioner just like a cat with its mouse.[18]

Time possessed characteristics in common with the Light of Nature. Both needed to be treated with respect and watchfulness. Also, both inspired wonderment because they reflected fundamental aspects of the character of the Creator, whose works were characterized by such features as lucidity, depth and ingenuity, all legitimately rendered by the term *scharpf*, or *scharpfsinnig*. It was perhaps not accidental that Paracelsus titled his major work, *Astronomia magna*, alternatively known as *Philosophia sagax* or *Scharfsinnige philosophie*.[19]

Understandably, the interpretation of the impact of time was one of the most ambitious of his undertakings. Given the seriousness of this responsibility, he considered it essential to establish that his thinking about prophecy was consistent with the Word of God. Biblical references were frequently intended to remind the reader of Paracelsus's apocalyptic frame of reference. An instance was provided by the contrast that he drew between himself and the medical establishment when he invoked the greening and barrenness of fig trees.[20] He asserted that the curse of the barren fig trees would fall upon the medical establishment, echoing Israel's unresponsiveness to God or the faithlessness of those who rejected the message of Christ.[21] His enemies were like a farmer trying to thresh grains from empty straw. The full weight of their sins was about to be hung around their necks. The axe would be applied to the rotten trunks of these fruitless trees.[22] By contrast, the future would witness a flourishing or greening of his own reputation, a construction which self-evidently connected with the biblical text describing the destruction of the unregenerate exemplified by the old Jerusalem and greening of the fig trees as the first indication of summer, which showed that the kingdom of God was at hand, a promise that Jesus deliberately addressed to his own generation.[23]

Taking the cosmic picture as a whole, Paracelsus drew the analogy between the human life cycle and the grand cycle of cosmic history. Among humans, every stage of life was characterized by its particular diseases, down to the final point of death. The cosmos was going through exactly the same developmental process, with the constitution of the heavens changing as it aged and moved towards its predestined end. Doctors acted in vain when they drew upon remedies that originated during the childhood of civilization. Instead, they should take account of the changed situation when dealing with the latest stage in the succession of monarchies, in which the firmament and the elements were in a state of old age. Failure to respond to this evolving pattern was the vice of the medical establishment, who were as a result destined to face the same ignominious end as the one that threatened the people of Nineveh. Accordingly, the doctors would live to see their wealth turned to ashes.[24]

The conditions for decrepitude were created by the explosion of population and by people's unparalleled mobility, not to mention their preoccupation with lusts of the flesh. This represented a crisis of biblical proportions, a level of distress among nations (*pressura gentium*), the like of which had never previously been witnessed. Accordingly it was necessary to adopt an entirely novel system of medicine, which of course was a main part of the mission that Paracelsus set for himself. Although his scriptural references tended to be fleeting, his readers would have recognized his reliance on the apocalyptic discourse of the gospels. Changes in the heavens and physical cataclysms in the seas would prefigure great distress (*pressura magna, pressura gentium*)[25] throughout the earth. People would be afflicted on many fronts, and many would be put to the sword. Paracelsus believed that the advent of fearful new diseases like the French disease were indicative of this situation. The old Jerusalem would come to an end. But hope was on the horizon. After the severe oppression of the saints, the tenure of the false Christians would be over and the times of nations would thereby be fulfilled.[26] The greening of fig trees would be the first signal of this revival. Then, betokening the emergence of a new heaven, the Son of Man would be carried down on a cloud and the kingdom of heaven would be at hand.[27]

On account of the relevance of the fig tree passage, Paracelsus located for himself a modest but distinctive part in the apocalyptic drama. First, his new system of medicine was purpose-made for the massive challenges that would arise amid the ruins of the apocalyptic age. Through his efforts, first aid would be available to believers awaiting the return of the Messiah. Secondly, as astronomer and magus, he was among the small elite of experts in a position to monitor and interpret the portentous signs and messages from angelic beings that God provided in such special situations. The interpretation of these signs, about which Christ himself had spoken, was intended to bring relief to believers, because they conveyed assurance that the damned were about to receive their just reckoning. The only persons who would be privileged to understand these portents, or 'celestial meteorology', were drawn from the thin ranks of the redeemed and, among this group, were those only with special knowledge granted by God.[28]

Participation by Paracelsus in celestial meteorology reflected his belief that he possessed precisely the right credentials for this sensitive assignment. His outlook was also coloured by his own experiences, which induced acute awareness of the current tragedy. His gloomy analysis underlined the irony of the situation reached in Christian civilization. God through His creation and Christ through his suffering on the cross had made sacrifices intended to bring peace to humankind. Yet humanity had ended up in precisely the opposite condition. Indeed, things had visibly deteriorated in the course of the last generation until everything was in a state of discord. There was no escape from the conclusion that the German nation was sliding into a crisis of biblical proportions, in which disease played a major part. The mounting chaos represented a state of war of all against all (*nichts anderst dan einer wider den andern*), just what Paracelsus concluded about the state of affairs in the animal kingdom. As a result, no one was safe in their bed or at their work. It was as if everybody were pursued by a tormenting spirit (*fegteufel*). Degeneration was also evident in knowledge and all of the arts, which had blossomed in the youth of civilization but had subsequently declined. Learning had remained within narrow confines and had not expanded with the proliferation of population. With evident feeling, Paracelsus declared that this gloomy portrayal of events was confirmed by his own experience. He was never free from trouble but had always been forced to bear his cross, for instance by willingly exposing himself to constant harassment on account of his philosophy.[29]

Notwithstanding the seemingly desperate state of world affairs and his own personal circumstances, Paracelsus was not despondent. He took heart from the prophetic assurances that those who contravened the ordinances of God would see their labours frustrated and ultimately face damnation. On the other hand, those who pursued their callings with humility would be richly rewarded. The cedar of Lebanon was held out as their model. Whatever the hazard of its environment, the cedar went from strength to strength and was destined to continue flourishing and fruiting (*grünen und blühen*). Appropriate rewards would be forthcoming in the fields of astronomy, philosophy and medicine for those who approached nature in the spirit of righteousness. There was also every reason to believe that the greatest achievements of all lay in the near future. The scriptures offered many instances where the greatest fruitfulness had occurred at a late stage in personal or historical affairs. On the basis of such prefigurations (*vorbild*), it was reasonable to expect a phase of renewed fruitfulness and regeneration (*geblüh und unser sprossen*) in the current advanced age of the world. Such rewards were within the grasp of those who faithfully followed the ordinances of God,[30] albeit on condition of rejecting the many temptations of materialism and accepting the tenets of poverty, chastity, marriage, rectitude and reversion to the simplicity of childhood.[31] The chastity of youth (*jungfraustand*) was also often invoked by Paracelsus as a condition of the future blissful existence.[32] If the proposed rehabilitation was successful, the last would become the first, and God would not be satisfied until the poor were in good comfort and were counted among His immediate companions. It seemed improbable that God was capable of producing such a radical transformation, but since He could make slag into gold, all other changes came easily to the Creator. God would establish Himself as the shepherd of his sheep-stall, and His flock would subsist in a state of rectitude. Their place of abode would truly become a city of righteousness, or even a paradise.[33]

The flourishing of Paracelsus's own philosophy and reputation comfortably fitted into this pattern of late flowering. Such promises of hope enabled him to minimize the significance of adversity, and even to pronounce with confidence that history was taking a turn for the better. He was sure that the appointed time had arrived for a momentous change in fortunes, integral to which would be the weeding out of good from bad. Comfort was taken from biblical passages conveying assurances that the future lay with the few and the oppressed.[34] He saw such texts as confirmation that the disputatious establishment would be confounded and condemned to the fate of the Pharisees. Paracelsus felt justified in standing apart from the noisy rabble and concentrating on his writings, which were conceived according to his own exacting standards of independence of judgement (*fadenrecht*). He was committed to purifying these works in the same way that gold was purified seven times by fire. His other model was the rose, which nature caused to bloom at exactly the right moment. He had been patient and content to await his time, since only error was produced if works were released before their time. It seemed that his own undertakings were now sufficiently well tested for his thoughts about the wisdom of celestial events to be suitable for public consumption. By this means he hoped to make his contribution to the understanding of the process of renewal that would come about, possibly during his own times.[35]

A Galaxy of Prophets

The speculations of Paracelsus about time, as well as his sense of living at the end of historical time, represented his response to a major preoccupation among his contemporaries.[36] Owing to the prevalence of such concerns, those possessing or pretending to relevant skills were drawn to trying their hand at prophecy. Their main products, commonly known as prognostications or *practica*, established themselves as one of the most buoyant sections of the new *Flugschriften* market. Prognostications were complemented by many types of related writing such as reports of disasters or strange events, which also connected in some way to prophecy. Such popular expositions were merely the most marketable of the various prophetic products, being parasitic on a more serious literature: astrology, chronology, prophecy and biblical hermeneutics. The scale of this literary effort indicated the existence of a readership that was hungry for intelligence on such issues and self-evidently in a state of deep anxiety about the future.[37]

In opting to engage in divination, Paracelsus was intruding into a crowded market-place. Many writers owed their success to their exploitation of the rich reservoir of materials inherited from the medieval apocalyptic tradition. The libraries of Germany contained a profusion of apocalyptically inclined treatises, most of which were the product of the last three hundred years and were accordingly recognized as pertinent to the condition of the early sixteenth century.[38] One of the dominant elements in these collections comprised the writings of Joachim of Fiore and his Franciscan imitators.[39] Prominent among the contributors to this genre were Arnold of Villanova and Johannes of Rupescissa, both known to Paracelsus also as medical and alchemical authors. Indeed, as indicated by the early fifteenth-century *Das Buch der Heiligen Dreifaltigkeit*, the symbolism of alchemy and of the apocalypse had many points in common.[40] Among the medieval prophetic writers, Arnold of Villanova and Johannes of Rupescissa were conspicuous for lending their authority to the idea of the enjoyment by the saints of a substantial period of Sabbath rest on earth before the Last Judgement.[41] As in the medieval period, in the sixteenth century medical doctors were prominent players in the apocalyptic dialogue. Through their intervention, new disasters such as syphilis were identified as part of the prophetic scheme and were thereby accorded an even higher profile than they had already attained.[42]

In the sixteenth century there was little direct knowledge among the general readership of recondite and inaccessible medieval sources, but an idea of their content was conveyed by some keen synthesizers. One of the attractions of the medieval sources was their attention to both socio-political criticism and prophecy.[43] In the process of recycling, the old polemic was harnessed for whatever purposes seemed most pressing. At one extreme, groups connected with the Taborites absorbed apocalyptic elements into manifestos that were designed for political and religious purposes, thereby constituting something of a precursor of the articles produced in connection with the German Peasants' War. There is little evidence concerning the influence of the Taborite apocalypticists, but it is doubtful whether they were known to Paracelsus, who proceeded to reinvent this socially orientated vein of prophetic commentary.[44]

The early decades of printing coincided with the lead up to the year 1500. Printing permitted full insight into the mood of ominous expectation associated with this date. In the field of prophecy, the most successful popularizer was Johannes Lichtenberger, whose *Pronosticatio* appeared in Latin in 1488 and in German shortly afterwards.[45] The success of Lichtenberger was partly due to his compendious text, but almost as much to the inclusion of large and impressive woodcut illustrations by Hans Hesse. The *Pronosticatio* constituted an inelegant but encyclopaedic conspectus of medieval prophetic sources, combined with recent astrological speculations, particularly those stimulated by the 'great conjunction' of Jupiter and Saturn in the sign of Scorpio that occurred in 1484. This conjunction was universally recognized as a major portent that was expected to work itself out over the course of the ensuing decades.[46]

Lichtenberger's work was promoted on account of his subscription to the Last Emperor myth, which was reworked by Lichtenberger and his successors to promote the idea that a Roman emperor would defeat the Ottoman Turks, oversee a general repentance, reform the institutions of state and church, and generally usher in a new age of peace and prosperity.[47] The *Pronosticatio* also seemed relevant to the times because of its prophecy that a new religious leader would emerge and institute a fresh order among the clergy. Lichtenberger played his part in fuelling an outburst of artistic and intellectual apocalyptic initiatives, among which the most brilliant expression was Albrecht Dürer's publication containing his *Apocalypse* (1498) sequence of fifteen woodcuts, his most ambitious undertaking to that date.[48] The next major outburst of pamphleteering related to the next predicted ominous conjunction, timed for 1524, this time in the sign of Pisces. When this latter conjunction failed to generate anything more than the usual level of flooding, rather than a catastrophe on the scale of the great Flood of Noah, this might have been a setback to the reputation of the experts, and indeed for the whole *practica* genre. Concentration of modern attention on the *Sintflut* episode rather gives the impression that after 1524 the prognostications had exhausted themselves and the genre had in the immediate future nothing of interest to say. But this was not the case. The débâcle of 1524 proved to be a momentary interruption in the flow of astrological, prophetic and apocalyptic speculation. Even the participants in the *Sintflut* debate were not particularly disconcerted. Like professional vaticinators before and after, they shrouded their forecasts in suitably defensive ambiguity. It was even possible to claim success with respect to various disasters in 1524, while in due course the disasters associated with the German Peasants' War of 1525 could be firmly ascribed to roots in 1524. In the event, the experts emerged from the *Sintflut* escapade without a stain on their reputation.

Reflecting their sensitivity to popular preoccupations, leaders of opinion like Luther and Zwingli displayed a morbid fascination with the omens. Despite their own apparent success in carving up the Roman church, both remained deeply pessimistic about the trend of events. Luther was in no doubt that his generation was witnessing the very signs in the heavens that were indicated in Luke 21: 25 as premonitions of the second coming. It was not possible to interpret the wrath of God exactly, but it was clear from the exceptionally common occurrence of eclipses or other signs cropping up on earth and in the heavens that a great commotion (*eyn großer wyrbell*) was imminent.[49] Luther's friends and followers, such as Melanchthon and Carion, between them ensured that their leader received intelligence about all varieties of astrological literature.[50] For the remnants of the peasant activists and militant Anabaptists, the disasters of the German Peasants' War and the persecution in its aftermath merely served to heighten their apocalyptic convictions. One indicator of the continuing obsession with prophecy was the rate of appearance of new editions of Lichtenberger, where the peak of demand was reached between 1526 and 1530. Editions were produced in no fewer than five German towns in 1526 and 1527, the most famous being the Wittenberg edition by Stephan Rodt, with a Foreword by Martin Luther.[51] Luther's intervention indicates the degree of sensitivity with which this text was regarded. Reflecting the excitement aroused by these sources, Andreas Osiander complained that, among the people, Lichtenberger and similar prophetic texts had assumed greater authority than the Word of God.[52]

Excavation of the medieval archive continued to throw up new sources. For instance, the little Magdeburg prophecy was first available in print only in 1522, after which it was reprinted separately on a few occasions, but given much wider currency through inclusion in Johannes Carion's *Chronica* of 1532.[53] The anonymous Magdeburg prediction dated from the thirteenth century, but seemed just as pertinent nearly three hundred years later. It announced that the cedars of Lebanon would be felled; Mars would prevail over Saturn and Jupiter; within eleven years there would be one order of faith and one monarchy; the sons of Israel would be liberated; there would be many battles in the world; mutations would occur in faith, laws and kingdoms; and the land of the Saracens would be destroyed.[54] Every one of these aphorisms connected with the cares of the public at the time of Luther, and they were obviously assimilable into the pattern of evidence apparent in other documents. Establishing the exact significance of sources such as the Magdeburg prophecy was a challenge that the most expert minds could not resist.

The *Sintflut* protagonists were by no means the only fish in the water. As the Magdeburg prophecy indicates, planetary conjunctions remained objects of concern, but they failed to establish any kind of exclusivity. Most authors agreed with Lichtenberger that conjunctions were just one source of wisdom among many. As the young Paracelsus was accustoming himself to the subject area, expertise was becoming enlivened from all sides. While in Salzburg, he must have been aware of the presence of

Berthold Pürstinger, a leading moderating influence in the archdiocesan hierarchy, whose *Onus ecclesiae* had been published anonymously in 1524. This impressive study both made the case for reform of the church from within and was conducted within an apocalyptic framework. Berthold possessed a fine command of medieval sources. His work may well have served as a convenient quarry for Paracelsus on Joachimite chronology, or with respect to the prophecies of Birgitta of Sweden or Hildegard of Bingen. Paracelsus would also have recognized much common ground with respect to the corruptions of the church and would have agreed with Berthold that sectarianism, especially in its Lutheran form, was not likely to improve the situation. More than Lichtenberger, Berthold's *Onus ecclesiae* mobilized the apocalyptic context to unearth and recycle potentially explosive critiques of the church, without incurring the obloquy that normally greeted authors who voiced similar complaints in contemporary *Flugschriften*.[55] Quite unintentionally, at this most sensitive moment, when the reformers were getting out of hand and the peasants had reached the edge of rebellion, the reforming bishop gave as much succour to radical critics as to his own reforming party within the old church. No doubt incipient radical voices like Paracelsus also detected the protective value of the use of prophecy as a medium of expression. As Lerner commented on earlier times, dissenters 'did not feel free to express their criticisms and hopes forthrightly but vented them without inhibition when they employed the vehicle of prophecy'.[56]

If not familiar with prophetic and astrological sources during his time in Salzburg, Paracelsus would have rapidly made up the deficit during his stays in Strasbourg, Basel and Nuremberg. In Basel, Pamphilus Gengenbach, the inveterate publisher, pamphleteer and literary figure, reached a wide audience with a *Fastnachtsspiel* that incorporated elements from many of the main medieval prophetic sources.[57] Gengenbach also made effective use of prophetic elements in some of his other dramatic presentations.[58] He died shortly before the arrival of Paracelsus in Basel, but his writings remained popular. In Strasbourg, Paracelsus may have been acquainted with Martin Borrhaus (Cellarius), who also arrived there as a refugee in 1526. Borrhaus provided a direct link with the Zwickau prophets. Just after the departure of Paracelsus from Strasbourg, Borrhaus produced an analysis of scriptural prophecies that attracted wide attention. The imminent future seemed to offer the prospect of calamity and suffering, but afterwards, he was sure, there would be a universal renovation. With respect to the current situation, Borrhaus was confident he was living in an age that was witnessing a great outpouring of the Holy Spirit, although believers should be prepared to see their progress obstructed by the forces of Antichrist, headed by the papacy. No doubt with recent catastrophes experienced by the peasants in mind, he rejected violent resistance and advocated patience. Like Paracelsus, he believed that God would in due course ensure that the saints were suitably compensated in the form of an age of peace and justice.[59]

A similar analysis was current among the Anabaptists. Within this group some of the leading opinion formers committed themselves to a specific and highly telescoped chronology of end times. For instance, Hans Hut and Leonhard Schiemer evolved chronologies envisaging a countdown to Pentecost beginning in 1521 and ending in 1528. The Last Judgement was expected to be preceded by all manner of catastrophes.[60] Both were executed before they could witness the outcome of their predictions, but they were outlived by Melchior Hoffman, in whose thinking predictions about end times occupied a central place from about 1525. His commentary on Daniel was published in 1526. In the same year he started work on his commentary on the Book of Revelation. After various false starts he settled in Strasbourg which, consistently with some notable earlier prophecies, he designated as the spiritual New Jerusalem.[61] In 1530 Hoffman published his commentary on Revelation. For him all the evidence converged to suggest that the age of apostolic witness had dawned, for which purpose God was pouring out the blessing of the Holy Spirit so plentifully that sons and daughters would be granted the gift of prophecy and the old would experience visions and revealing dreams. Fulfilment of this prophecy of Joel was just one sign that the long age of darkness was over, that the eternal light was breaking through and announcing the dawn of the final age. Sons, daughters, young and old were granted free access to this light, enabling them to learn about the future New Jerusalem to which they would soon gain entry.[62] Hoffman's scheme reassigned Pentecost to 1533, and when this prophecy was not fulfilled his forecast was revised, but without abandoning his ideas of living in end times.[63]

Strasbourg was host to the entire spectrum of religious and political opinion. Otto Brunfels was a prolific writer, whose pamphlets reflected similar perspectives to those of his fellow physician Paracelsus on issues of social justice. Just before the latter's arrival in Strasbourg, Brunfels produced an almanac, anti-astrological in spirit, but regarding the omens of the times as indications of an eschatological crisis. Like Paracelsus, he was critical of the clerical and secular establishment, sympathetic to the oppressed classes, and sceptical about the pretensions of the Lutherans.[64] Among conservative voices was the versatile and entrepreneurial Lorenz Fries, who established himself as a writer on geography, astronomical instruments, astrology and various aspects of divination. Twenty-seven of his sixty titles relate to these areas of practical mathematics.[65] As previously mentioned, Fries was something of a model for Paracelsus as a popular writer and for a short time the two were on friendly terms. The writing programme of Fries indicates the interweaving of commercial and ideological considerations. His very first publishing effort in 1513 was a broadsheet on a monstrous birth near Rome, which was used to stir up alarm, but also to induce consolation on account of the accession of Leo X.[66] Fries emerged as an argumentative defender of the astrological approach to prophecy, and he was one of the astrologers who warned in 1523 of an imminent flood catastrophe, while opposing the prevailing pessimistic responses to the prospect of this event.[67]

Leaders of opinion in Nuremberg indicate the pervasiveness of the appeal of prophecy and the apocalyptic. As a theologian, Andreas Osiander used the Foreword to his edition of a letter by Argula von Grumbach to draw attention to the prophecy from Joel 3: 1–4. Osiander believed that Argula's letter provided evidence that hitherto disenfranchised groups such as women were emboldened 'in these last days' to attack the 'blind Pharisees', in this case the Catholic academic theologians of Ingolstadt. Such emancipation represented a revival of the condition of the apostolic age, when the gift of interpretation of the scriptures was open to young and old, unlearned as well as learned, and women as much as men.[68] In order to emphasize the importance of female voices in final times, Osiander also produced an edition of the prophecies of Hildegard of Bingen.[69]

Also in Nuremberg, Hans Sachs, the famous writer and shoemaker, used his dialogue between the canon and the shoemaker to mount a robust defence of the lay person's independent ability to interpret the scriptures. He took a dim view of the intellectual standing of his betters. Those trained in the high schools were likely to be more of a hindrance than a help. After all, Jesus drew his disciples from among the humble people; and the important gospel of John came from the pen of a fisherman. Any doubts about the capacities of the laity were dispelled by precisely the same text of Joel that was cited by Osiander. In the last days, God pronounced that He would pour out His spirit on all flesh.[70] Given some common denominators of outlook and indicating their opportunism as writers, Osiander and Sachs teamed up to produce an edition of one of the most famous series of medieval apocalyptic images, a project that was calculated to attract the widest interest and was naturally also commercially attractive. Paracelsus too recognized that this source was an ideal basis on which to establish his rival claims as an interpreter of medieval prophetic sources.

A Prophet in Troubled Times

It is evident that the prophetic and apocalyptic obsession of the early sixteenth century lost none of its salience after the German Peasants' War. On account of his particular combination of interests and skills, Paracelsus was perfectly poised to take advantage of this situation. He operated from a position of advantage owing to being a fresh voice, able to benefit from hindsight concerning the course of recent catastrophic events. He was also free from involvement in the affair of the 'watery conjunction' of 1524 and able to benefit from the mistakes of some of his less prudent competitors who had become victim to their excesses of enthusiasm and committed themselves to prophecies that quickly turned out to be contradicted by events.

Paracelsus gained his first access to the printing presses only in 1529. Understandably, his first priority was finding an outlet for his accumulating medical writings; it was natural that he should select syphilis as the area to demonstrate his abilities as theoretician and therapist. In making this choice, he was perhaps guided by the example of Fries.[71] Friedrich Peypus, the respected and successful printer, took on a first short pamphlet on syphilis and was prepared to publish its much longer sequels. As previously mentioned, the medical establishment successfully blocked this plan, causing Paracelsus to leave Nuremberg in a spirit of disillusionment. Peypus was also receptive to the idea of launching Paracelsus as a writer of prognostications, making a start with the little *Practica gemacht auf Europen 1530–1534*.[72] This modest pamphlet was an instantaneous success; Sudhoff records at least seven separate early printings.[73] Building on this auspicious launch, Paracelsus continued to find no difficulty in locating publishers willing to take on his short commentaries on astronomical and meteorological phenomena. A new publication of this sort was produced almost every year between 1529 and 1538. At the time of his death, sixteen of his twenty-three publications fell into this category.[74] To the extent that his reputation relied on publications, he was mainly known as a specialist in the *practica* market, a genre that constituted a significant test of skill in the handling of politically sensitive issues.

Contrary to his pugnacious instincts but consistently with his prudential policy, Paracelsus proved adept at handling this challenge. His writings were sufficiently original and challenging to command attention, but also statesmanlike enough to avoid the risk of punishment or ridicule. No doubt with the example of the Anabaptists in mind, he astutely avoided commitment to specific and unambiguous forecasts.

He frankly accepted that, even to adepts such as himself, the course of events was such a deep secret that truths about the future only became fully evident after the event. Humans were privileged to know their general fate, but they were denied access to the precise chronology. Nevertheless, it was a fundamental duty to interpret signs and wonders. Collective effort on this front was bound to provide some understanding of the likely course of end times.[75] On these issues of great public interest, Paracelsus was judicious without being evasive. He was inclined to adopt an accelerating apocalyptic sequence, but he was also philosophical about the precise pace and course of the cataclysmic process.

The seriousness of his commitment to this variety of journalism is indicated by the survival of various unpublished drafts of similar type. He must have appreciated that, as a medium, the *practica* offered too little scope for the realization of his full ambition. Probably during his visit to Nuremberg, Paracelsus concluded that the best chance to make an impact in the field of prophecy lay with the Lichtenberger model of publication. He was especially drawn to material containing visual images possessing the kind of magical significance that was likely to be overlooked by his competitors. Interpretation of what he called 'magic figures' called for the input of a magus, precisely the skills that he himself possessed. In this sphere Paracelsus conducted three major exercises, but only one of them achieved publication during his lifetime.

First, in all likelihood shortly after 1527, he embarked on a commentary on Lichtenberger, which survives only in a fragmentary form but is still the most detailed critique of Lichtenberger that was ever produced.[76] It is possible that Paracelsus abandoned this project, perhaps appreciating that demand was being satisfied by the glut of rival editions of Lichtenberger. Perhaps he concluded that a lengthy commentary on Lichtenberger's old book was an over-complicated exercise. In view of the Habsburg ascendancy in Germany, making an attack on Lichtenberg's alleged pro-French sentiment the centrepiece of his own commentary was not likely to stir up much interest.

With his usual perversity, Paracelsus seems to have taken no interest in the Lichtenberger chapters that attracted most interest during the late 1520s owing to their alleged prediction that Luther would be the prime mover in the revival of the church. Such an invitation to pass comment on the status of Luther in the prophetic scheme would not readily have been ignored by Paracelsus. Perhaps he tackled this subject, but the relevant part of his commentary has not survived. For whatever reason, Paracelsus abandoned his tract on Lichtenberger and sought alternative ways of expressing his own point of view on the issues of contention.

For his second project, he turned to one of the most famous sets of medieval prophetic images, the Papal Prophecies, in the edition supervised by Andreas Osiander.[77] The latter provided a short prose commentary on each of the thirty images; complementary verses were supplied by Hans Sachs, while a complete set of well-executed woodcut illustrations is attributed to Erhard Schön. The Papal Prophecies had been available in an Italian edition since around 1515, but the Osiander edition was the first to be published in Germany. Osiander's book was an instant success. Among its admirers were Luther and Melanchthon, who were impressed by its consistent Lutheran slant. Paracelsus recognized his chance to make a mark with a rival commentary written from an independent perspective. Although he failed to find a publisher for this undoubtedly marketable product, his concise prose commentary survived and was published more than twenty-five years after his death.[78] Perhaps Paracelsus had completed his commentary on the Papal Prophecies by the date of his arrival in Nuremberg. There he would have discovered that the Osiander edition had been confiscated on account of vague suspicions about over-friendliness to radical sentiment.[79] Owing to its obviously more radical perspective, the commentary by Paracelsus ran an even greater risk of condemnation by the authorities. In the atmosphere of suspicion and tension over his work on syphilis, he may well have decided to freeze work on the Papal Prophecies and search for yet another alternative method of exploiting the magic figure as a basis for prophecy.

In his third attempt, no doubt dissatisfied by the restrictions imposed by reliance on recycling medieval sequences of magic figures, Paracelsus devised his own series of images and subjected them to commentary, which enabled him to describe an outcome more congenial to his own thinking about the final times. With this third project he was fortunate to discover a publisher. On this occasion, as earlier in Nuremberg, the publisher agreed to take on both a substantial medical work and his prophetic figures. As already noted, Heinrich Steiner of Augsburg was a publisher with distinct radical credentials, who was willing to invest in the costly *Grosse Wundarznei* and in the ambitious prognostication containing the customary illustrated title-page and no fewer than thirty-two woodcuts, together with their brief accompanying text.[80] Such an undertaking was well within the competence of Steiner, who possessed extensive experience in the publication of lavishly illustrated books of many kinds. Steiner's genuine enthusiasm for the Paracelsus prophetic project is indicated by the production of a simultaneous Latin edition. All of these proved to be successful publishing propositions. Accordingly, the association with Steiner was one of the few harmonious and productive interludes in the publishing career of Paracelsus.[81] Although an aesthetically successful publication, the text of the Steiner *Prognostikation* was in some respects perfunctory, perhaps suggesting that Paracelsus was at his best in situations where the catalyst of controversy was exercising its stimulus. Paracelsus himself realized that he risked underselling his illustrations, which prompted him to add an appendix elaborating his interpretations to some extent. Despite the brevity and untidiness of his package, his remarks were well chosen, and they certainly attracted attention. A set of marginal annotations by a contemporary sympathizer, unearthed by Milt, indicated that contemporaries were quite capable of extracting the most radical message from the aphorisms of Paracelsus and the images of his illustrator.[82]

As is evident from his prophetic writings as a whole, Paracelsus was sceptical about the abilities of his competitors and determined to impose his authority as an independent reforming voice. Since he was already a seasoned religious and medical controversialist, it was merely a matter of importing ideas from these fields and applying his established mode of attack to the relevant aspects of divination. As always, he distanced himself from virtuosi among the popular practitioners. He expressed suspicion about the practices of popular soothsayers, who tried their hand at foretelling the future using all kinds of methods of divination: crystal spheres, divining rods and so on. He granted that they would meet with some success, for instance in detecting treasure, but Paracelsus was convinced that their positive results were obtained only through consorting with demons. Since such practitioners elevated these demons into gods, they were propagators of idolatry. As a consequence, such popular auguries should be recognized as a nest for the machinations of the Devil and his agents.[83]

Confident about avoiding such pitfalls on account of his confidence in the Holy Spirit and the Light of Nature, his own commitment to magic remained undiminished. The Light of Nature, the God-given vehicle for instruction, permitted the liberal use of dreams, the value of which was increased by their regulation by diet and regimen, both of which were standard elements in the theurgical discipline of the Neoplatonists. Such confidence in dreams and visions was of course also evident in other parts of the radical movement.[84] On account of the extra freedoms available when the body was resting, sleep provided an auspicious occasion for accessing influences from angels or sidereal spirits. The power of dreams had been definitively confirmed by the example of Daniel in the Old Testament, whose dreams were particularly appealing to Paracelsus and other radicals because of their apocalyptic content. In other classic instances angelic beings had provided insights during sleep, as for instance in the case of Joseph, the husband of the Virgin Mary. Such angels could provide direct insight into future happenings, providing intelligence that was not available from any other source. Because of their complexity and outlandish symbolism, the understanding of various types of dream and vision represented a difficult challenge. Paracelsus was not fazed by such problems and announced that he would give some model explanations that would act as a key to the understanding of standard dreams and visions.[85] He attached importance to certain words and characters that commonly featured in dreams, which he believed possessed the stamp of heavenly authority and were amenable to being apocalyptically handled with the help of angels.[86] There were thus manifold opportunities for divination of all kinds and indeed for making ambitious predictions. At this point he advocated prudence. Speculations about the future, or insights into secrets such as alchemy, required careful preparation and complex procedures. Access to such secrets would only emerge at the right time and would be available only to those possessing the highest spiritual probity. Only the latter would be able to resist the abundant invitations to engage in futile interventions.[87]

Paracelsus warned about the misuse of astronomy. This science should limit itself to the regularities of the heavens and related natural phenomena. Alluding to the *potentia ordinata* and *potentia absoluta* distinction, he concluded that it was inappropriate to subsume under astronomy events which were of supernatural causation. The latter should be regarded as the province of magic and interpreted appropriately as interventions of God. Such supernatural events had 'inner' rather than 'outer' significance. They coincided with the phenomena described by Christ as signs (*zeichen*), which he intended as serious moral warnings and omens for the benefit of humankind.[88] It was necessary to be vigilant to detect such signs, which were often manifest as strange happenings, for instance the large meteorite that fell at Ensisheim, Alsace in 1492. Along with many others, Paracelsus insisted that such wonders were not routine events; special consideration should be given to their likely supernatural significance. Paracelsus highlighted the case of the Magi who attended the infant Christ in Bethlehem as the most auspicious example of a supernatural celestial occurrence. The star was a particularly clear instance when God had restricted understanding of a celestial wonder to a select body of sincere believers. It suggested that in his own turbulent age the interpretation of celestial portents would again be restricted to a similar small nucleus of upright and convinced believers.[89]

On the strength of the testimony of the scriptures and the Christian message, it was the will of God that the art of divination, especially those aspects relating to prediction, would be revealed to a select band of experts. In order to equip themselves for receipt of such blessings, believers needed to acquire the requisite skill and also take full advantage of the Light of Nature and relevant guiding spirits. They would then be in a position to understand all the changes of human fortune, including the effects of the punishment deriving from humans' fall from grace, changes within religion and within secular orders, the passing away of kingdoms and structures of authority, indeed, every kind of suffering and destitution. It was an essential part of the Christian mission to bring sense to these various revelations of the Creator's power and intentions.[90]

The most striking feature of the commentary of Paracelsus on the current situation and prospects for the immediate future was its prevalent mood of pessimism. This applied also to his *practicas*, his commentaries on Lichtenberger and Osiander, or many of his relevant theological, social and ethical expositions. Certainly, his rivals also habitually supplied lurid accounts of the decadence of their times, but they tended to offer easy formulas for a better future. Some demanded reversion to stricter compliance with the old faith; others offered inspiring prospects conditional on affiliation to new churches or sects. Others again placed their hopes for salvation in one or other of the secular princes or civil leaderships.

By contrast, Paracelsus detected few grounds for optimism. The whole structure of institutional authority in all of its permutations seemed to him to be characterized by fundamental defects. The increasing wealth that was being generated was engrossed by the few. There was casual regard for social justice in the civil sphere and a collapse of the moral authority of the church. It was evident from the recent historical record and the witness of his own lifetime that in every direction there was instability, oppression and anarchy. In all of its variants, the system operated to consolidate the power of the tyrant, the exploiter and the oppressors of the poor.

Paracelsus warned the little band of believers who possessed the gift of the fiery tongue not to be misled by the vain promises of false apostles. He was confident that magic would expose the errors of those who prophesied about the future beyond 1524 and portrayed themselves as divinely appointed to overcome evils such as the papacy. It is tempting to regard this warning as being directed against the militant

Anabaptists, since they were committed to specific prophecies concerning the immediate future. In fact, the context suggests that the rival 'sects' portrayed by Paracelsus were the Catholics and Lutherans. In his view, both had failed to emancipate themselves from corrupt practices and moral decadence; neither could claim to be a reliable guide to salvation or to the blessed existence.[91] They were no better than the wild beasts of the Apocalypse. On the analysis of Paracelsus there was every reason to believe that the future belonged not to the powerful rulers, but to the oppressed and the poor. Although the immediate future offered nothing but continuation of suffering, the approach of the end of time would bring about reward for their life of patient sacrifice.

The commentary on Lichtenberger provided little comfort to secular princes. For the most part Paracelsus ignored the customary partisan uses of Lichtenberger to inspire support for either the French or the Habsburg ascendancy, although at one point he allowed for a Kaiser to supplant the existing papacy. Instead he concentrated on warnings of dire consequences for princes who allowed themselves to fall under the power of the stars through their rapacious struggle for supremacy over their neighbours. He appreciated that his appeals for princes to live in the spirit of repentance, peace and wisdom were unlikely to be heard sympathetically.[92] Significantly, the real climax of his Lichtenberger commentary is the discussion of Jeremiah's sermons on the destruction of the Temple of Jerusalem. Paracelsus saw no immediate prospect of relief deriving from the strife and anarchy of the peasants' uprisings. As a class, the peasants were free from the influence of the stars and therefore untainted by the corruption that infected their betters. They remained in this state as long as they were committed to simplicity, but their leaders sacrificed this virtue when they joined the ranks of the monks or *nollbrüder*.[93]

Since medieval times, the main conflict upon which prophetic tracts focused was between eastern Agarenes and the Christian west. The Agarenes were conventionally identified as the Saracens or Turks. At the time of Paracelsus the Ottoman Turks were making their furthest incursions into western Europe, and even threatening to annex Vienna. Accordingly, prophetic and apocalyptic commentary, especially from Habsburg sources, was strongly geared to working up anti-Ottoman hysteria. The Lutherans were anti-Ottoman, but manipulated their analysis to ensure that the blame for the current military catastrophe was placed at the door of the papists. Some others, notably Michael Sattler and Paracelsus, adopted an entirely different interpretation of the Agarenes. Sattler identified the Agarene enemy, not as any external threat, but as those responsible for corrupting Christianity from within. At his trial in 1527 he called such Christian reprobates 'Turks after the Spirit'; Paracelsus said that it was right to apply the Turkish label to the idle and arrogant false Christians of all the existing established churches, or to the affluent classes and all those who exploited the poor. He attacked such debased rulers and the church for allowing themselves to fall under the influence of the stars. In this condition they continued to fill up their churches, but the true Temple of God stood empty. Paracelsus reflected the mood of Jeremiah by dwelling on the devastating punishments imposed by God on corrupt rulers and on the decadent churches. The power of the Agarenes would end only when humans broke free from the hold of the stars and heeded the call for repentance and a new religion of the spirit.[94]

Just as Paracelsus refrained from contributing supportively to the generally held myth of the Last Emperor, his commentary on the Papal Prophecies decisively rejected Osiander's bid to represent Lutheranism as the agency that would bring about decisive reform of the papacy. Neither Osiander nor Paracelsus took much trouble to identify the individual popes, but Paracelsus at least recognized that the final five images in the thirty-strong series represented a transition to a time of renovation and a future realm of Angelic Popes. He repeatedly invoked magic as the key to understanding the papal figures, especially on account of their elaborate use of animal imagery. His commentary was an implied censure of Osiander for his ignorance about such symbolism. Adoption of a broader perspective on the papal figures enabled Paracelsus to draw up a much fuller and more colourful catalogue of invective against the papacy than was attempted by the Osiander–Sachs partnership. Paracelsus also visited the sins of the papacy on the magisterial reformers.

With respect to the eighth figure depicting the pope in the company of two women, both Osiander and Paracelsus considered this an attack on the dissolute lives of the popes. Osiander regarded the women as representing the alterative life of righteousness, whereas Paracelsus saw them as symbols of the prevalence of vice in both the old and the new 'sects'. Furthermore, as usual with his references to sexual vice or adultery, Paracelsus took these terms as surrogates for corrupt practices in general and in this case emphasized the misuse of alms and the exploitation of the poor.

In commenting on the ninth, thirteenth and twentieth figures, Osiander underlined the optimistic expectations for the Lutheran church and even suggested that the monk featuring in the twentieth figure offered a premonition of the reforming mission of Luther himself. By contrast,

Paracelsus identified the churches in general as the barren fig tree destined to be consigned to the flames. He found the twentieth figure entirely consistent with this negative judgement on the state of the church and its clergy. Noticeably, he offered absolutely no support for the view that Luther should be regarded in more favourable light than the detested papists.

The climax of the disagreement between Osiander and Paracelsus turned on images twenty-three and twenty-four, where Osiander employed particularly impressive and realistic images of Worms and Nuremberg. Worms was taken to represented the papist past, while Nuremberg depicted the Protestant future. Paracelsus rejected this reading. He identified the first as the sack of Rome. While conceding that the second was Nuremberg, he regarded the imperial city as the new centre of idolatry, destined to repeat all the basic faults of the discredited papacy. On the construction of Paracelsus, the new Lutheran regime was decisively not a vehicle for peace, but was destined to foster yet further misery.[95] No doubt communicating this verdict gave Paracelsus some personal satisfaction, since it could be taken as representing his own experience of the situation in Nuremberg.

In the hands of Paracelsus, the Papal Prophecies communicated a uniform and depressing tale of wantonness, corruption and suppression on the part of all of those in a position of power within church and state. The tyranny of both Catholics and incipient Protestants was blamed for the regime of suffering imposed on believers and the poor. The Papal Prophecies series therefore stood in stark contrast to the slightly earlier *Passional* series of Cranach, utilized for Illustrations 1 and 3, which prepared the way for Osiander's stark contrast between the Catholics and Lutherans. The much darker story presented by Paracelsus was enlivened by only a few glimpses of light relating to the present, but much more optimistic prospects for the future. The great secular and ecclesiastical powers were destined to disintegrate and break down into small entities, which themselves would collapse under the weight of their falsehood. The Word of God would then come into its own and persist for ever.[96] Just as the end of night and beginning of the new day was announced by the crowing of the cockerel, it was inevitable that false Christians of all kinds, with their negative associations, would, like night itself, pass away. Afterwards true Christians would control the day and enjoy the full benefits of the light.[97] First, the papacy would be overcome by its ghastly enemies, after which the latter also would be eliminated. The blessed, golden age would then dawn and the faithful would live in love and righteous expectation.[98] Three of the last images in the papal series were appropriately devoted to spelling out expectations for the golden age (*güldenen welt*) that represented a just reward for the faithful.[99] As additional comfort for the oppressed, the concluding sections of the Papal Prophecies emphasized the consensus between Paracelsus's own magical analysis and other authentic sources of prophecy. Such convergence of authority is indicated in the two parts of Illustration 7. All the signs suggested that the moment of retribution was approaching, when all manner of false Christians, including the worldly rulers and their clientele, would face ruin and destruction.[100] Everything pointed to the imminence of this conclusion, although Paracelsus warned believers to be patient and expect in the short term yet further misery and suffering (*das ellent facht aber erst an*).[101]

The 1536 Prognostication conveyed a similar mixed message of despair and hope. Entering into the spirit of the commentary of Paracelsus, his annotator interpreted this tract as an attack on the Emperor, Prince Ferdinand, and the Lutherans. The secular rulers would face indictment particularly for their merciless persecution of dissidents and Anabaptists. On this account they would face fearful retribution. No merit was recognized in the Lutheran innovations. The future lay in the religion of the heart and spirit, and in religious toleration. Paracelsus had deliberately avoided precise commitment to the date of the future golden age, but his annotator was certain that the author had 1560 in mind as the fundamental turning point of history, the date when Christ would return and God would reveal His most profound secrets.[102]

The Golden Age

Amid all the pessimism about the crisis in church and state, anxiety about imminent catastrophes, and fears of future judgement on mankind, there were distinct notes of optimism, especially strong in some quarters of opinion, reflecting belief in temporary respite, or even some more substantial phase of amelioration.

In some intellectual circles, especially among the Italian Neoplatonists, there was already a firm belief that they were at the centre of a great cultural revival, which merited the epithet 'golden age'. There was no difficulty in listing remarkable achievements in all spheres of learning and the practical arts. The astrologer, Paul of Middelburg, who was one of the main sources for Lichtenberger, placed Florence at the centre of the revival, but also acknowledged the significance of Germany with respect to modern inventions in the field of printing. He was in no doubt that his age had witnessed a secular cultural shift from darkness to light and that they were already living in a *seculum aureum*.[103] On the basis of their astrological analysis, Rabbi Yohanan Alemanno, the most notable Jewish adviser of the Florentine Neoplatonists, was also confident that the time was ripe for a notable upturn in intellectual fortunes.[104] With such prospects in mind, the youthful Giovanni Pico plunged into his massive schemes for a new philosophy with what can only be described as apocalyptic fervour in the short period before his untimely death.[105] This sense of positive achievement echoed around the humanists and grew in influence, strengthening the position of the innovators in the ancients versus moderns debate that rumbled along for more than a century in all parts of Europe.[106] The idea of an imminent golden age helped to offset the pessimism of the times. Representing the joint efforts of Konrad Celtis and Albrecht Dürer, Illustration 2 encapsulates the spirit of positive expectation being cultivated among the German humanists. Notwithstanding the many legitimate reasons for pessimism, it seemed that the groundwork was being laid for a great and positive cultural transformation.

As already noted, Paracelsus agreed with the humanists only to a limited extent. He was certainly not inclined to be sympathetic to their preoccupation with the culture of classical antiquity, but he agreed with the importance attached by humanists such as Celtis to the reorientation of philosophical outlook and to their greater valuation of magic and the applied arts. His own programme was conceived as a logical continuation of the general process of innovation that had taken root among artisans and artist engineers in many sectors of the economy. With respect to his expectations for the longer term, the attitudes of Paracelsus, like those of other radicals, were predominantly determined by reference to the messianic expectations of the Old Testament, which promised an age of peace and plenty to be enjoyed on earth by the chosen people. Old Testament constructions were an active inspiration for the radicals, since they provided a firm indication of future expectations for the persecuted community of saints. The importance of these ideas for Paracelsus is shown by many of his writings, particularly by the closing sections of his commentary on the Psalms of David.

The project of Paracelsus embodied the expectation that the saints would be rewarded for their sacrifices at the end of the historical process. Hence they would witness a period of Sabbath rest before the second coming.[107] No doubt intentionally, his writings were imprecise about the chronology or duration of the Sabbath renewal, but he firmly indicated that this was an imminent expectation. Potential rewards were outlined in terms consistent with the realities of the current social system, rather than reflecting objectives that could only be realized in some transcendent context. Paracelsus accordingly held out the expectations of a distinct improvement in conditions of life, even comprehensive social renewal and ambitious achievements in the technical arts and sciences. Such an approach constituted a marked contrast with that of figures like Hans Hut, who gave only the most slender consideration to the practicalities of life for the saints at the time of the Sabbath rest, relying instead on vague apocalyptic imagery. Paracelsus was also inclined to intersperse his exhortations with apocalyptic symbolism, but this was a subsidiary element. It is absolutely clear from the structure of his presentations that he believed that the moment was approaching when God would intervene to create conditions for the realization of the practical objectives for which he and like-minded planners had been making such conspicuous sacrifices.

Tentative ideas about expectations for the new age were included in the *Prologus in vitam beatam*. This brief essay was conceived as the introduction to a sequence of writings on the theme of the *selige leben*, the blissful existence briefly discussed in the previous chapter. The *Prologus in vitam beatam* should therefore be viewed as an important statement. While the *vita beata* was not a specifically apocalyptic conception, in the case of Paracelsus it was clearly conceived as integral to the apocalyptic sequence.

Paracelsus accepted that he had misjudged events. God had granted an appointed time for the growth and maturity of every being. It was admitted that he had mistakenly placed his energies in alchemy and geometry, thinking that these disciplines were about to experience genuine fruition. In the event such optimistic expectations were disappointed and these vain human endeavours had proved to be pervaded by *fliegenden geisten*.[108] Reflecting on the fundamentals of faith, he had turned away from these vanities. From firmer ground, he was certain that the appointed time for renewal had arrived and that summer was near.[109] But he also warned that the time and circumstances surrounding the arrival of the summer season of our history were inscrutable to humans. Many would undertake the sowing, but others would harvest and thresh, while others again would undertake the milling and baking, and finally yet others would consume the bread.[110] Given the repeated failure of recent apocalyptic expectations, such expression of caution was entirely understandable. Nevertheless, the whole of Paracelsus's construction was premised on the assumption that his own generation was witnessing the dawn of a fresh enlightenment and that his own project was evidence of this new state of affairs. Indeed, as already noted, his own 1536 *Prognostikation* contained the broad hint that the second coming would take place within his own expected lifetime. The timetable he envisaged was not as compressed as those proposed by Hans Hut or Melchior Hoffman, but he was expecting a distinct acceleration in the pace of cultural transformation. His prognosis for the immediate future appropriately reflected this expectation of escalating change.

With respect to the fields of knowledge in which he had participated, such as geometry, 'artisterei' and philosophy, the tenure of established authorities had completely run its course. The moment had come for the old arts to be supplanted and for all of their works to melt away. Reminiscent of the call of Grebel and Karlstadt for an end to the 'sparing' approach of the Lutherans, Paracelsus in this context insisted that sparing the old disciplines would obscure the new light that was dawning.[111] Already he detected signs of a general collapse in authority, for instance as indicated by monks deserting their posts and fleeing to remote places to escape the authority of false Christians. His rivals were warned that they would be damned unless they, along with their allies among the rich, including the secular and religious hierarchies, all submitted to a new birth and committed themselves to total poverty and simplicity of life and outlook.

It was boldly announced that the time was ripe for the ascendancy of his own works (*Die zeit meines schreibens ist zeitig*).[112] He was confident that the labours to which he had turned his hand were inspired by a light ignited by God. The Creator undertook nothing in vain and would see to it that later times were enlightened by His chosen disciples. It seemed evident that the long time of waiting and suffering was over. In this new age, the ephemeral would be replaced by a blissful and eternal state of existence, which included the experience of wonders such as the production of more than one kind of fruit on cultivated plants and trees.[113]

Having prepared the ground during the long winter, they were now awaiting a new dispensation, a time of general renewal, which Paracelsus described as the May season of the world.[114] God would release all the abundant benefits of nature, which previously had been reluctantly withheld on account of the crippling sinfulness of humans. Those who continued in the many ways of wickedness that were still rampant would of course be denied these benefits and ultimately they would face fearful retribution. Spelling out the misdeeds of the rich and powerful persisted as one of his dominant themes; there was no excuse for complacency and every reason for continuing alertness and vigilance concerning the menace of such degenerates.[115] God would take delight in restoring nature to its full potentialities for the sake of those who applied themselves according to the spirit of God's wisdom. Apart from the benefits available through the Light of Nature that He had ignited, God would see to it that humans had access to all the arts and crafts that contributed to human welfare.[116] Providing this work was pursued in a spirit of humility, praise and recognition that God was the master and humans His vassals, then the benefits of this May season would prevail for as long as humans remained on earth.[117] Paracelsus gave full expression to this expectation of a goodly season of reward for all the sacrifice, assiduity and hard work of the saints. However, such optimistic prospects needed to be tempered in light of the apocalypse as recorded in the Book of Revelation, which underlined the resilience of Antichrist and his agents on earth. It was impossible to ignore this alarming perspective which, among other things, made it unlikely that the forces of Antichrist would be dispatched without dramatic intervention by an outside agency.

Producing a convincing account of the final destiny and reward of the saints, consistent with the apocalyptic drama, was a problem that could not be ignored. In outlining the course of these concluding events, Paracelsus avoided the temptation to concentrate on the pungent imagery of the Book of Revelation. Although, unavoidably, the events were traumatic, he adopted a line of interpretation that allowed the elect to experience an element of continuity in the course of their ultimate fate. Consistently with this optimistic projection for later times, he drew on the familiar imagery of the golden age. His conception of the future had a limited amount in common with the *seculum aureum* of the humanists. He remained steadfastly convinced about the fundamental shortcomings of the scholarly disciples, in line with his general scepticism concerning the possibility of reviving any of the existing institutions of church or state. By contrast with the medieval authorities and their recent followers, Paracelsus had few expectations for emancipation through any kind of charismatic religious or secular leaders of the types that were currently on offer. Any glorious end to history would certainly not be mediated through an Angelic Pope or Last Emperor. All such rulers and hierarchies had been found wanting and would continue to be completely discredited.

Regardless of such negative factors, Paracelsus remained convinced that the apocalyptic machinery was capable of overcoming any obstacles imposed by human perversity and Satanic interference. He was confident that, reflecting the bounteous generosity of God, the practical arts would continue to flourish and eventually provide abundantly for all needs, taking to a logical conclusion the revolutionary developments in the practical arts that were already taking place. All the positive benefits of the future dispensation would eventually be at the disposal of the community of saints, whose monarchy would take effect after their long apprenticeship of resignation to poverty and oppression. The oppressed minority would witness the withering away of the weeds that hitherto had strangled their efforts, and would at last be able to enjoy in abundance the fruits of their labours. Essential to this final stage of history would be a fading away of temporal powers and the extension of the rule of God from heaven to the whole earth. After their long period of suffering, the poor would live in perfect harmony and joy in an untroubled environment for as long as the world remained in its existing physical state.[118]

The End of Time

In speculating about the future, Paracelsus was at his most comfortable with the Old Testament conception of the final vindication of the people of God and their survival to witness an age of harmony and bliss. His own priorities were consistent with such a progression. In the first place the monarchy of his scientific and medical ideas, which was an imminent expectation, represented a decisive contribution to relief in the current age of misery, discord and oppression. Immediate circumstances indicated the likelihood of a continuing demand for relief from every kind of medical emergency. Compared with any of its rivals, Paracelsianism, in its technical and ethical dimensions, seemed better equipped to meet such exigencies. Perhaps on account of the unremitting gloom of the immediate prognosis, like other leaders of opinion in the radical movement ,Paracelsus held up the expectation of a decisive turn for the better in the not too distant future. At this point the saints would experience all the benefits of an age of peace and tranquillity. In this context, the need for medical intervention would recede and the other side of the mission of Paracelsus would come into its own. His programme for the *vita beata*, or *selige leben*, laid down principles of governance that seemed remote from the experience of his day but were entirely appropriate to the new age that was on the horizon. Explicit guidance on prospects for this concluding phase of history was accordingly not merely a utopian literary exercise; it was essential for completing the message of hope and for preserving morale among the oppressed body of believers with whom Paracelsus identified.

Although the main point of emphasis in the writings of Paracelsus related to the end stages of the historical period, inevitably he also engaged with the eschatological transition to a new earth and new heaven. Such deliberations necessitated attention to the apocalyptic forecasts of the New Testament, about which he wrote relatively little and reached no settled opinion. Nevertheless, at many points in his writings, Paracelsus touched upon these final events; in a few cases he provided a summary of the entire process, including the second coming, the general resurrection of humanity, the Last Judgement and the final physical transformations of the macrocosm and microcosm.

Reflecting his habitual caution about calculating timetables for final times, he repeated the gospel strictures about predicting dates for the second coming or the Day of Judgement. These most sensitive of secrets rested entirely in the possession of the Father and would not be revealed.[119] As already noted, his reticence to make dogmatic forecasts about questions of chronology did not detract from the sense in his writings that the final apocalyptic sequence was in progress and was gathering pace. Paracelsus also emerges as a cautious commentator with respect to events surrounding the second coming. He was faithful to the apocalyptic point of view, but was not attracted by the kind of elaborate and gruesome constructions adopted by those who relied on the Book of Revelation as their main point of reference. In general, Paracelsus abided by the simpler delineation contained in the gospels. The Matthew apocalypse provided his main guidance, which was appropriate since this text covered all the main points of contention. Confirming his high estimate of this gospel source, Paracelsus concluded his important *De secretis secretorum theologiae* with a short commentary on Matthew 24.[120] Apart from his close reading of the scriptural texts, the most obvious feature of the account by Paracelsus was the care he took with naturalistic detail, including drawing attention to the fact that the climax of the narrative was consistent with his ideas about the sacraments and his theory of matter. The main effect of this presentation was to impart an atmosphere of tranquillity to a situation that might well have stimulated the utmost alarm.[121]

Following medieval precedent, in this context Paracelsus adopted a tripartite view of history, which he saw as being divided into two 'generations', the dispensations of the Old Testament and the New Testament. The third generation would be marked by the second coming of Christ. The Son of God would duly arrive in great majesty, but not, as usually depicted, with the symbols and the regalia of office of secular princes.[122] These artefacts were duly listed in order to draw attention to the contrast with the reality of the second coming of Christ, whose body would bear all the scars inflicted at the time of his crucifixion. To emphasize the contrast between Christ and secular monarchs, these physical humiliations were summed up by Paracelsus in forensic detail, which was helpful for his construction, although not supported by the relevant scriptures.

Continuing to stress the simplicity of the occasion, Paracelsus noted that Christ would not be surrounded by a troop of horsemen and associated paraphernalia such as drums.[123] On this occasion he was consistent with the text in stating that only four angelic trumpeters would be present. Their trumpets would then emit a fearful sound directed to the four parts of the world, to summon up all the living, revive the recently deceased and raise the long dead from their graves and their sleep.[124]

At the sound of an order, the peoples would be summoned to the final judgement of God.[125] Participating in the judgement would be twelve apostles, who would be seated on stools made from clouds. Such assistance was needed to dispense justice to the twelve tribes of Israel.[126] Further assistance would be provided by angels, who were assigned to separating out the good from the bad: the lambs blessed by God would be placed to the right and the evil-smelling billy goats (*stinketen böck*), who merited damnation, to the left.[127] The elect would rise like eagles or smoke from a fire,[128] whereas the condemned would descend like stones or lead.[129] Satan and his allies would at last be consigned to the fires of hell that had been awaiting this use since the fall of these reprobates from heaven.[130]

Paracelsus relied on the Revelation narrative for the fate of Satan, but he ignored the final sections of the biblical apocalypse comprising the eloquent description of the New Jerusalem. Instead, repeating the emphasis of the Matthew apocalypse, he concentrated on the selection criteria for the chosen people. As elsewhere in the writings of Paracelsus, the emphasis was placed on humility and service, especially expressions of love of one's neighbour. Had they given food to the hungry, drink to the thirsty? Had they displayed compassion towards the sick, the imprisoned, the helpless and the naked? Had they provided these needy with support, consolation, clothing and a roof over their head?[131] If this generosity was not forthcoming, God would not reciprocate with His mercy. Those who had fulfilled their duties in the spirit of generosity would be counted among the elect and be admitted into the house of the Father, prepared at the beginning of time for the reception of angels and the regenerate.[132] This house contained many dwellings made ready for the saints.[133] When all of these things were accomplished, the scene would be set for all elemental bodies to revert to their *materia prima*, expressed in its highest sacramental form, which was a completely enlightened and clarified state of being (*erleucht, clarificirt*). Believers were at last in a position to praise their Creator from the vantage point of certain salvation, and this state of affairs would persist from world to world and from eternity to eternity.[134]

In bringing his end-time narrative to a complete conclusion, Paracelsus needed to give consideration to the possibility of some kind of personal reign of Christ with his elect on earth, which thus embodied the ideal of a New Jerusalem in its most advanced form. The final two chapters of the Book of Revelation formed the obvious basis for such suppositions. On various occasions Paracelsus incorporated relevant elements from Revelation concerning such an interlude into his narrative.[135] Mammon and his allies would succumb slowly, but ultimately they would be routed and eliminated.[136] Only at this point would the saints finally witness the dissolution of all those religious and secular establishments that had long been the targets of Paracelsus's criticisms. The holy city would then be free of weeds.[137] Only then would it be safe to gather the elect from far and wide into the City of God, the New Jerusalem or the earthly paradise. Such constructs are revealing because they indicate that Paracelsus tended to emphasize continuity with the state of affairs at the end of the historical period. The earthly paradise even featured the need for an advanced state of learning, still reliant on the Light of Nature, ignited by God, but now exploited more effectively to attain an even higher plane of knowledge than before. In the case of the arts and handicrafts, knowledge would come direct from God. Human wisdom would flourish, unimpeded by its previous limitations, and would at last bring about the return of human dominion over nature.[138]

Such a concept was faithful to the prophecy of Daniel that a transcendent state of wisdom and righteousness would be reached, but it was understood that such achievements were dependent on the continuing guidance of the small band of *maskilim*, who were the appointed guardians of enlightenment.[139] Such inspired teachers would have the capacity to shine with the brightness of the firmament. To those around them they would act like stars lasting into eternity and they would lead believers towards righteousness.[140] The *maskilim* in turn were seen both by Paracelsus and in the early Christian era as the forerunners of the wisest teachers of apostolic times.[141] The passage of Daniel concerning the *maskilim* was also seen by Paracelsus as a firm forecast of a future Christian era which would fulfil Daniel's 'age of knowledge' when many would 'run to and fro, and knowledge shall be increased'.[142] Also at this point Paracelsus introduced his favourite imagery of the seasons and growth, portraying the pre-Christian era as the winter, the birth of Christ as the inauguration of the spring season and the inception of an inevitable progression of events that would soon end with a season of eternal bliss.[143]

The rectitude of the patriarchs and prophets, the miraculous intervention of the Magi and the culminating achievements of the apostles[144] acted as inspiration to those who took up the gospel commission to preach, baptize and heal during the heroic period, when the radical movement was in its infancy. Like others in his situation, Paracelsus was inspired by all of these earlier models. Also from the apostolic era he absorbed a strong sense of operating at the end of time. The many-sided mission in which he was engaged was given unity and purpose by his sense of satisfaction that his various labours were making a proportionate contribution to the final summer of fruitfulness and to the messianic age that seemed to be on the very verge of realization.[145]

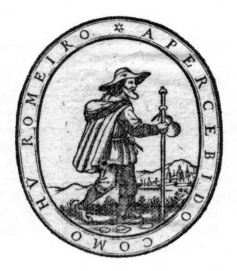

CONCLUSIONS
THE WAY TO GOD

dan in zwen wege seind die werk grottes geteilt, in die werk der natur, das die philosophia begreift, und in die werk Christi, das theologia begreift. In denen sollen wir verzeren die zeit, so wir auf erden zu verzeren haben, damit wir mit friden sterben.[1]

Paracelsus repeatedly insisted that the 'philosophical' (scientific and medical) and 'theological' (religious, ethical and political) aspects of his mission were inseparable and mutually supportive. Exploring the various dimensions of this integrated programme has been one of the main objects of this study. The vast body of his writings demonstrate the seriousness with which Paracelsus pursued his central objectives. From the moment his works became available to the wider public it was clear that he had succeeded in making a substantial and distinctive contribution over a remarkably broad front. However, the task of interpretation was never straightforward: indeed it appeared ever more daunting as the large scale and intractable content of the modern editions became evident. Engaging with the writings of Paracelsus was therefore never a task for the fainthearted.

Notwithstanding the self-referential writing habit of Paracelsus, it is quite obvious that he was operating in isolation from his intellectual environment. Many years ago Walter Pagel illustrated this conclusion by reference to the pronounced Neoplatonic element in the thinking of Paracelsus. The present study attempts to shed further light on relevant intellectual associations, and this contextual perspective has unavoidably also involved attention to the troubled times in which he lived. This raises the question of the links of Paracelsus with radical religious movements during the early Reformation and the German Peasants' War, issues that were marginal to the investigations of Walter Pagel and more recently have only been considered in the most limited respects.

In common with other radical activists of his day, in every sphere of his speculations Paracelsus deferred to his carefully conceived religious commitments. He was therefore unwilling to contemplate any course of action unless it was consistent with the dictates of the spirit and with the 'ways' laid down in the scriptures, both of which he regarded as providing immutable guidelines for the necessarily painful ascent towards the kingdom of heaven.

In setting such demanding standards for himself, Paracelsus realized that he was stepping out of line with the prevalent norms of society. He was by no means alone in expressing profound disenchantment with the existing state of affairs. Within his generation, the arrival of the date 1500 was perceived as a crisis and ominous turning point in the history of Christian civilization. Evidence from every direction gave reason for anxiety and uncertainty about the future and grounds for anticipation of continuing turbulence in both the religious and the secular spheres.

Those in positions of influence pursued their agenda for change according to their own perception of the ongoing crisis and undoubtedly in their own interests. Dissatisfied with the self-serving approach of the establishment, the young Theophrastus von Hohenheim aligned himself with those adopting the most adverse judgement on prevailing institutions and demanding the most complete break with the past. His drift in the radical direction arguably reflected his personal experience at the margins of the professions, where he was evidently distressed by the unprincipled scramble for wealth among his contemporaries, which he believed was conducted at the expense of the poor, with whose plight he strongly identified.

From this marginal perspective, he was inclined to blame all the existing institutions for conniving in squandering the rich legacy that the divine plan had granted for the amenity of modern civilization. Already, pre-capitalist society seemed to be in the iron grip of a culture of commodification which tended to commercialize all transactions, greatly to the detriment of the least privileged members of the community. In the areas that related to him personally, the church and professions seemed to have lost their moral authority through their avarice, distorted values and failure to comply with the basic standards of probity laid down in the gospels. His repeated experience of adverse relations with priests and physicians confirmed this pessimistic analysis. Like his radical counterparts, Paracelsus believed that he was witnessing a spiralling decline, the effects of which were evident throughout society. Such a situation, he felt, was unsustainable, as was clear from the mounting evidence of manifestations of divine retribution.

The above social criticisms were elaborated at length in the writings of Paracelsus and were communicated at every opportunity, usually in a spirit of urgency, evident anger and bitterness, no doubt reflecting his frustration that basic and genuine grievances of the poor were ignored and remained unaddressed. His disenchantment with the magisterial reformers was connected with their cultivation of endemic social grievances for the purposes of their own advancement, but when in power they seemed to be no improvement on the bankrupt regime of the old church that they had superseded. The magisterial reformers were therefore not applauded for the benefits stemming from their break with the bondage of Rome, but were denounced as false prophets serving the purposes of the Devil in the hectic final stages of apocalyptic confrontation between the forces of good and evil.

Accidentally, the magisterial reformers had served a positive purpose by helping to diagnose the diseases of church and state, thereby preparing the ground for activists more willing to pursue problems to their logical conclusion and contemplate solutions that were intolerable to the emergent reform establishment and their powerful backers. Once called into existence, this radical thinking tended for a short period to run out of control. The early maturity of Paracelsus coincided exactly with the brief flowering of this social and religious radicalism, which was at its height between 1520 and 1525. Not surprisingly, the outlook of Theophrastus approximated with that of other radical activists, many of whom were of his own age and disposition. Often they were skilled artisans, a class that Theophrastus identified as a model for the rehabilitation of his own profession. In view of these radical affinities, it is understandable that the first reliable information about Theophrastus relates to his emergence among the ranks of the itinerant preachers and peripatetic medical practitioners. At this point he was also a propagandist on the social and religious grievances of the day, making his own minor but distinctive contribution from the sidelines as an ideologue of the German Peasants' War.

The radical environment of this early thinking is important because from the outset of his literary career, notwithstanding his situation of disadvantage, the young Theophrastus was fired with confidence about the feasibility of making a decisive impact both as a critic and as an architect of change. In this false dawn, he committed himself to working for the decisive betterment of both church and state. For this purpose his writings increasingly appeared under the concocted name of Paracelsus. Owing to rapid reversion to the normalities of intolerance and repression, it was not possible for either Paracelsus or other radical voices to exercise anything like the influence to which they aspired. However, they tried to build up a constituency of support and wrote persuasively about their programmes for religious and social change.

Although Paracelsus, like all of his reform-minded contemporaries, was inevitably influenced by Luther and Zwingli, it is entirely inappropriate to regard him as one of the wayward followers of these magisterial reformers. In almost every aspect of his outlook, Paracelsus belongs among the critics of Luther and Zwingli, rejecting the whole magisterial approach to reform and adopting a theological perspective that the magisterial establishment would have regarded as alien and subversive. Paracelsus resolutely rejected identification with specific sects, but he subscribed to a generalized separatist point of view, placing his confidence in the ideal of a loose federation of lay-dominated congregations of believers, tolerant of adult baptism and adopting an interpretation of the Lord's Supper that was confined to dissenting circles. Although Paracelsus never contemplated joining any kind of Anabaptist congregation, this study has demonstrated that he was, nevertheless, extremely close to the spiritualist Anabaptists in his basic religious and secular outlook. Furthermore, in the course of his career, Paracelsus showed no retreat from his early radicalism; if anything his nonconformist instincts became more firmly entrenched as time went by and as his bitter experiences multiplied.

When it emerged that the ecclesiastical and civic authorities of all colours rejected a pluralistic approach to reform, many of the leading radical voices among the contemporaries of Paracelsus discovered that the pursuit of a radical agenda was the passport to prison and an early grave. Paracelsus was more fortunate. Owing to his medical commitments he was able to switch gear and satisfy his reformist ambitions in this specialized professional context. While his incorrigible nonconformity exposed him to permanent insecurity and discomfort, he was good enough as a doctor never to be short of wealthy and influential patients. Such patronage conferred a certain immunity from harassment. Also, it is likely that he was perceived as operating in a civic sideshow and thereby seemed to offer no threat as an agent of sedition.

Because of his notorious tenacity and appetite for industry, Paracelsus overcame the disadvantages of disruption and achieved the remarkable feat of executing an ambitious writing programme, surveying not only major parts of medicine and natural philosophy but also, in more fragmentary outline, many aspects of theology, ethics and politics. Since his overt controversial activity was limited to medicine, and his wider radical opinions allowed only limited airing in brief digressions in the medical writings or in the protected environment of prophetic tracts, the full range of his speculations and extent of his radicalism were obscured from both the broader public and the policing authorities. Fortuitously, despite continuous disruption and many other adversities, Paracelsus managed to bequeath a literary legacy on the scale of most of the other major figures in the early modern scientific movement. The fourteen volumes of the Sudhoff edition establish his credentials as a challenging innovator within the scientific movement. Much more unusual is the insight into the broader framework of his thinking provided by the non-scientific writings which equal the Sudhoff edition in their extent.

In his attacks on the professions and in his wider social critique, Paracelsus was subscribing to widely shared opinions. However, he was the sole activist to demand root and branch change in the medical profession, its related specialisms and indeed the whole body of learning upon which they depended. Unconvinced by the aura of altruism cultivated by the humanist doctors, Paracelsus accused all the professions relating to medicine of being participants in the prevalent regime of exploitation that he believed was exercising a destructive effect on the whole social fabric. He was determined that medical doctors and their cherished institutions of higher education should bear proportionate blame for the injustices and social discontent that were highlighted in his writings and which it became part of his mission to address.

Paracelsus must have been familiar with the major intellectual disputes among the humanists and he will have realized that the learned world was alive with proposals for reform in the fields of philosophy and medicine. Not uncommonly, leaders of opinion advocated educational and institutional reforms; they also commonly announced that they were advocates of some kind of new philosophy. Paracelsus was more extreme in his demands. He insisted that compliance with gospel principle required a more decisive break with the past and a different spirit of enquiry. Just as he exceeded the boundaries of tolerance of the magisterial reformers in the area of religion, in his 'religion' of medicine and natural philosophy he pursued a radical course that was well outside the limits of tolerance of the humanistic elite. Such reckless disregard for the past was an affront to the cherished cohesive values of the educated classes. It must have seemed both gratuitous and perverse that Paracelsus should break ranks with all of his humanistic colleagues and embark on an impassioned assault on their programme to revitalize ancient systems of knowledge. Perhaps the humanists had themselves to blame. Their taste for internecine disputes and habit of blanket rejection of everything outside their personal avocations inevitably undermined confidence in the whole humanist enterprise at the popular level and thereby prepared the ground for the radical intervention by Paracelsus.

Even in the iconoclastic spirit of the times, it was never going to be easy to undermine confidence in a system of values and knowledge that had taken more than a thousand years to construct and which was still being vindicated by powerful intellectual authority. Even more daunting was the design of a credible alternative in the space of a few years by a single person. Few were likely to mount a constructive challenge of this kind, however much they were fired with a sense of evangelical confidence.

Paracelsus took on the tasks of demolition and reconstruction without any fear of the daunting scale of the operation. The ongoing root and branch reappraisal of all institutions of church and state provided an ample supply of arguments that were transferable for use in the critique of philosophy, the sciences and medicine. Destructive criticism therefore presented few problems and a growing constituency was predisposed to be sympathetic to the distrust of entrenched establishments and their ramshackle systems of knowledge. With respect to the presuppositions of the new approach, the basic orientation of Paracelsus was determined with reference to his sources of religious inspiration. This study has indicated in detail the extent to which his conceptual preferences and use of language possessed self-evident theological and scriptural associations. Such roots were readily recognizable to his readership and would have added to their confidence in his vantage point.

The various religious sources that contributed to the basic outlook of Paracelsus provided a rich reservoir of insights that could be mobilized for other purposes. The new wave of Paracelsus research is fully alert to the significance of the religious dimension. Indeed, in an excess of enthusiasm, some commentators are tempted to discount the influence of philosophical factors such as Neoplatonism and play down the role of technical traditions. However, it is premature to reach such conclusions. As indicated at many points in this study, it is self-evident that scriptural insights were of limited relevance and that a fuller explanation of necessity involved the importation of information from the technical sphere, which was interpreted in the light of generalized principles derived from Neoplatonic sources. Consistent with his abhorrence of pagan philosophy, Paracelsus avoided reference to particular authorities, adopted theories in a schematized form, and even devised his own terminology, gratuitously encouraging the impression that his theories were freshly devised for each specific purpose. It has taken the archaeological exercises conducted by Pagel and his contemporaries to reveal that the ideas of Paracelsus can be related to currents of philosophy that were exercising profound influence during his formative years.

Such conclusions are by no means detrimental to the reputation of Paracelsus as an innovator. Even at their most derivative, his writings avoided the compilation model that was the staple of Sebastian Frank, and also Cornelius Agrippa's famous *De occulta philosophia*. Paracelsus was so averse to imitation and so committed to innovation that his compositions tended not only to be unconventional, but also idiosyncratic, and even impenetrably obscure. In some notable instances, such as his tripartite conception of matter, his ontological theory of disease or his homoeopathic therapeutics, Paracelsus demonstrated an impressive capacity to draw discriminatingly on a diverse blend of religious, Neoplatonic, alchemical and technical resources. In such cases he proved capable of contributing impressive insights in important areas of scientific theory.

Further evidence of his Neoplatonic leanings derives from his attachment to magic and kabbalah. This commitment to magic clearly connects with a parallel trend among his Neoplatonic contemporaries. Indeed the joint promotion of magic and kabbalah may well derive from Giovanni Pico. However, the approach of Paracelsus remained distinctive and he resisted the temptation to elevate magic into a refined esoteric art, the exclusive property of some inner circle of an erudite elite. Notwithstanding his exalted aspirations, the magic of Paracelsus was regarded as universally accessible, subject to the important condition applying to every other aspect of his system that the magical arts should be pursued in the spirit of complete evangelical commitment. The path to magic required full submission to the Light of Nature; this in turn was open only to those who were receptive to the Light of the Holy Spirit and accepted the demanding disciplines associated with spiritual regeneration. Like his learned counterparts, Paracelsus assumed that magic and kabbalah were the property of a small elite, but his group was defined very differently from the class of esoteric virtuosi to which the Florentines subscribed. The Paracelsus elite was to be recruited from his community of saints. The highest achievements of magic were not conditional on the accumulation of erudite credentials. Indeed, as in the case of the *schriftgelehrten* in religion, esoteric virtuosity was viewed as a hindrance rather than an aid to the magical discipline. Paracelsus therefore translated magic and kabbalah into a form consistent with the values of the Radical Reformation, thereby in principle opening up universal access to the exciting opportunities offered by these arts. Magic and kabbalah now fell within the sphere of aptitudes and artisan skills that were already prevalent among the common people. In magic as in matters of faith, the future lay in the hands of the select minority of this laity who possessed the capacity and foresight to take on the momentous challenge with which they were now presented.

On account of the massive ambition of his labour, Paracelsus was unable to complete more than a fraction of his writings. Much of what he bequeathed is no more than a sketch. But the scale of his achievement is truly impressive. Few scientific writers have ever worked with such effect on such a wide canvas. The writings of Paracelsus give the impression of a race against time, of a person working against the current of declining health and ever mindful of the imminent expectation of the end of time. The fragmentary compositions, many of them frustratingly near to publishable form, were then abandoned owing to changed circumstances and the need to move on to some distant and uncertain assignment. He seems to have borne these multiple disappointments with stoical resolve; no obstacle was allowed to stand in the way of yet further and expansive plans for elaborating his ideas. Such a high level of motivation can only be explained by reference to his deeply entrenched sense that he was participating in a great mission and by the fact that he pursued his career in a spirit of dedicated pilgrimage.[2]

The whole way of life of our reformer during his later years seems profoundly dysfunctional to the modern observer, but Paracelsus may well have regarded the uncertainties of his life as being in keeping with common assumptions concerning final times. After all, despite his cautious stance about prophecy, it seems he believed that the Last Judgement was on the horizon and would occur during the expected term of his own lifetime. His early death prevented him from discovering that providence had a more extended timetable in mind. Such ominous expectations must have heightened his state of dismay at the condition of the Christian west, including the treatment of sincere souls harbouring views not dissimilar to his own but whose fate was to be hunted down, apprehended and brutally executed. To be spared the extremes of persecution and to have had the opportunity to contribute so fully to the causes of social justice and spiritual regeneration must have been a distinct consolation. Whatever his thoughts about the apocalyptic future of the Christian west, he must have been satisfied that he had fulfilled his own calling in an exemplary manner and therefore had every right to die in a spirit of contentment.

NOTES

Abbreviations

The main abbreviations used in this study relate to editions of the writings of Paracelsus. These abbreviations are indicated in Part I of the Select Bibliography. Other abbreviations are given here:

CWE	*Collected Works of Erasmus* (Toronto: University of Toronto Press, 1974–).
Osiander Gesamtausgabe	Gottfried Seebaß and Gerhard Müller (eds), *Andreas Osiander d.Ä. Gesamtausgabe*, 10 vols (Gütersloh: Gütersloher Verlagshaus Gerd Mohn, 1975–97).
WA	*D. Martin Luthers Werke. Kritische Gesamtausgabe*, 65 vols (Weimar: Verlag Hermann Böhlaus Nachfolger, 1883–1965).
Wander	Karl Friedrich Wilhelm Wander, *Deutsches Sprichwörter-Lexikon*, 5 vols (Leipzig: F.A. Brockhaus, 1867–80).

Chapter I: Life and Labour

1. P I, 8, 38. 'Why are you so full of hatred for me that I must be labelled as Luther when I am Theophrastus and not Luther. Let Luther be responsible for himself and I will see to my own affairs.'
2. Henry E. Sigerist, *Grosse Ärzte* (Munich: J.F. Lehmanns Verlag, 1932), 77–86.
3. See especially draft material to *Paragranum*, c. 1529, P I, 8, 38, 43, 44, 47, 63.
4. The names of Paracelsus attract a great deal of curiosity. This issue is further considered in Chapters II and IV. For present purposes it is sufficient to note that *Theophrast*, the abbreviated form of the first name, seems not to have been used during his life, Benzenhöfer, *Paracelsus*, 20–1.
5. Christian Heck (ed.), *Le Retable d'Issenheim et la sculpture au nord des Alpes à la fin du Moyen Age: Actes du colloque de Colmar, 1987* (Colmar: Unterlinden Museum, 1989); Peter Thurmann, *Symbolsprache und Bildstruktur. Michael Pacher, der Trinitätsgedanke*

und die Schriften des Nikolaus von Kues (Bern: Peter Lang, 1987); Barbara Rommé, *Henrick Douwerman und die niederrheinische Bildschnitzkunst an der Wende zur Neuzeit* (Bielefeld: Verlag für Regionalgeschichte, 1997). See also Baxandall, *Limewood Sculptors of Renaissance Germany*, including on the organization and economic importance of this sector of the art market.

6. Andrée Hayum, *The Isenheim Altarpeice. God's Medicine and the Painter's Vision* (Princeton, NJ: Princeton University Press, 1989), 13–52; Manfred Mohr, *Die heilige Wolfgang in Geschichte, Kunst und Kult. Ausstellungs des Landes Oberösterreich* (Linz: Amt der Oberösterreichen Landesregierung, Kulturabteilung, 1976).

7. In listing famous names associated with Nuremberg in 1512, Johannes Cochlaeus specified only five, all craftsmen who were in the European public eye for their recent work: Dürer of course, also, predictably, Peter Vischer the bronze worker, and, in addition, Johann Neuschel the brass musical instrument maker, Erhard Etzlaub the compass maker and cartographer, and Peter Henlein, who had just invented the portable, spring-powered watch capable of running for forty hours without rewinding, Cochlaeus, *Brevis Germaniae descriptio*, ed. Karl Langosch (Darmstadt: Wissenschaftliche Buchgesellschaft, 1960), 88–91.

8. For an important expression of this partnership, see Illustration 2 and the related explanatory text.

9. Jeffrey Chipps Smith, *Nuremberg, A Renaissance City, 1500–1618* (Austin, TX: University of Texas Press, 1983), 63–4 for examples of collaboration involving goldsmiths. For some twenty examples of elaborate retables displaying what the author terms the 'florid' virtuosity of sculptors, Baxandall, *Limewood Sculptors of Renaissance Germany*, 62–9.

10. Another of Schedel's main associates in this project was Hieronymus Münzer (1437–1508), the Nuremberg physician and cosmographer: Klaus Herbers, 'Nürnberg und Nürnberger auf der Iberischen Halbinsel', in Helmut Neuhaus (ed.), *Nürnberg. Eine europäische Stadt in Mittelalter und Neuzeit* (Nürnberger Forschungen, 29), (Nuremberg: Selbstverlag des Vereins für Geschichte der Stadt Nürnberg, 2000), 151–83; Reinhard Stauber, 'Hartmann Schedel, der Nürnberger Humanistenkreis und die "Erweiterung der deutschen Nation"', in Johannes Helmrath, Ulrich Muhlack and Gerrit Walther (eds), *Diffusion des Humanismus. Studien zur nationalen Geschichtsschreibung europäischer Humanisten* (Göttingen: Wallstein Verlag, 2002), 159–85.

11. Rolf Kiessling, 'Das gebildete Bürgertum und die kulturelle Zentralität Augsburgs im späten Mittelalter und der frühen Neuzeit', in Bernd Moeller, Hans Patze and Karl Stackmann (eds), *Studien zum städtischen Bildungswesen des späten Mittelalters und der frühen Neuzeit* (Göttingen: Vanderhoeck & Ruprecht, 1983), 553–85, at 565–6; Gensthaler, *Das Medizinalwesen in der Freien Reichstadt Augsburg*, 44–6, 93–7 and passim.

12. Immediately after the death of Fries, Brunfels took over as editor of his successful medical handbook the *Spiegel der Artznei*. Karl Bittel, 'Die Elsässer Zeit des Paracelsus'; Josef Benzing, 'Bibliographie der Schriften des Colmarer Arztes Lorenz Fries'.

13. For the last twenty years of his life Etzlaub was known as much as *Arzt* as *Kompaßmacher*. The link between the mathematical and medical sides of his profession was provided by calendars and almanacs. Although primarily a medical author, Fries was active in astrology and for a few years he was also engaged in cartographical publishing.

14. For an exemplary study of this competitive situation, Pelling, *Medical Conflicts in Early Modern London*. See also Robert Jütte, *Ärzte, Heiler und Patienten. Medizinischer Alltag in der frühen Neuzeit* (Munich: Artemis & Winkler, 1991), 17–32.

15. For a sound and succinct account of the life, providing full references to earlier and relevant specialized sources, see Udo Benzenhöfer, *Paracelsus*.
16. Commentary on Psalm 118 (119), P II, 6, 109.
17. Goldammer, 'Die geistlichen Lehrer des Theophrastus Paracelsus' (1957), in *Paracelsus in neuen Horizonten*, 58–86, for the most detailed exposition of the positive case. The single paragraph upon which this construction rests served primarily to underline the availability of good libraries in distant Carinthia, partly owing to the named clerical luminaries. As Sudhoff eventually conceded, the Sponheim reference may well have been to the Spanheim family's patronage of the important Carinthian Benedictine abbey of St Paul in Lavanttal, which was appropriate to Paracelsus's theme on account of its celebrated library. There are no other grounds to suggest that Paracelsus was ever in direct contact with the famous kabbalist and cryptographer Johannes Trithemius who, in any case, ceased to be abbot of Sponheim (in the Rheinland Palatinate) in 1506 and died in Würzburg in 1516. Noel L. Brann, on his own grounds, is sceptical about links with Paracelsus: see his *Trithemius and Magical Theology* (Albany: State University of New York Press, 1999), 181–5, summarizing his article in *Sixteenth Century Journal*, 10 (1979), 70–82. The relevant autobiographical remark was published in the second part of the *Grosse Wundarznei* (1536), P I, 14, 354.
18. Bittel, 'Die Elsässer Zeit des Paracelsus'.
19. Basel Protocol dated 21 May 1527, transcribed in full in Blaser, *Paracelsus in Basel*, 68–9.
20. The heading of his *Intimatio*, dated 9 June 1526 (P I, 4, 3), and the dedication of his *De gradibus et compositionibus receptorum* to Christoph Klauser, 10 November 1526 (P I, 4, 71), used *utriusque medicinae doctor*; while in the introduction to the *Spital-Buch* (1529) he merely called himself *Doctor Theophrastus* (P I, 7, 369).
21. For representative lists of places with which Paracelsus claimed acquaintance, see *Spital-Buch* (1529), (P I, 7, 374–5), and *Grosse Wundarznei* (1536) (P I, 10, 19).
22. In the introduction to his *Spital-Buch* (1529) he claimed experience in the military context in six diverse countries and direct medical experience in twice as many, P I, 7, 374–5.
23. *Entwürfe, Notizen* (1528*)*, P I, 6, 180; *Von blattern lähme*, P I, 6, 329–30, where Paracelsus relates his trouble with his Siebenbürgen competitors to their jealously over his *Opodeldok* treatment. See note 58,and Peter Mario Kreuter in *Forschungen zur Volks-und Landeskunde*, 50 (2007) 147–57.
24. *Septem punctis*, P II, 3, 5.
25. Draft Preface to *Paragranum* (*c.* 1529/30), (P I, 8, 34). At exactly the same period, Cornelius Agrippa von Nettesheim experienced even more serious difficulties over fees at the court of Louise of Savoy in Lyons.
26. Blaser, *Paracelsus in Basel*, 22–8.
27. Hohenheim, *Intimatio*, P I, 4, 3; Sudhoff, *Paracelsus* (Leipzig: Bibliographisches Institut, 1936), 27–30.
28. A suitable date in view of the ancient magical associations of this feast date and its importance for the collection and use of herbal remedies. The identity of the offending volume is not known, but in all likelihood it was a student crammer, perhaps a summary of Avicenna.
29. Franck, *Chronica, zeytbuch und geschychtbibel* (Strasbourg: Balthasar Beck, 1531), 253. For reference to this event by Paracelsus, see the draft Foreword to his *Paragranum*, P I, 8, 58.This Johannisfeur was symbolically relevant, since it was traditionally associated with the driving out of evil spirits. For books that were possible candidates for burning, see Sudhoff, *Paracelsus*, 30–1.
30. Franck, *Chronica, zeytbuch und geschychtbibel*, 253.
31. *Von der franzosischen krankheit* (1529), P I, 7, 70.

32. Stromer was no doubt suspicious of the interventions of Paracelsus on syphilis on account of his proprietary interest in Ulrich von Hutten's famous *De guaiaci medicina et morbo gallico* (1519), which praised Stromer and placed confidence in guaiacum treatment in a way that was bound to meet with the disapproval of Paracelsus. For an excellent review of the guaiacum question, Claudia Steiner, *Die Behandlung der Franzosenkrankheit in der frühen Neuzeit am Beispiel Augsburgs* (Stuttgart: Franz Steiner, 2003).
33. *Paragranum* draft, P I, 8, 41–50.
34. Sudhoff, *Versuch*, I, 6–7, No. 2.
35. Sudhoff, *Versuch*, I, 13–14, No. 10.
36. *Schlussrede*, dated 1533, Sudhoff, *Versuch*, I, 292.
37. Benzenhöfer, *Paracelsus*, 94.
38. Sudhoff, *Versuch*, I, No. 15.
39. Sudhoff, *Versuch*, I, No. 20. Joachim Telle, 'Wolfgang Talhauser'.
40. Künast, '*Getruckt zu Augspurg*', 9–11, 69–71, 107–9, 204–11, 231–48 demonstrates that, despite his aptitude to controversy, Steiner was the most prolific and impressive Augsburg publisher of his generation.
41. For the copper engraving by AH, see Frontispiece. The traditional attribution to Augustin Hirschvogel is unlikely, see Ingonda Hannesschläger, 'Echte und vermeintliche Porträts des Paracelsus', in Dopsch and Kramml, *Paracelsus in Salzburg*, 217–50, and Webster, 'A Portrait of Paracelsus'.
42. *Astronomia magna*, P I, 12, 403. He complained bitterly about his experience of humiliation owing to dependence on his patrons, which he described as being chained like a dog (*hundsketten*), *An der pest an Sterzingen*, P I, 9, 561. He employed similar terminology for the habitual humiliation of the poor by the rich, *De felici liberalitate*, P II, 2, 12.
43. *anno scilicet 1541 Salisburgae, ubi honorifice sepultus est laudabili ad posteritatem commendatus epitaphio*: Blaser, *Paracelsus in Basel*, 67.
44. Udo Benzenhöfer, 'Zum Brief des Johannes Oporinus über Paracelsus'. Johannes Weyer is usually regarded as the sole recipient of the letter, but Benzenhöfer suggests that it was produced for the benefit of a group of humanist physicians in Cologne who were in controversy with the Paracelsian Georg Phaedro (Fedro). This view is consistent with evidence from Konrad Gessner, who charted the progress of Fedro between 1562 and 1565 with alarm: Webster, 'Conrad Gessner and the Infidelity of Paracelsus', 17–18. Sudhoff firmly dates the letter to 1555, but if it is connected with the Fedro affair, then 1565 is more probable. Phaedro was also attacked as an impostor by Bodenstein: Wilhelm Kühlmann and Joachim Telle, *Der Frühparacelsismus*, especially 415, 491.
45. Bernhard Milt, 'Conrad Gesner und Paracelsus', *Schweizerische Medizinische Wochenschrift*, NS 10 (1929), 488.
46. For a convenient source for the letter, Sudhoff, *Paracelsus*, 46–9.
47. Bittel, 'Die Elsässer Zeit des Paracelsus', 178.
48. Ulrich von Hutten's strictures on drink in his *De guaiaci medicina et morbo gallico* (1519) were reflected in Sebastian Franck, *Vonn dem grewlichen laster der trunckenheit so in disen letsten zeiten erst schier mit den Frantzosen auffkomen* (Augsburg: H. Steiner, 1528 and 1531), for which see Andreas Wagner, 'Das Falsche der Religionen bei Sebastian Franck', 278–90. Reflecting the popular criticism of indulgence in drink by clergy, Schwenckfeld caricatured them as *bierprediger*, *Ermanung ahn alle bruder in Schlesien* (1524), in *Corpus Schwenckfeldianorum*, vol. 2 (Leipzig: Breitkopf & Härtel, 1911), 70. Attack on drinking habits of the clergy also commonly featured in literary sources, for instance Georg Wickram's *Das Rollwagenbüchlin* (1555), Chapter 3. Criticism of the debauchery of the clergy was a main theme of this satire, Elisabeth Endres, *Nachwort* to Johannes Bolte (ed.),

Georg Wickram. Das Rollwagenbüchlin (Stuttgart: Reclam, 1968), 192. Wickram may have known Paracelsus, since he was from Colmar. Wickram's father was a dedicatee of one of the surgical writings of Paracelsus. See also Fritz Blanke, 'Reformation und Alkoholismus', *Zwingliana*, 9 (1949), 75–89. For Petrarch's reservations about drink, see Klaus Bergdolt, *Arzt, Krankheit und Therapie bei Petrarca*, 126–7, 293–4. In his dialogue *Die Anschauenden*, Hutten took a more sanguine attitude to German drinking customs and recommended the proverb *Abends zechen, morgens ratschlagen*: Peter Ukena (ed.), *Ulrich von Hutten, Deutsche Schriften*, 146.

49. *Septem punctis*, P II, 3, 3–4.
50. Ibid., P II, 3, 6, 8–9.
51. See Frontispiece.
52. Webster, 'A Portrait of Paracelsus'.
53. Scribner, *For the Sake of Simple Folk*, 228–39; Christiane Andersson, 'Popular Imagery in German Reformation Broadsheets', 140–3.
54. Fries, *Prognostication auf 1531*, quoted from Bittel, 'Die Elsässer Zeit des Paracelsus', 168–9.
55. Kühlmann and Telle, *Der Frühparacelsismus*, 597–8 for a summary of the demonic accusations. Perhaps Erastus calculated that live attacks on Paracelsus would be helpful in his own defence against accusations of anti-Trinitarianism.
56. In the course of his indignant rejection of the accusation that he had reverted to anti-Trinitarian and heathen beliefs, Paracelsus insisted on being known as a Christian and not a heathen and as a German, not a foreigner: *Astronomia magna*, P I, 12, 9–10. Pantheism arose because of the tendency to make God coexistent with the infinite Neoplatonic universe.
57. Wilhelm Kühlmann, 'Das häretische Potential des Paracelsismus gesehen im Licht seiner Gegner', in Hartmut Langhütte and Michael Titzmann (eds), *Heterodoxie in der Frühen Neuzeit* (Tübingen: Max Niemeyer Verlag, 2006), 217–42.
58. Sudhoff, *Paracelsus*, 46. Even Paracelsus's famous *Opodeldok* cure turns out to be a minor variant of a standard medieval preparation. The seemingly bizarre rebranding by Paracelsus was nothing more than a shorthand list of main ingredients, see Michael Kuhn, *De nomine et vocabulo*, 190–1. See also Chapter II, note 55.
59. Benzenhöfer, 'Zum Brief des Johannes Oporinus', 59. These testimonies to the clinical abilities of Paracelsus echo the epitaph on his gravestone, which was included in a preface of one of his publications in 1554 and thereafter frequently reprinted, Sudhoff, *Versuch*, I, No. 33. In his biographical entry Gessner criticized Paracelsus for excessive reliance on opiates; opiates were also mentioned by Oporinus, but in a favourable light.
60. Goltz, 'Paracelsus as a Guiding Model', in Grell, *Paracelsus*, 98–9; Weeks, *Paracelsus*, 46–7.
61. For a lively introduction to scornful expressions at this date, Norbert Schindler, *Widerspenstige Leute. Studien zur Volkskultur in der frühen Neuzeit* (Frankfurt am Main: Fischer, 1992), 78–120, 329–43.
62. Pamphilus Gengenbach, *Gouchmatt*, 1520, and similarly the anonymous *Murarus Leviathan* Günter Hess, *Deutsch-lateinische Narrenzunft*; Heike Talkenberger, *Sintflut: Prophetie und Zeitgeschehen in Texten und Holzschnitten*.
63. Haas, *Der Kampf um den Heilige-Geist. Luther und die Schwärmer*, for a review of the exchanges between Luther and Karlstadt.
64. Ukena brackets Paracelsus with the humanists, especially Regiomontanus and Celtis, and also includes Hutten in this group: Ukena, *Ulrich von Hutten, Deutsche Schriften*, 343.
65. Harder, *Sources of Swiss Anabaptism*, 552–3.

66. Stafford, *Domesticating the Clergy*, 195–200; Chrisman, *Conflicting Visions of Reform*, 65–90.
67. For interventions by aristocratic patrons on behalf of unauthorized practitioners, Pelling, *Medical Conflicts in Early Modern London*, 234–45.
68. Lambert Wacker noted that such was the scale of opposition and persecution Paracelsus experienced that he intentionally concealed his writings pending the arrival of better times, Sudhoff, *Versuch*, II, 299.
69. For examples from this sequence, see Illustrations 1 and 3 from Lucas Cranach d.Ä. *Passional Christi und Antichristi* (Erfurt: Mathes Maler, 1521/22). This series was probably inspired by older sets of antitheses emanating from John Wyclif and Hussite sources. Luther, Melanchthon and Schwertfeger were all directly involved in plans for the Cranach *Passional*.
70. For a representative example of Cranach's cruel caricature of the papacy, see Illustration 3.
71. Lucas Cranach d.Ä., Eleventh Woodcut, from the Sixth Antithesis, Cranach's *Passional Christi und Antichristi* (Erfurt: Mathes Maler, 1521/22), fol. B2v. See Koepplin and Falk, *Lukas Cranach. Gemälde, Zeichnungen, Druckgraphik*, 319–31 & passim; Hildegard Schnabel (ed.), *Lucas Cranach d.Ä. Passional Christi und Antichristi* (Berlin: Union Verlag, 1972).
72. John 6: 10–14.
73. Luther, *Das Evangelium am Tage der heyligen drey Künige*, WA 10, *Erste Abteilung, 1 Hälfte*, 559–69.
74. Krautwald's *Novus Homo* was composed in 1529 but not published until 1542: Schantz, *Crautwald and Erasmus*, 133–56.
75. Vetter, *Die Predigten Taulers*, No. 66, on Matt. 6: 33, 364. For the medieval advocacy of the apostolic model, see Herbert Grundmann, *Religiöse Bewegungen im Mittelalter*, 2nd edn (Hildesheim: Georg Ohms Verlag, 1961), 503–13. For the pilgrimage ideal, see Illustration 8 and Conclusions, note 2.
76. Grebel to Müntzer, 5 September 1524, Harder, *Sources of Swiss Anabaptism*, 286.
77. Quoted from Baylor, *The Radical Reformation*, 177.
78. Schlaffer, *Ein kurzer Unterricht zum Anfang eines RechtChristlichen Lebens* (1527), in Müller, *Glaubenszeugnisse*, 87.
79. Matt. 28: 19–20; Mark 16: 15–16.
80. Mark 16: 15–20.
81. Schäufele, *Die missionarische Bewußtsein und Wirken der Täufer*, 75–9; for a different perspective on the commission, Friesen, *Erasmus, the Anabaptists, and the Great Commission*.
82. Jakob Hutter, 1535, addressing Erbmarschall Johann von Leippa, Müller, *Glaubenszeugnisse*, 163.
83. Lotzer, *Ain hailsame ermanunge* (1523), in Alfred Goetz, *Sebastian Lotzers Shriften* (Leipzig, Teubner, 1902), 27: 25–9.
84. Kurt Goldammer, 'Aus den Anfängen evangelischen Missionsdenkens. Kirche, Amt und Mission bei Paracelsus' (1943), in Goldammer, *Paracelsus in neuen Horizonten*, 9–33. Goldammer's article coincided with the first part of Wiswedel's 'Die alten Täufergemeinden und ihr missionarisches Wirken', in *Archiv für Reformationsgeschichte*, 1943. See also Hans Kasdorf, 'Anabaptists and the Great Commission in the Reformation', *Direction*, 4 (1975), 303–18; idem, 'Zur Mission der Täufer: Verständnis und Verwirklichung im Reformationsjahrhundert', in Hans Kasdorf and Friedemann Walldorf (eds), *Werdet meine Zeugen: Weltmission im Horizont von Theologie und Geschichte* (Neuhausen-Stuttgart: Hänssler, 1996), 181–200.
85. *Astronomia magna*, P I, 12, 12; Commentary on Psalm 109, P II, 5, 116. Goldammer, 'Aus den Anfängen evangelischen Missionsdenkens', 23.

86. *Prologus in vitam beatam*, Matthießen, 75, 84, Goldammer, *RSSchr*, 3, 6.
87. This important issue is further considered in Chapter V.
88. Paracelsus, *De auctoritate sanctorum*, P I, 14, 341.
89. Paracelsus, *De genealogia Christi*, P II, 3, 161.
90. Lambert Wacker noted with satisfaction that Paracelsus was 'no server of princes', Sudhoff, *Versuch*, II, 299.
91. For Paracelsus's justification for sacrifice of family ties among the apostolic elect, Sudhoff, *Versuch*, II, 247–8, 277, 289.
92. Schwenckfeld, *Vom christlichen Streit und Ritterschaft Gottes* (1533), in Laube et al., *Flugschriften vom Bauernkrieg*, vol. 2, 1110–14, 1110. See also *Ermanung ahn alle bruder in Schlesien* (1524), in *Corpus Schwenckfeldianorum*, vol. 2, 46, 52, 80–2. *Vom christlichen Streit* was conceived in the spirit of Erasmus's *Enchiridion*.
93. *Septem punctis*, P II, 3, 3–5.
94. *Vorredt uber die vier Evangelisten*, Sudhoff, *Versuch*, II, 438.
95. *De martyrio Christi*, Matthießen, 180–4, Goldammer, *RSSchr*, 50–3, Sudhoff, *Versuch*, II, 257.
96. *De genealogia Christi*, P II, 3, 132–4, 159.
97. *Astronomia magna*, P I, 12, 136.
98. *zeit und ziel*, Commentary on the Fifth Commandment, P II, 7, 153–6; Ps. 39: 4. For fuller discussion, see Chapter VII.
99. Commentary on the Fifth Commandment, P II, 7, 167–8. For discussion of other sources containing expressions of this antagonism to martyrdom and suicide, Goldammer, ' Der cholerische Kriegsmann und der melancholische Ketzer' (1958), in *Paracelsus in neuen Horizonten*, 177–88.
100. *Prologus in vitam beatam*, Matthießen, 78–9, Goldammer, *RSSchr*, 4.

Chapter II: The Power of Print

1. For source, see note 124. The year 1517. With respect to this year Lichtenberger predicted that three innovations would come to pass: (1) through Dr Luther in religious practice; (2) through Theophrastus in medicine; (3) through Albrecht Dürer in all manner of the arts.
2. Sudhoff, *Versuch*, I, 60–596.
3. Sudhoff, *Versuch*, I, 3–35.
4. Biegger, *Paracelsus und die Marienverehrung*, 24–7.
5. Sudhoff, *Versuch*, I, 3–4, discusses the fate of this broadsheet, the original of which is not listed in his bibliography and was not accessible to Sudhoff.
6. This tract was known to Gessner because it was published in Zürich, as he points out in his *Bibliotheca Universalis* (Zürich: Froschauer, 1545), 614v.
7. Blaser, *Paracelsus in Basel*, 117–21.
8. Gessner, *Bibliotheca Universalis*, 614v.
9. For the *gross/klein* distinction in surgeries and texts in competition with the surgery of Paracelsus, Habermann, *Deutsche Fachtexte der frühen Neuzeit*, 429–67.
10. For relevant sources, including estimates offered by Valentius de Retiis/Valentius Antrapassus Sileranus in about 1562, and for other relevant detail, see Kühlmann and Telle, *Der Frühparacelsismus*, 584–620.
11. Eckhard Bernstein, 'From Outsiders to Insiders: Some Reflections on the Development of a Group Identity of the German Humanists between 1450 and 1530', in James V. Mehl (ed.), *In laudem Caroli: Renaissance and Reformation Studies for Charles G. Nauert Jr.* (Kirksville, MO: Thomas Jefferson University Press, 1998), 45–64.
12. Similarly, Dirk van Ulsen was known as Theodericus Ulsenius.

13. Similarly, Georg Bauer, the physician and writer on mining, was known as Agricola; the prolific writer on popular astronomy and medicine and professorial colleague of Fuchs in Marburg, Johannes Eichmann, was known as Dryander.

14. Tannstetter originated from Rain am Lech in Bavaria. His Latin name combines *collis* with *limes*, the latter meaning '*rain*' or '*rein*', indicating some kind of boundary path often extending along the side of a hill.

15. *Chordus/cordus*, an uncommon usage in classical times, signifying a second crop, or anything in nature that was late born.

16. Ukena, *Ulrich von Hutten. Deutsche Schriften*, 288. For evidence of the long-standing adversity attached to Hinz, Kunz, etc., see Vetter, *Die Predigten Taulers*, No. 24, 101.

17. Cornarius, *Hippocratis libri omnes* (Basel: Froben & Episcopus, 1538); Fuchs, *Hippocratis ... aphorismorum* (Basel: Oporinus, 1544), aa5r. No doubt 'rabid dog' was intended to recall 'dogrose', a pun on the vernacular of the name of Cornarius.

18. Cornarius, *Vulpecula excoriata* (Frankfurt am Main, 1545); Fuchs, *Cornarius furens* (Basel, 1545). This was not the end of the exchanges, see Frederick G. Meyer, E.E. Trueblood and J.L. Heller (eds), *The Great Herbal of Leonhart Fuchs* (Stanford: Stanford University Press, 1999), 804–15. For the taste for polemic among the medical humanists, Maclean, *Logic, Signs and Nature in the Renaissance*, 18–22.

19. Benzenhöfer, *Paracelsus*, 21–3 for the various components of the name.

20. *Paragranum*, P I, 8, 55.

21. Blaser, *Paracelsus in Basel*, 21, 42, 68–9.

22. Ibid., 82–102 for full exegesis of this text.

23. There is just a possibility that the author was Cornarius himself. According to his own testimony, he arrived in Basel shortly after the death of Johann Froben the elder, therefore in October 1527 or shortly later. Hieronymus Froben permitted Cornarius to visit Italy, after which he remained in Basel until September 1529, working mainly on his Hippocrates edition. *Manes Galeni* claims that Theophrastus was not fit to carry the chamber-pot of Hippocrates. No other ancient authority is mentioned in the verses themselves. Twice and prominently, Theophrastus is accused of plagiarism; on one of those occasions he is called a crow (*cornicula*), which could imply stealing from Cornarius himself. Paracelsus opens his own reply by asking about the '*cornuten*' or tiros of his profession. At this point he insisted that none of his ideas had been stolen from others, P I, 8, 56.

24. Josef Strebel made the ingenious suggestion that the new name was adopted to escape the difficulty Italians and others experienced in the pronunciation of the three 'Hs' in Hohenheim, *Paracelsus. Sämtliche Werke* (St Gallen, Verlag Kollikofer, 1944), I, 42.

25. The 'Eight Books of Medicine' of Celsus were readily available in print, but the first edition published in Germany was not produced until 1528, and the first German vernacular translation appeared in 1531, shortly after the adoption by Theophrastus of his Paracelsus identity: Habermann, *Deutsche Fachtexte der frühen Neuzeit*, 379–428.

26. Sudhoff, *Versuch*, II, 335. See also Sebastian Franck, *Paradoxa ducenta octoginta* (Ulm, 1534). For earlier use in the medical context, Symphorien Champier, *Paradoxa in artem parvam Galeni* (1516), perhaps prompting his rival, the commercially minded Leonhard Fuchs, to adopt the title *Paradoxorum medicinae libri tres* (1535) for a new edition of a work published under a different title in 1530.

27. *De vera influentia rerum*, P I, 14, 237–47; *Sieben defensiones*, P I, 11, 126, 128, 150.

28. Weiß, *Die deutschen Mystikerinnen und ihr Gottesbild*, vol. 1, 499–507.

29. Ps. 137: 6, 'though the Lord be high, yet he hath respect for the lowly'.

30. Suggesting that the name Paracelsus had gained currency by the date of his death,

despite being attached to only a handful of mostly obscure writings, the first printed biographical notice by Konrad Gessner, *Bibliotheca Universalis*, 614v, was headed *Theophrastus Bombast ex Hohenheim ... alicubi se Paracelsum vocat.*

31. Sudhoff, *Versuch*, I, No. 1, 4–5. In his tract on comets (1531), the name became shortened to *Herren Paracelsus* (Sudhoff, *Versuch*, No. 10, 13–14). Of his two commentaries on prophetic figures, the first, on the Nuremberg Figures (1529), used the name *Theophrastus von Hohenheim*, while the later one, the Prophecy on the next Twenty-four years (1536), used the name *Herrn Doktor Paracelsus.*

32. Franck, *Chronica, zeytbuch und geschychtbibel*, 253.

33. Sudhoff, *Versuch*, I, No. 1, 4–5.

34. Sudhoff, *Versuch*, I, No. 7, 10–11. At the end of the main title is the mysterious insertion 'para.', which Sudhoff understandably suspects was meant to be expanded into Paracelsus.

35. Sudhoff, *Versuch*, I, No. 66, 104–5.

36. *Paragranum*, P I, 8, 31–50 and 51–68.

37. Ibid., P I, 8, 56–7.

38. Of course there were no sharp lines of demarcation between sectors of the book trade. For instance, humanist editors commonly produced eclectic digests and compilations largely derived from classical authorities but containing some original material. These were usually first produced in Latin but soon afterwards translated into the vernacular, as for instance the herbals produced by Brunfels and his successors. This class of publications is discussed by Habermann in her *Deutsche Fachtexte der frühen Neuzeit.*

39. Albrecht Dürer, Allegory of Philosophy, from Conrad Celtis, *Quatuor libri Amorum secundum quatuor latera Germanie* (Nuremberg: Sodalita Celtica, 1502), fol. A6v. For extensive amplification of this theme, Peter Luh, *Kaiser Maximilian gewidmet*; Jörg Robert, *Konrad Celtis und das Projekt*, and Dietter Wuttke, 'Humanismus als integrative Kraft'.

40. For a history of the book aspects of medical humanistic publishing, Maclean, *Logic, Signs and Nature in the Renaissance*, 36–67.

41. Joachim Knape, *Dichtung, Recht und Freiheit. Studien zu Leben und Werk Sebastian Brants 1457–1521* (Baden-Baden: V. Koerner, 1992). The identity of the Petrarca Meister responsible for the 261 illustrations is a matter of dispute, the favoured candidate being Hans Weiditz, the illustrator of the Brunfels herbal.

42. For fuller insight into the rich culture of medical humanism from representative perspectives, see Klaus Bergdolt, *Zwischen 'scientia' und 'studia humanitatis'. Die Versöhnung von Medizin und Humanismus um 1500* (Nordrhein-Westfälische Akademie der Wissenschaften Vorträge G.379) (Wiesbaden: Westdeutscher Verlag, 2001); Timo Joutsivuo, *Scholastic Tradition and Humanist Innovation. The Concept of Neutrum in Renaissance Medicine* (Annales Academiae Scientiarum Fennicae, Humaniora, 303, 1999); Maclean, *Logic, Signs and Nature in the Renaissance*; Overfeld, *Humanism and Scholasticism in Late Medieval Germany*; Nancy G. Siraisi, *Medieval & Early Renaissance Medicine. An Introduction to Knowledge and Practice* (Chicago: University of Chicago Press, 1990).

43. For rival efforts, Janus Cornarius, *Universae rei medicae compendiae tractata* (Basel: Johannes Froben, 1529), and Leonhart Fuchs, *Compendiaria in medendi artem introductio* (Hagenau: Johann Setzer, 1531), both of which went into further editions. For the wider context, see Maclean, *Logic, Signs and Nature in the Renaissance*, 56–7.

44. Nancy G. Sirasi, 'Oratory and Rhetoric in Renaissance Medicine', *Journal of the History of Ideas*, 85 (2004), 191–211; Sachiko Kusukawa, *Philipp Melanchthon, Orations on Philosophy and Education* (Cambridge: Cambridge University Press, 1999).

45. Peter G. Bietenholz, 'Printing and the Basle Reformation, 1517–65', in Gilmont, *The Reformation and the Book*, 235–63, 244–5.
46. Frank Hieronymus (ed.), *Griechischer Geist aus Basler Pressen. Katalog der frühen griechischen Drucke aus Basel in Text und Bild* (Basel: Bibliothek der Universität, 2003).
47. Ibid., No. 316.
48. Ibid., No. 317.
49. Ibid., Nos 319, 321. Among those assisting with important manuscripts, Cornarius thanked Adoph Occo of Augsburg.
50. See for instance the introduction to his edition of Aetius of Amida from 1533: ibid., No. 319.
51. Chrisman, *Lay Culture, Learned Culture*, 34–6.
52. Chrisman estimates that of her 77 printers in Strasbourg, only 10 originated from the city, ibid., 13.
53. C. Jäcker, *Christian Egenolff 1502–1555. Ein Frankfurter Meister des frühen Buchdrucks aus Hadamar* (Limburg: Glaukos-Verlag, 2002).
54. Künast, '*Getruckt zu Augspurg*', 71; Sudhoff, *Versuch*, I, Nos 24 and 34.
55. Chrisman, *Lay Culture, Learned Culture*, 187–8. Paracelsus indicated his debts to the manuscript *Manual* by Hans Seiff von Göppingen (*c.* 1440–1518), P I, 5, 337, 339, 524. For Seiff, see Manfred Gröber (ed.), *Das Wundärztliche Manual des Meisters Hans Seiff von Göppingen* (Göppingen: Kummerle, 1998), 416, 419 for connection with Paracelsus's *Opodeldok*.
56. For Gersdorff and Brunschwig, see Habermann, *Deutsche Fachtexte der frühen Neuzeit*, 468–74, 487–502. For Fries, Benzing, 'Bibliographie des Lorenz Fries', No. 27; Chrisman, *Lay Culture, Learned Culture*, 136.
57. Benzing, 'Bibliographie des Lorenz Fries', Nos 28–41 records one or more editions of the *Spiegel* in 1519, 1529, 1532 and 1546.
58. Ibid.
59. Josef Benzing, 'Walther H. Ryff und sein literarisches Werk. Eine Bibliographie', *Philobiblon*, 2 (1958), 126–54, 203–26; Chrisman, *Lay Culture, Learned Culture*, 179–80; Habermann, *Deutsche Fachtexte der frühen Neuzeit*, 428–87.
60. Schwitalla, *Deutsche Flugschriften 1460–1525*, 6–8 for a brief review of *Flugschriften* estimates.
61. For relevant specialized studies of *Flugschriften* in the religious sphere, Thomas Hohenberger, *Lutherische Rechtfertigungslehr*, Alejandro Zorzin, *Karlstadt als Flugschriftenautor*.
62. Volker Honemann et al. (eds), *Einblattdrucke des 15. und frühen 16. Jahrhunderts. Probleme, Perspektiven, Fallstudien* (Tübingen: Max Niemeyer, 2000) and Heike Talkenberger, *Sintflut: Prophetie und Zeitgeschehen*, 15–26 for reviews of *Flugschriften* as a mass medium.
63. Christiane Andersson, 'Popular Imagery in German Reformation Broadsheets', 121; Lorraine Dasten and Katherine Park, *Wonders and the Order of Nature 1120–1750* (New York: Zone Books, 1998), 180–9; Irene Ewinkel, *De Monstris. Deutung und Funktion von Wundergeburten auf Flügblattern im Deutschland des 16. Jahrhunderts* (Tübingen: Niemeyer, 1995); R. Po-chia Hsia, 'A Time for Monsters: Monstrous Births, Propaganda and the German Reformation', in L.L. Knoppers and J.B. Landes (eds), *Monstrous Bodies/Political Monstrosities in Early Modern Europe* (Ithaca, NY: Cornell University Press, 2004), 67–92; Jennifer Spinks, 'Wondrous Monsters: Representing Conjoined Twins in Early Sixteenth-Century German Broadsheets', *Parergon*, 22 (2005), 77–112.
64. Scribner, *For the Sake of Simple Folk*, 125–38; Andersson, 'Popular Imagery in German Reformation Broadsheets', 120–50.
65. W. Hübner, 'Astrologie in der Renaissance', in Bergdolt and Ludwig,

Zukunftsvoraussagen in der Renaissance, 253. Other authors give variant, but similar estimates for these publications. For further discussion of the Pisces conjunction, see Chapter VII.

66. Theodericus Ulsenius, *Vaticinium in epidemicam scabiem* (Nuremberg, 1496). Catrien Santing, *Geneeskunde en humanisme. Een intellectuele biografie van Theodericus Ulsenius (c.1460–1508)* (Rotterdam: Erasmus Publishing, 1992), 175–89.

67. Webster, 'Paracelsus: Medicine as Popular Protest'.

68. *Grosse Wundarznei*, P I, 10, 96.

69. The evidence of Master Simon, a surgeon, recorded in the diary of Johannes Rütiner: Meier, *Paracelsus*, 52.

70. *Liber de fundamento*, P I, 13, 307.

71. For typical examples: the proverb *Witz kein Kaufmannschatz* was employed to indicate the incompatibility between the trade mentality and true wisdom (P II, 2, 139, Wander, 4, 1230); *Die Stüle auf die Benke wöllen* warned the peasantry of the corrupting influence of false political aspiration (P II, 2, 131, Wander, 4, 937, Cornette, *Luther*, 207); the saying about training dogs with a stick rather than a sausage was invoked to defend the hard life of the apostle against the soft existence of the clergy (P II, 4, 284, Wander, 3, 1415); the familiar *Gleich und gleich gesellt sich gern* was invoked by both Paracelsus and Luther to support their ideas about sympathy and antipathy (P I, 14, 30, Cornette, *Luther*, 62, Wander, 1, 1714–15). Proverbial expressions often punctuate the argument, as for instance in his *Paragranum* (P I, 8, 66–7), when Paracelsus attacked his critics, lamenting that these grimy kitchen hands were as subversive to progress as the Devil in the lenten altar cloth or *hungertuch* (Wander 2, 921, citing Luther making a similar point); these incompetent practitioners were like tiros trying to be carpenters, while equipped only with bread knives; and, like a cat circling round its boiling broth, they were incapable of reaching the essence of their discipline (Wander, 2, 930, Cornette, *Luther*, 161). Paracelsus told them to try harder; then, like the goat, the higher they went the better the quality of their feed (Wander, 5, 576). The seriousness with which proverbs such as *Gleich und gleich*, or *Gelehrt-verkehrt*, were taken is evident from later chapters of this study.

72. For further remarks about *alterius non sit* and its sources, see Chapter IV. What has come to be known as the motto of Paracelsus was derived from Aesop. He made just one direct reference to Aesop, *Von den natürlichen dingen*, P I, 2, 95.

73. Webster, 'Paracelsus and Demons: Science as a Synthesis of Popular Belief'.

74. The basilisk is discussed further in Chapter V.

75. For a helpful review of the status of fable and proverb at this date, Barbara Bauer, 'Die Philosophie des Sprichworts bei Sebastian Franck', in Müller, *Sebastian Franck*, 181–221.

76. Hut, *Von dem geheimnus der tauf*, in Müller, *Glaubenszeugnisse*, 17–18. The gospel of creatures is further considered in Chapter VI.

77. Adapting Aesop, Eckhart cited the contest between the snake and the weasel to reinforce his conclusion of a sermon about wisdom and the power of sympathy, Steer et al., *Lectura Eckhardi I*, 100–101.

78. *De fundamento scientiarum*, P I, 13, 312–24.

79. Ibid., P I, 13, 314.

80. *Elf tractat*, P I, 1, 142.

81. Fragment on *Ens astrale*, P I, 1, 237–8.

82. *De felici liberalitate*, P II, 2, 13.

83. *De vera influentia*, P I, 14, 246. The bear in its winter posture features in Figure XI of the *Prognostikation auf 24 zukünftige jahre*, the text of which identifies this as a case of punishment for improvidence, P I, 10, 595.

84. *De inventione artium*, P I, 14, 266–72. For further discussion see Chapter VI.

For a virtuoso listing of animal lore underlining the theme of universal discord, the long Foreword and extraordinary associated double-page woodcut by the Petrarca-Meister, see Eckhard Keßler (ed.) and Rudolf Schottlaender (trans.), *Petrarca, Heilmittel gegen Glück und Unglück* (Munich: Wilhelm Fink Verlag, 1988), 151–85.

85. For the ubiquitous fascination with dogs, Keith Thomas, *Man and the Natural World* (London: Allen Lane, 1983), 100–8. The hunting dog was the animal most often invoked by Johannes Tauler: Vetter, *Die Predigten Taulers*, No. 9, 44, No. 11, 51–4, No. 60f., 312–16. The climax of Pico's Oration contained a couple of dog metaphors, comparing his critics to dogs barking at things they do not understand, Garin, *De dignitate*, 155–6. For ancient precedents, C. Joachim Classen, *Untersuchungen zu Platons Jagdbildern* (Berlin: Akademie-Verlag, 1960).

86. *De inventione artium*, P I, 14, 267. *De virtute humana*, P II, 2, 101 cites competitiveness for food among hungry dogs to indicate the human tendency to ruthless competition.

87. *Labyrinthus medicorum errantium*, P I, 11, 186.

88. *Paragranum*, P I, 8, 101.

89. *Sieben defensiones*, P I, 11, 159.

90. *De felici liberalitate*, P II, 2, 12, Matthießen, 173, Goldammer, *SSSchr*, 172. For the uncontainable greed of dogs, also *De virtute humana*, P II, 2, 101.

91. *De generatione hominis*, P I, 1, 298.

92. *De caduco matricis*, P I, 8, 365–6: *dan dieweil der arzt nichts ist als ein leithund*. Paracelsus's *leithund* is perhaps the *roten leithund*, the bloodhound, used in hunting boar and deer.

93. Commentary on Psalm 77 (78), P II, 4, 80, and Ps. 22: 24.

94. *De martyrio Christi*, Matthießen, 184.

95. *Buch der erkantnus*, *BdE*, 20–1. To Tauler, lack of inner faith was the dominance of *hündischer Mensch*; this state was compared to a smelly dog for whom the only outcome was to be dispatched, Vetter, *Die Predigten Taulers*, No. 45, 199: 8–21; No. 420: 78, 20–25.

96. Jürgen Helm, 'Die Galenrezeption in Philipp Melanchthons *De anima* (1540/1552)', *Medizinhistorisches Journal*, 31 (1996), 288–321.

97. For Paracelsus's strictures on Fries, draft Foreword to *Opus Paramirum*, P I, 13, 3.

98. *De modo pharmacandi*, P I, 4, 454.

99. *Paragranum*, P I, 8, 76–7, 144–5

100. *Prologus in vitam beatam*, Matthießen, 76, Goldammer, *RSSchr*, 3: *dann nit ein Apostel oder dergleichen bin ich, sondern ein Philosophus nach der teuschen Art*.

101. *Herbarius*, P I, 2, 3–6.

102. Vetter, *Die Predigten Taulers*, No. 37, 144: 23.

103. *Astronomia magna*, P I, 12, 10.

104. Habermann, *Deutsche Fachtexte der frühen Neuzeit*, 99, for a tabular presentation of the basic data on Latin and German editions of leading herbals, and 98–167 for fuller discussion of the structure of these herbals.

105. With respect to the ambitious *Astronomia magna*, Book 3, entitled *Die astronomie des glaubens oder des neuen Olymps*, is completely missing.

106. C.G. Jung, *Alchemical Studies* (Princeton, NJ: Princeton University Press, 1967), 120.

107. For the wider context of these polemics, Maclean, *Logic, Signs and Nature in the Renaissance*, 18–22.

108. E. Wickersheimer, 'Laurent Fries et la querelle de l'arabisme en médecine', *Les Cahiers de Tunisie, Revue de Sciences Humaines*, 2 (1955), 96–103.

109. Franck, *Chronika, zeytbuch und geschychtbibel*, 253.

110. For the context to Agrippa, Christiane Lauvergnat-Gagnière, *Lucien de Samosate et*

le Lucianisme en France au XVI siècle: Athéisme et polémique (Geneva: Droz, 1988). Suitably attached to *De incertitudine et vanitate* was Agrippa's *Encomium asini*, which artfully suggested that perhaps those designated as the lowest might with justice be regarded as the highest.

111. Barbara Könneker, 'Vom "Poeta laureatas" zum Propagandisten. Die Entwicklung Huttens als Schriftsteller in seinen Dialogen von 1518 bis 1521', in J. Lefebvre and J.-C. Margolin (eds), *L'Humanisme allemand (1480–1540)*, (Munich/Paris: Fink/Vrin, 1979), 303–19.

112. Werner Lenk (ed.), *Die Reformation im zeitgenössischen Dialog* (Berlin: Akademie-Verlag, 1968), 254. Within a year ten editions had been issued; the authorship remains a matter of dispute. Hutten is one of the candidates.

113. Paracelsus may also have known about a satirical fable by Zwingli entitled *Das Labyrint*, published in 1516, which employed animal types to symbolize current social and political evils.

114. *Spital-Buch*, P I, 7, 391, for an attack on the sects of *Scotisten, Thomisten, Albertisten, Modernis*, etc.

115. Sudhoff, *Versuch*, I, 4.

116. Sudhoff, *Versuch*, I, 6.

117. Sudhoff, *Versuch*, I, 16; *Practica Teutsch*, 1535.

118. Sudhoff, *Versuch*, I, 84; *Von ersten dreyen principiis*, 1563.

119. Sudhoff, *Versuch*, I, 170; *Archidoxae*, 1569.

120. Sudhoff, *Versuch*, II, 300.

121. *Astronomia magna: oder die gantze philosophia sagax der grossen und kleinen welt* (Frankfurt am Main, 1571), Sudhoff, *Versuch*, I, No. 131, 219–21. The Foreword to Book 4, ends *Finis Philosophiae Magnae sagacis*.

122. Sudhoff, *Versuch*, I, 218–19, 'illustrious, experienced and definitive German Philosopher and Physician'.

123. Sudhoff, *Versuch*, I, No. 131, 219–21, Dedication signed Strasbourg, 1 March 1571.

124. See quotation at the head of this chapter. R.E. Reuss (ed.), *Les Collectanées de Daniel Specklin, chronique strasbourgeoise du seizième siècle* (Strasbourg: J. Noiriel, 1890), No 2212, 487. The date of this entry cannot be ascertained, but 1589 is the latest date possible. Specklin was extrapolating from Johannes Lichtenberger's *Pronosticatio*, published originally in 1488; four of the earliest editions were published in Strasbourg; reissues were particularly frequent between 1526 and 1530; a 1527 edition included a Foreword by Luther himself. The prophecy concerning 1517 was arrived at by Lichtenberger by the common device of taking the text *tibi cherubin et seraphin incessabili, voce proclamant* and extracting the letters equivalent to roman numerals.

125. Albert Fischer, *Daniel Specklin aus Straßburg (1536–1589). Festungsbaumeister, Ingénieur und Kartograph* (Sigmaringen: Jan Thorbecke, 1996). Close links between Basel and Strasbourg are evident from the Paracelsus editions. After 1560, the leading Basel editor was Adam Bodenstein, whose pupil Michael Schütz (Toxites) performed the same service in Strasbourg.

126. Dieter Harmening, *Superstitio* for the evolution of opinion. Adolf Franz, *Die kirchlichen Benediktionen im Mittelalter* for the concessions allowed in practice.

127. For context, Hans Peter Broedel, *The Malleus Maleficarum and the Construction of Witchcraft: Theology and Popular Belief* (Manchester: Manchester University Press, 2003); Peter Segl (ed.), *Der Hexenhammer. Entstehung und Umfeld des Malleus maleficarum von 1487* (Cologne: Böhlau, 1988). The alleged authors of *Malleus maleficarum* were not named until 1519, in the Nuremberg edition published by Friedrich Peypus, who ten years later emerged as the first publisher of the writings of Paracelsus.

128. Klaus Deppermann, 'Judenhass und Judenfreundschaft im frühen Protestantismus', in Bernd Martin and Ernst Schulin (eds), *Die Juden als Minderheit in der Geschichte* (Munich: Deutscher Taschenbuchverlag, 1981), 110–30; R. Po-chia Hsia, *The Myth of Ritual Murder. Jews and Magic in Reformation Germany* (New Haven, NJ: Yale University Press, 1988); Heiko A. Oberman, *Wurzeln des Antisemitismus: Christenangst und Judenplage im Zeitalter von Humanismus und Reformation* (Berlin: Severin & Schneider, 1981); Overfeld, *Humanism and Scholasticism in Late Medieval Germany*, 247–97.
129. Concerning the vast literature on this subject area, the older work by W.-E. Peuckert, D.P. Walker and Frances Yates is reviewed by Stuart Clark, *Thinking with Demons. The Idea of Witchcraft in Early Modern Europe* (Oxford: Clarendon Press, 1997); Christoph Daxelmüller, *Zauberpraktiken. Eine Ideegeschichte der Magie* (Zürich: Artemis & Winkler, 1993); Wolf-Dieter Müller-Jahncke, 'Magie als Wissenschaft im frühen 16. Jahrhundert. Die Beziehungen zwischen Magie, Medizin und Pharmazie im Werk des Agrippa von Nettesheim' (Doctoral dissertation, Phillipps-Universität Marburg/Lahn, 1973); idem, *Astrologisch-magische Theorie und Praxis in der Heilkunde der frühen Neuzeit*; Paola Zambelli, *L'ambigua natura della magia: filosofi, streghe, riti nel Rinascimento* (Milan: Il Saggiatore, 1991).
130. Gessner to Crato, 16 August 1561, *Epistolarum medicinalium libri III*, ed. C. Wolf (Zürich, 1577), 1r–2v.
131. Robert, *Konrad Celtis und das Projekt*, 378–94.
132. D.P. Walker, *The Ancient Theology: Studies in Christian Platonism from the Fifteenth to the Eighteenth Century* (London: Duckworth, 1972), 3–10. Indicative of the low profile of the Bethlehem Magi in the writings of the Italian Neoplatonists, these magi are little mentioned in the writings of Walker and Frances Yates.
133. Stephen M. Buhler, 'Marsilio Ficino's *De stella magorum* and Renaissance Views of the Magi', *Renaissance Quarterly*, 43 (1990), 348–71. The Bethlehem Magi perhaps impressed themselves on Ficino owing to the activities of a powerful Florentine fraternity devoted to their veneration.
134. Farmer, *Syncretism in the West*, 4.
135. Hugo Kehrer, *Die heiligen drei Könige in Literatur und Kunst*, 2 vols (Leipzig: Seemann, 1908–9); Martin Hengel and Helmut Merkel, 'Die Magier aus dem Osten und die Flucht nach Ägypten im Rahmen der antiken Religions-geschichte und der Theologie des Matthäus', in Paul Hoffmann et al. (eds), *Orientierung an Jesus. Für Josef Schmitt* (Freiburg im Breisgau: Herder, 1973), 139–69; Manfred Becker-Huberti, *Die Heiligen Drei Könige. Geschichten, Legenden und Bräuche* (Cologne: Greven, 2005).
136. Richard C. Trexler, *The Journey of the Magi. Meanings in the History of a Christian Story* (Princeton: Princeton University Press, 1997).
137. Sylvia Harris, 'The *Historia trium regum* and the Mediaeval Legend of the Magi in Germany', *Medium aevum*, 28 (1959), 23–30. The Hildesheim legend was popularized in pamphlet form, for instance in a Cologne *Pilgerbuch* dating from 1520.
138. See particularly Luther, *Das Evangelium am Tage der heyligen drey Künige*, WA 10, *Erste Abteilung, 1 Hälfte*, 559–69.
139. Sudhoff, *Versuch*, II, 240. See also a fragment of the same text, Sudhoff, *Versuch*, II, 442. For magic in the later Matthew commentaries, see Miller-Guinsberg, 'Paracelsian Magic and Theology. A Case Study of the Matthew Commentaries'.
140. Sudhoff, *Versuch*, II, 391–6; quoted from Biegger, *Paracelsus und die Marienverehrung*, 189. Gause, *Paracelsus*, 169–73.
141. *Aus der philosophia super Esaiam prophetam*, P I, 12, 506–7.
142. Biegger, *Paracelsus und die Marienverehrung*, 189–91. Biegger discusses the questions

raised by the presence of this concluding section in only one of the manuscripts of this tract, accepting that it genuinely represents the views of Paracelsus.

143. *Astronomia magna*, P I, 12, 27, 83, 85, 125, 278, 370; *Erklärung der ganzen astronomie*, P I, 12, 463, 476.

144. *De vita longa*, P I, 3, 258. For the exploitation of the magus idea in later spurious works, see the opening chapter of *Aurora philosophorum*, a work excluded from the Sudhoff edition.

145. Ulinka Rublack, *Reformation Europe* (Cambridge: Cambridge University Press, 2005), 1–4. The pamphlet by Melanchthon and Luther was concerned with the Monk Calf and Papal Ass; the latter came to assume great importance in Lutheran propaganda, Andersson, 'Popular Imagery in German Reformation Broadsheets', 122–9; Scribner, *For the Sake of Simple Folk*, 127–36.

146. Biegger, *Paracelsus und die Marienverehrung*, 190; *Aus der philosophia super Esaiam prophetam*, P I, 12, 507. Dieter Wuttke, 'Sebastian Brant und Maximillian I. Eine Studie zu Brants Donnerstein-Flugblatt des Jahres 1492', in Otto Herding and Robert Stupperich (eds), *Die Humanisten in ihrer politischen und sozialen Umwelt* (Boppard: Boldt, 1976), 141–76; Andersson, 'Popular Imagery in German Reformation Broadsheets', 121–3. Similar attention was attracted by the conjoined twins born near Worms in 1495. These twins were immediately publicized in broadsheets by Brant and others: Moriz Sondheim, *Thomas Murner als Astrolog*, 96–9; Dieter Wuttke, 'Wunderdeutung und Politik. Zu den Auslegungen der sogenannten Wormser Zwillinge des Jahres 1495', in Kasper Elm et al. (eds), *Landesgeschichte und Geistesgeschichte. Festschrift für Otto Herding zum 65. Geburtstag* (Stuttgart: W. Kohlhammer Verlag, 1977), 217–44; and Spinks, 'Wondrous Monsters', 81–91.

147. *Astronomia magna*, P I, 12, 130.

148. Ibid., 136–7.

Chapter III: The Sources of Dissent

1. *Das Buch der Erkanntnus des Theophrast von Hohenheim gen. Paracelsus*, ed. Kurt Goldammer (Texte des späten Mittelalters und der frühen Neuzeit, Heft 18) (Berlin: Erich Schmidt Verlag, 1964), 43. 'My disciples are without possessions or riches, but false disciples will emerge; they will be so provided with property, women, mistresses, rents, possessions, and proceeds from benefices, from which they have no desire to turn away; so they will only preach what their clientele finds agreeable, and therefore they will not forfeit their money, staff or purse.' A similar sentiment was reflected in the Franciscan rule for itinerants: *sollen sie kein provision, zehrsack, seckel, gelt, oder stecken mit sich tragen, Der Croniken der Minderen Brüder* (Constance: 1603), Part I, Chapter 12: *Von der Regel die S. Franciscus gemacht hat*, cap. 14. Both Paracelsus and the Fransciscans were consciously echoing Matt. 10: 9–10 and Luke 9: 3, which explicitly forbade even a staff, although this concession was allowed in Mark 6: 8. For the relevance of Illustration 3 and the Cranach woodcut sequence, see note 8.

2. Sudhoff, *Paracelsus*, 48.

3. Ute Gause, *Paracelsus (1493–1541). Genese und Enfaltung seiner frühen Theologie* (Tübingen: J.C.B. Mohr (Paul Siebeck), 1993); Katharina Biegger, '*De invocatione beatae Mariae virginis*'. *Paracelsus und die Marienverehrung* (Stuttgart: Franz Steiner, Verlag, 1990).

4. *Außlegung aus der propheten weissagung*, Sudhoff, *Versuch*, II, 275.

5. *Septem punctis*, P II, 3, 55; Theophrastus gives the title of this work as *De viribus veteris testamenti*.

6. Sudhoff, *Versuch*, II, 276.

7. *De martyio Christi*, Matthießen, 185–6.
8. Lucas Cranach d.Ä., Twenty-Second Woodcut, from the Eleventh Antithesis. From Cranach's *Passional Christi und AntiChristi* (Erfurt: Mathes Maler, 1521/2), fol. C4r. The associated text, I Tim. 4: 1, warns that in 'latter times some shall depart from the faith, giving heed to seducing spirits, and doctrines of devils'. The illustration shows the pope sitting on a rich throne, dressed in his full garb, wearing his tiara and carrying a papal staff. His admiring audience consists entirely of church functionaries, which Cranach takes as indicating that there is no real place for the laity. The next papal woodcut, the Twenty-Fourth, gives prominence to the filling of clerical purses from the proceeds of indulgences.
9. Commentary on Daniel, in Matheson, *Collected Works of Müntzer*, 235.
10. *Septem punctis*, P II, 3, 3–57.
11. For a recent analysis, Walter Brunner, 'Aufrührer wider Willen'.
12. Obvious sources included Luther's *Ninety-Five Theses* (1517), *To the Christian Nobility of the German Nation*, *Babylonian Captivity*, and *Christian Freedom* (all 1520), Karlstadt's *On the Removal of Images* (1522), and Zwingli's *Sixty-Seven Articles/ Schlussreden* (1523). Also, among Luther's prolific output, it is quite possible that Theophrastus was acquainted with some of his sermons such as the one on the Epiphany (1522), since these included lengthy digressions on abuses within the church, covering most of the points included in *Septem punctis*. See Luther, *Das Evangelium am Tage der heyligen drey Künige* (1522), WA 10, *Erste Abteilung, 1 Hälfte*, 624–5, 637–9.
13. Steven Ozment, 'The Revolution of the Pamphleteers', in Antonio Rotondò (ed.), *Forme e destinazione del messaggio religioso*, 1–18, 9.
14. Hamm, 'Geistbegabte gegen Geistlöse', in Dykema and Oberman (eds), *Anticlericalism*, 379–440.
15. For further evidence in Sachs and other artisan writers on themes relevant to Paracelsus, Martin Arnold, *Handwerker als theologische Schriftsteller*, 56–105.
16. Hamm, 'Geistbegabte gegen Geistlöse', 437–40, for bibliographical details.
17. On the authority of Sudhoff, the authenticity of this letter has often been disputed, but without good reason; see Rudolph, 'Einige Gesichtspunkte zum Thema "Paracelsus und Luther"'. As the leaders of the Wittenberg movement, Luther and Melanchthon were obvious choices for correspondence, but Bugenhagen less so. Interestingly, Luther and Melanchthon head the list of fourteen theologians designated to pronounce on divine law, which was appended to the Memmingen Federal Constitution finalized in March 1525. Bugenhagen is not included, but just one manuscript of the constitution, from the monastic library of St Paul im Lavanttal, mentioned in Chapter I, contains 'pomeranus', the only name given as an addition, which is an interesting coincidence: Seebaß, *Artikelbrief, Bundesordnung und Verfassungsentwurf*, 114–15. Unabashed by any rejection among the high-ups, Paracelsus directed some of his later religious writings to Pope Clement VII.
18. Commentary on Matthew 1–5, Sudhoff, *Versuch*, II, 238–45, No. 83, Görlitz MS, fols 169–249.
19. Harder, *Sources of Swiss Anabaptism*, 282–4.
20. *Septem punctis*, P II, 3, 3. Variant lists feature on pages 29–30, 31, 37 and 48.
21. For a similar listing perhaps from the same date, *De martyrio Christi*, Matthießen, 187, Goldammer, *RSSchr*, 53, Sudhoff, *Versuch*, II, 256–7; for objections to ceremonials in the context of the mass, *Buch außlegung aus S. Paulo*, Sudhoff, *Versuch*, II, 275.
22. Cranach's text associated with Illustration 2 listed as offensive preccupations 'vestments, clothing, church plate, feastdays, benedictions, benefices, orders, monks and priests'.
23. Erasmus listed: vigils, fasts, tears, prayers, sermons, study, sighs, toil, humiliations

and a thousand other unpleasant hardships in his caricature of contemporary piety: *Moriae encomium*, CWE, 27, 115, 138, 149

24. John L. Flood, 'The Book in Reformation Germany', in Gilmont, *The Reformation and the Book*, 79; for a similar list, *De martyrio Christi*, Matthießen, 187, Goldammer, *RSSchr*, 53, Sudhoff, *Versuch*, II, 256–7.
25. Wolfgang Capito, *Was man halten und antwurten soll* (1525), quoted by Ozment, *The Reformation in the Cities*, 81.
26. Hans Sachs, *Die Wittenbergisch Nachtigall*, lines 120–50, cited from Seufert, *Die Wittenbergisch Nachtigall*, 20–21. For a further attack on chapel proliferation, Johann Eberlin von Günzburg, *Mich wundert, daß kein Geld im Land ist*, in Ludwig Enders (ed.), *Johann Eberlin von Günzburg, Ausgewählte Schriften*, 3 vols (Halle: Max Niemeyer, 1896–1902), vol. 3, 147–81, 175–8.
27. It will be observed that '*punctis*' was used in the title and '*artikel*' in the text. In contemporary usage, the two terms were interchangeable, both denoting a self-contained section, often in a connected series, such as a legal, theological or academic argument. '*Thesis*' possessed a similar connotation.
28. *Septem punctis*, Introduction, P II, 3, XXVII. For a recent discussion of the tension between four and seven symbolism in early Christian sources, J.A. Whitlark and M.C. Parsons, ' "The Seven Last Words": A Numerical Motivation for the Insertion of Luke 23.34a', *New Testament Studies*, 52 (2006), 188–204.
29. Jörg Haugk von Jüchsen, *Christliche Ordnung*, 1526, in Laube et al. (eds), *Flugschriften vom Bauernkrieg*, vol. 1, 667–86.
30. *De secretis secretorum theologiae*, P II, 3, 204.
31. Isa. 11: 2–3. Vetter, *Die Predigten Taulers*, No. 26, 106–10; Jörg Haugk von Jüchsen, *Christliche Ordnung*, 1626, in Laube et al. (eds), *Flugschriften vom Bauernkrieg*, vol. 1, 667–8.
32. *Septem punctis*, P II, 3, 41 mentions the holy virtues, but, following biblical rather than patristic precedent, he listed them as six.
33. Ibid., P II, 3, 57.
34. Beissel, *Geschichte der Verehrung Marias*, 404–13, 524–5; Barbara Rommé, *Henrick Douwerman und die niederrheinische Bildschnitzkunst an der Wende zur Neuzeit* (Bielefeld: Verlag für Regionalgeschichte, 1997), which is largely concerned with the patronage and design of shrines to the Virgin Mary revolving around the theme of the seven sorrows.
35. Schleitheim was one of various sets of articles discussed among Anabaptists at this date, many of them being seven in number. For detail, see Robert Friedmann, 'The Nicolsburg Articles'. In the secular context, in April 1523 the Gräubunden peasantry expressed their aspirations in their 'Sieben Artikel des Grauen Bundes', while in April 1525 the citizens and peasantry in the Bamberg area also expressed their grievances in seven articles.
36. Schwitalla, *Deutsche Flugschriften 1460–1525*.
37. Sylvia Weigelt, *Otto Brunfels. Seine Wirksamkeit in der frühbürgerlichen Revolution unter besonderer Berücksichtigung seiner Flugschrift 'Vom pfaffenzehnten'* (Stuttgart: Verlag Hans-Dieter Heinz, 1986).
38. Franz, *Quellen zur Geschichte des Bauernkrieges*, 295–309.
39. Melchior Spach, a witness to the will of Paracelsus in 1541, was an important dignatory in Hallein. Spach was briefly a leading figure in the local regional peasant movement and author of one of the statements of grievance. It is possible that his link with Paracelsus might have originated in 1525: Heinz Dopsch, 'Paracelsus in Salzburg – Das Ende eines Mythos?', in Dopsch and Kramml, *Paracelsus und Salzburg*, 181–2; Sallaberger, *Kardinal Matthäus Lang*, 339, 372.
40. Harder, *Sources of Swiss Anabaptism*, 284–92. For full context, Goertz, 'A Common Future Conversation'.

41. Text contained in Vögeli, *Jörg Vögeli*, vol. 1, 478–519. For relevant background information, vol. 3, 973–91. For a full discussion of Vögeli, Berndt Hamm, 'Laienthologie zwischen Luther und Zwingli', in Nolte, Tompert and Windhorst, *Kontinuität und Umbruch*, 222–332. The *Schirmred* is briefly outlined in Ozment, *The Reformation in the Cities*, 79–82.
42. Zell's *Christliche Verantwortung*, probably published in the summer of 1523, is an extended form of his reply to these articles. This book was referred to by Brunfels as Zell's 'Artikelbuch': Stafford, *Domesticating the Clergy*, 7–46, 237–41. Just before the Zell episode, also in Strasbourg, Tilman von Lyn produced a short manifesto comprising six articles criticizing current church practices and calling for specific reforms, Marc Lienhard and Jean Rott, 'Die Anfänge der evangelischen Predigt in Strassburg', in de Kroon and Krüger (eds), *Bucer und seine Zeit*, 54–73. For the social context to the writings of Brunfels and Zell, Lienhard, 'La Percée du mouvement évangélique à Strasbourg'; Looß, 'Reformatorische Ideologie und Praxis'.
43. Gottfried Seebaß, *Das reformatorische Werk des Andreas Osiander*, 114.
44. The spread of information about Idelhuser's case is suggested by the reference to him in Marschalck, *Spiegel der Blinden*, in Laube, et al. (eds), *Flugschriften der frühen Reformationsbewegung*, vol. 1, 201.
45. Sallaberger, *Kardinal Matthäus Lang*, 326–9.
46. Tauler, on Matt. 6: 33, Vetter, *Die Predigten Taulers*, No. 66, 359–60.
47. Luther, *Disputatio pro declaratione virtutis indulgentiarium/ Die 95 Ablass-Thesen* (1517), theses 27 and 28, WA 1, 233–8.
48. Luther, *Von weltlicher Oberkeit* (1523), WA 11, 265.
49. Karlstadt, *Von Anbetung und Ehrerbietung der Zeichen des Neuen Testaments* (1521), cited from Furcha, *The Essential Carlstadt*, 49.
50. Karlstadt, *Von Gelübden Unterrichtung* (1521), cited from Furcha, *The Essential Carlstadt*, 85.
51. Karlstadt, *Von Abtuhung der Bilder* (1522), cited from Furcha, *The Essential Carlstadt*, 126.
52. Hutten, *Klag und Vormahnung* (1520), in Ukena, *Ulrich von Hutten, Deutsche Schriften*, 206–7.
53. Sachs, *Die Wittenbergisch Nachtigall*, in Seufert, *Die Wittenbergisch Nachtigall*, 22–5. For a similar line of argument against the church locally and with special condemnation of Rome, Johann Eberlin von Günzburg, 'Mich wundert, daß kein Geld im Land ist', in Enders (ed.), *Johann Eberlin von Günzburg*, vol. 3, 147–81, 175–8.
54. Commentary on Matthew 1–5, Sudhoff, *Versuch*, II, 240–1. For Luther's use of *höllküchlein*, Cornette, *Proverbs in Luther*, 155, *hölle* indicating both hell and oven.
55. At this date one gulden was worth 480 heller.
56. *De caduco matrices*, P I, 8, 322–3.
57. *Septem punctis*, P II, 3, 39; *De caduco matrices*, P I, 8, 322–3. Elsewhere alms to the poor were described as chaff and bran, enabling the wealth of the church to be used for idolatrous purposes: *De felici liberalitate*, P II, 2, 12.
58. For example, *gottsgaben fresser, bettelfresser* (devourers of gifts to God and the proceeds of begging), as well as hypocrites, profiteers, etc.: *Septem punctis*, P II, 3, 38–9.
59. *De caduco matrices*, P I, 8, 322–3.
60. *Septem punctis*, P II, 3, 8–9.
61. *De martyrio Christi*, Matthießen, 182–3.
62. *Buch der Erkanntnis*, BdE, 52–3.
63. Thomas N. Tentler, *Sin and Confession on the Eve of the Reformation*.
64. Erasmus, *Enchiridion*, CWE, 66, 13.
65. Erasmus, *Moriae encomium*, CWE, 27, 138.

66. Zwingli and Grebel, reply to the Bishop of Constance, 22–23 August 1522: Harder, *Sources of Swiss Anabaptism*, 182–3, 636–7.
67. Stafford, *Domesticating the Clergy*, 28–31.
68. Commentary on Matthew 1–5, Chapter 2, Sudhoff, *Versuch*, II, 241–2. 1 Cor. 13: 3. The three virtues occupied a prominent place in the conclusions of his *Prologus in vitam beatam*, Matthießen, 85–6, Goldammer, *RSSchr*, 6–7.
69. *De confessione, poenitentia et remissione peccatorum*, P II, 2, 379–404; *Liber de poenitentiis*, P II, 2, 405–19.
70. *Septem punctis*, P II, 3, 6, 8–18, 33, 42, 54.
71. *De martyrio Christi*, Matthießen, 188–9, Goldammer, *RSSchr*, 53, Sudhoff, *Versuch*, II, 257.
72. *Septem punctis*, P II, 3, 11–14.
73. For further development of his attack on pride (*hoffart*), portrayed as the most unforgivable of the sins and as the antithesis to humility (*demut*), see *De virtute humana*, P II, 2, 95–107. This tenet was treated as an article (*puncten*) (p. 96).
74. *Liber de poenitentis*, P II, 2, 414–15; *Liber de iustitia*, P II, 2, 155–6.
75. *Liber de iustitia*, P II, 2, 153–63.
76. *Septem punctis*, P II, 3, 4.
77. Ibid., P II, 3, 4–6.
78. *Liber de iustitia*, P II, 2, 159–60, 163; Biegger, *Paracelsus und die Marienverehrung*, 43. Paracelsus made frequent reference to 2 Cor. 3: 6, in which Paul calls on the ministers of the new covenant not to follow the letter (*buchstabens*) but the spirit (*geistes*), for the letter kills, but the spirit gives life. This verse had long exercised influence and Paracelsus must have appreciated its importance among the mystics, spiritualists and radicals. For further relevant discussion, see Chapter VI.
79. For the extended application of this critique, see Chapters IV and VI.
80. For representative attacks on Aristotle and the scholastics: by Erasmus, *Moriae encomium* (CWE, 27, 126–30), and his favour for Plato and Pythagoras against Aristotle, *Enchiridion* (CWE, 66, 69); and by Kettenbach, *Ein Gespräch*, in Laube et al. (eds), *Flugschriften der frühen Reformationsbewegung*, vol. 1, 202, Aristotle was called '*Narrenstultilem*' and '*Archistultilis*' by Kettenbach.
81. For a representative denunciation by Luther of the influence of Aristotle's natural philosophy in the universities, *Das Evangelium am Tage der heyligen drey Künige* (1522), WA 10, *Erste Abteilung, 1 Hälfte*, 567–70.
82. For instance, 'Judas Nazarei' in his *Von alten und nüen Gott* (1521) expresses the common concern that Aristotelianism in the universities was standing in the way of the correct teaching of the gospel. This view and its sources are discussed by Hofacker, '*Von alten und nüen Gott*', in Nolte, Tompert and Windhorst, *Kontinuität und Umbruch*, 148–9, 157.
83. *Septem punctis*, P II, 3, 52. For further elaboration on dress, clerical headgear and jewellery, *De virtute humana*, P II, 2, 97–8, underlining the incompatibility of these things with the teaching of Christ.
84. Commentary on Matthew 1–5, Chapter 4, Sudhoff, *Versuch*, II, 243. Erasmus shared this distaste for the extravagant dress of the upper echelons of the church, *Moriae encomium*, CWE, 27, 137–8. Illustration 4, at the lower left, makes satirical reference to the cardinal's hat and its tassels.
85. Könneker, *Wesen und Wandlung der Narrenidee*.
86. *Prologus in vitam beatam*, Matthießen, 83, Goldammer, *RSSchr*, 6.
87. For this important theme, Pauline Moffett Watts, *Nicolaus Cusanus. A Fifteenth-Century Vision of Man* (Leiden: Brill, 1982), 120–52; Könneker, *Wesen und Wandlung der Narrenidee*; Michael Screech, *Erasmus and the Praise of Folly* (London: Duckworth, 1980). Imagery of the fool was prevalent among reformers; for instance Luther repeatedly called both clerics and their clerical allies fools for attempting to

force the people into beliefs that were contrary to the Word of God, *Von Weltlicher Oberkeit*, WA 11, 245–81, 261–71.

88. *De desperatis morbis*, P I, 9, 356–9, Matt. 18: 3. Erasmus concluded his *Moriae encomium* with an advocacy of the worth of children, simpletons, etc., but in his characteristic satirical overtones, CWE, 27, 148–9.

89. *Astronomia magna*, P I, 12, 49–51; *De generatione stultorum*, P I, 14, 73–94. Cranefield and Federn, 'The Begetting of Fools', 56–74, 161–74.

90. For instance the husbandry analogy was elaborated at length in *Prologus in vitam beatam*, Matthießen, 69–80, Goldammer, *RSSchr*, 1–5, roughly based on Matt. 13: 36–40.

91. *Septem punctis*, P II, 3, 8, Matt. 13: 38.

92. Ibid., P II, 3, 8–9.

93. Ibid., P II, 3, 10.

94. For a recent relevant discussion of the Rheinland mystics, Alain de Libera, *Eckhart, Suso, Tauler, ou la divinisation de l'homme*. For further relevant sources, see Chapter VI.

95. Goertz, *Innere und äussere Ordnung*; Ozment, *Homo spiritualis*; Packull, *Mysticism and the Early South German-Austrian Anabaptist Movement*.

96. Hutten, *Klag und Vormahnung* (1520), in Ukena, *Ulrich von Hutten, Deutsche Schriften*, 235 (lines 1300–13).

97. Hutten, *Klag und Vormahnung* (1520), ibid. (lines 264–5, 997–8).

98. Carlos Gilly, 'Das Sprichwort "Die gelehrten die verkehrten" oder der Verrat der Intellektuellen im Zeitalter der Glaubensspaltung', in Rotondò (ed.), *Forme e destinazione del messaggio religioso*, 229–375.

99. Luther, *Von weltlicher Oberkeit* (1523), WA 11, 265.

100. Müntzer, *Hochverursachliche Schutzrede* (1524) in Franz, *Thomas Müntzer. Schriften und Briefe*, 322–43, 329: *den armen ackerman, handtwerckman und alles da lebet, schinden und schaben.*

101. Karlstadt, *Ob man gemach faren und des ergernüssen der schwachen verschonen soll* (1524), in Hertzsch, *Karlstadts Schriften*, vol. 1, 73–97.

102. Grebel to Müntzer, 5 September 1524, in Harder, *Sources of Swiss Anabaptism*, 284–92. Harder translates this expression as 'false forbearance', while Williams prefers 'false caution', both of which are acceptable.

103. Commentary on Psalm 139 (140), P II, 7, 25–38.

104. Hutten, *Klag und Vormahnung* (1520), in Ukena, *Ulrich von Hutten, Deutsche Schriften*, 227 (lines 1519–30).

105. *De caduco matricis*, P I, 8, 322–4.

Chapter IV: Call of the New

1. *De coena domini*, Sudhoff, *Versuch*, II, 281 (paraphrase). 'In the form of the old body inherited from Adam we cannot proceed to righteous works. The new body must transcend the old; then we will belong to God's own household, and in place of the old body will emerge a noble essence.' For the connection between fruitfulness, *anthera* and glorification, *De resurrectione*, Matthießen, 304–11.

2. 2 Cor. 5: 17, *Darum, ist jemand in Christo, so ist er eine neue Kreatur. Das Alte ist vergangen; siehe, es ist alles neu worden.*

3. *De virtute humana*, P II, 2, 98.

4. Lucas Cranach d.J., Additional Woodcut Title-Page, *Biblia Deudsch* (Wittenberg: Hans Lufft, 1544/45), not specifically relating to the prophetic books, but rather based on the woodcut and many variant paintings by Lucas Cranach d.Ä. on the theme 'Gesetz und Evangelium', dating from the 1529 onwards, and in turn

derived from one of the same artist's versions of the crucifixtion. The *Biblia Deudsch* version starkly sets out the choice between old and new, the left-hand side representing catastrophes stemming from the fall of Adam, the right the salvation offered through the sacrifice. Literature: Koepplin and Falk, *Lukas Cranach*, 505–9; 399–407; Friedrich Ohly, *Gesetz und Evangelium. Zur Typologie bei Luther und Lucas Cranach. Zum Blutstrahl der Gnade in der Kunst* (Münster: Aschendorff, 1985); Frank Büttner, ' "Argumentatio" in Bildern der Reformationszeit. Ein Beitrag zur Bestimmung argumentativer Strukturen in der Bildkunst', *Zeitschrift für Kunstgeschichte*, 57 (1994), 23–44.

5. Oration, Section 36; Garin, *De hominis dignitate*, 146.
6. Strauss, *Law, Resistance, and the State*, 3–30.
7. Ibid., 3.
8. Erasmus, *Moriae encomium*, CWE, 27, 107, 121–2.
9. Hutten, *Praedones*, in Eduard Böcking (ed.), *Hutten Opera*, 5 vols (Leipzig: Teubner, 1859–62), vol. 4, 363–406, for lawyers, 378–86.
10. Gerhard Rill, *Fürst und Hof in Österreich. Band 2: Gabriel von Salamanca, Zentralverwaltung und Finanzen* (Vienna etc: Böhlau, 2002), 161–207, 235–8.
11. Strauss, *Law, Resistance, and the State*, 10–13, 39, 50.
12. *De religione perpetua*, Sudhoff, *Versuch*, II, 248–9.
13. *Paragranum*, P I, 8, 151.
14. *Auslegung über die zehen gebott gottes*, P II, 7, 153–68.
15. Ibid., P II, 7, 197–202.
16. For typical examples of exploration of the vices of medical practitioners portrayed in popular dramas from Sterzing, see Werner M. Brauer (ed.), *Sterzinger Spiele. Die weltlichen Spiele des Sterzinger Spielarchivs*, vol. 6 (Vienna: Österreichischer Bundesverlag, 1982), 89–190. For the literary context, Andrea Carlino, 'Petrarch and the Early Modern Critics of Medicine', *Journal of Medieval and Early Modern Studies*, 35 (2005), 559–82.
17. Barbara Könneker, *Sebastian Brant. Das Narrenschiff* (Munich: R. Oldenbourg Verlag, 2002); Michael Rupp, *'Narrenschiff' und 'Stultifera navis'. Deutsche und lateinische Moralsatire von Sebastian Brant und Jakob Locher in Basel 1494–1498* (Münster, etc.: Waxmann, 2002), 144–209 for medical aspects, discussing Chapters 48 and 76.
18. Hutten, *Die Anschauenden* (1520), in Ukena, *Ulrich von Hutten. Deutsche Schriften*, 146.
19. Haug Marschalck, *Spiegel der Blinden* (1522), in Laube, et al. (eds), *Flugschriften der frühen Reformationsbewegung*, vol. 1, 133.
20. Paracelsus remarked that patients placed their faith in doctors regardless of their competence. Thus the professionals prospered and kept their kitchens well stocked, but this was a case of faith without works, or dead faith, *Paragranum*, P I, 8, 145.
21. *De morbis caducis*, P I, 8, 319–26; see also 333, 358–68.
22. *Paragranum*, P I, 8, 49.
23. Ibid., P I, 8, 55, 136. Paracelsus's *kothauer* (*kothhauer*) was probably alluding to Daniel 3: 29, where, after the ordeal of fire of Sadrach, Mesach and Abed-Nego, the houses of the idolaters were reduced into dunghills (Luther has *misthaufen*). For the three escapees, see also Haugk, *Christliche Ordnung*, in Laube, et al. (eds), *Flugschriften vom Bauernkrieg*, vol. 2, 677.
24. *Bertheonea*, P I, 6, 39–169; *Bertheonea* fragments, 169–206.
25. *Bertheonea*, P I, 6, 41–57.
26. As a result of the protection of God and the wonderful self-healing powers of the human body, recovery often took place. Indeed the peasantry was deceived into thinking that doctors were in possession of great skills, but in fact all their actions stemmed entirely from foolishness, *Paragranum*, P I, 8, 151–2.

27. Fragment on turpentine, P II, 2, 190. These abusive epithets were no doubt in common use, as suggested by *kelberarzt* in Johannes Weier, *De praestigiis*, 1575, vol. 1, 408. The links suggested by Paracelsus (*Grosse Wundarznei, III*, P I, 10, 433) between the story of Lazarus, his Hemmerlin character and the *Fastnachtsspiel* perhaps suggest his familiarity with the Zürich Lazarus play dating from 1529, which also features a heartless doctor: Josef Schmidt (ed.), *Das Zürcher Spiel vom reichen Mann und vom armen Lazarus* (Stuttgart: Reclam, 1969), 7–38, especially 22–3. For fuller discussion, Stephen L.Wailes, *The Rich Man and Lazarus on the Reformation Stage* (Selinsgrove: Susquelanna University Press, 1997), 66–92.

28. *Grosse Wundarznei, III*, P I, 10, 478–9. To his readers, the nickname Starwadel, like compounds involving *schwanz*, would possess obvious bawdy connotations.

29. *De modo pharmacandi*, P I, 4, 454.

30. *Schwirbelgeist*, also called at this point *idolum, magorina*: *Bertheona* fragments, P I, 6, 200; more commonly *fliegenden geister*: *Von der gebärung der empfindliche dinge*, P I, 1, 245 (*umbfliegenden geistern*); *De generatione hominis*, P I, 1, 245; *De modo pharmacandi*, P I, 4, 444; *De desperatis morbis*, P I, 9, 335–6 (*fliegende phantasei ... geist*); *Labyrinthus medicorum errantium*, P I, 11, 172; *Astronomia magna*, P I, 12, 65 (*fliegents*); *De vera influentia rerum*, P I, 14, 214; *Prologus in vitam beatam*, Matthießen, 80, Goldammer, *RSSchr*, 1, 4.

31. *De apostematibus*, P I, 6, 198.

32. Paracelsus called practitioners who failed to engage with nature *baretlisleute* or *hütlisman*. He advised that the red beret should be taken as a badge of ignorance, indicating that the doctor was on a level with the wandering mountebank, *Bertheonea*, P I, 6, 52, 54, 55, 57; *Bertheonea* fragments, P I, 6, 177, 198. Just as much as the mitre and tiara, the beret was taken as an expression of the sin of pride, *De virtute humana*, P II, 2, 98. For further discussion of the red beret and the distaste for ostentatious dress in the context of the AH portrait reproduced as our Frontispiece Illustration, Webster, 'A Portrait of Paracelsus'.

33. *Paragranum*, P I, 8, 152–4, 159–60.

34. *Elf tractat*, P I, 1, 150–2. Erasmus likewise complained that medicine as it was currently practised was just 'one aspect of flattery', *Moriae encomium*, CWE, 27, 107.

35. *Sieben defensiones*, P I, 11, 142–3.

36. Elsewhere Paracelsus uses *gugelnarr*, while Nikolaus Manuel prefers *gugelgans*. *Gugel* refers to the cowl and habit of a monk, or cap and habit of a fool.

37. *Paragranum*, P I, 8, 150.

38. *Sieben defensiones*, P I, 11, 136. Jonah, 3: 5–10.

39. *Paragranum*, P I, 8, 152–4, 159–60.

40. *Bertheonea* fragments, P I, 6, 177–8.

41. *Septem punctis*, P II, 3, 4. See Chapter VI for further discussion.

42. *Von den natürlichen dingen*, P I, 2, 95–6.

43. *De podagricis*, P I, 1, 311–12.

44. *Paragranum*, P I, 8, 151.

45. *Bertheonea*, P I, 6, 55; *Bertheonea* fragments, P I, 6, 170; *Paragranum* draft, P I, 8, 49.

46. *Bertheonea*, P I, 6, 53; *Bertheonea* fragment, P I, 6, 175.

47. *Bertheonea* fragment, P I, 6, 200.

48. *De mineralibus*, P I, 3, 42; *Astronomia magna*, P I, 12, 28–9.

49. *De felici liberalitate*, P II, 2, 6. For an example, drawn from the Sterling archive, of a doctor assiduously protecting the interests of his rich patron at the cost of the life of a sick pauper, see *Der reiche Mann und Lazarus*, in Walter Lipphardt and Hans-Gert Roloff (eds), *Die geistlichen Spiele des Sterzinger Spielarchivs*, vol. 5 (Bern: Peter Lang, 1980), 237–68, especially lines 450–71.

50. *De causis morborum invisibilium*, P I, 9, 251–2.
51. *Labyrinthus medicorum errantium*, P I, 11, 160–220.
52. For the positive case about direct links with these figures, Pagel, *Paracelsus*, 218–23, 284–9, 295–302; for greater reservation, Goldammer, *Paracelsus in neuen Horizonten*, 288–320.
53. Typical of respected authorities: Kilbansky et al. conclude that without Ficino and Agrippa 'the thought of Paracelsus could never have emerged', *Saturn and Melancholy* (London: Nelson, 1964), 267; Pagel describes Ficino and Agrippa as 'fixed points in the literary sources through which neo-Platonic and magical tradition came to Paracelsus', 'Paracelsus and the Neoplatonic and Gnostic Tradition', 158; and more recently a similar conclusion was reached by Carol V. Kaske and John R. Clarke, *Three Books on Life* (Binghamton, NY: Center for Medieval and Early Reaissance Studies, 1989), Introduction, 54–5.
54. Pagel, 'Paracelsus and Techellus the Jew'; Pagel and Winder, 'Gnostisches bei Paracelsus und Konrad von Megenberg'. *Das Buch der Natur* dates from about 1350; it is loosely based on the *Liber de natura rerum* of Thomas of Cantimpré, which dates from a century earlier; Dagmar Gottschall, *Konrad von Megenbergs Buch von den natürlichen Dingen: Ein Dokument deutschsprachiger Albertus Magnus-Rezeption im 14. Jahrhundert* (Studien und Texte zur Geistesgeschichte des Mittelalters, 83), (Leiden: Brill, 2004). Gottschall points out that Konrad is a possible source for Paracelsus's reports on raining frogs, fish and other alien objects, 368–9.
55. For a recent survey, Peter Binkley (ed.), *Pre-Modern Encyclopaedic Texts* (Leiden: Brill, 1997).
56. Gottschall, *Konrad von Megenbergs Buch von den natürlichen Dingen*, 244–52; Walter Blank, 'Mikro- und Makrokosmos bei Konrad von Megenberg', in Klaus Grabmüller et al. (eds), *Geistliche Denkformen in der Literatur des Mittelalters* (Munich: W. Fink Verlag, 1984), 83–100.
57. For reference to Aristotelian and Galenic ideas, see for example *Von der gebärung der empfindliche dinge*, P I, 1, 276–83; *De generatione hominis*, P I, 1, 303–5.
58. *Paragranum*, P I, 8, 148.
59. *Sieben defensiones*, P I, 11, 128–9.
60. *De modo pharmacandi*, P I, 4, 451–4.
61. *De genealogia Christi*, P II, 3, 73–4.
62. *Labyrinthus medicorum errantium*, P I, 11, 203.
63. *Bertheonea*, P I, 6, 47, 172.
64. Ibid., P I, 6, 47, 178.
65. *Spital-Buch*, P I, 7, 412; *Zwei bücher von der pestilenz*, P I, 8, 371. For two longer lists, which between them add three further names, Ugo Benzi, Bartolomeo da Montagnana and Michele Savonarola, see P I, 6, 459; P I, 8, 321.
66. Symphorien Champier, *Paradoxa in artem parvam Galeni* (Lyons, 1516).
67. For instance, *Paragranum*, P I, 8, 148–50. The alchemical works attributed to Lull were from many different hands and were produced after the lifetime of the supposed author, Michela Pereira, *The Alchemical Corpus attributed to Raymond Lull* (Warburg Institute Surveys and Texts, 18) (London: The Warburg Institute, 1989).
68. Suggestive parallels with Johannes de Rupescissa are found in the early *Neun Bücher Archidoxis* and *De gradibus*, raising the possibility that Theophrastus was drawing on a relevant manuscript source: Udo Benzenhöfer, *Johannes' de Rupescissa 'Liber de consideratione quintae essentiae omnium rerum'* (Stuttgart: Franz Steiner, 1989), 75. More likely Theophrastus used some other printed intermediate source containing similar ideas, such as the Lullian *De secretis natura, seu de quinta essentia* (1514 etc). Pagel, Keil and others tend to assume the influence of *Das Buch der Heiligen Dreifaltigkeit*, the first German alchemical work, relevant to Paracelsus for its synthesis of alchemy, mysticism and apocalyptic symbolism. However, despite

the existence of numerous copies of the manuscript, there is no real evidence that it was known to Paracelsus or employed in his work: Pagel, *Paracelsus*, 212, 269, Barbara Obrist, *Les Débuts de l'imagerie alchimique (XIVe – Xve siècles)* (Paris: Le Sycomore, 1982), 126–40, 261–75. For Keil, see Chapter V, note 38.

69. *Paragranum*, P I, 8, 148, 190.

70. *Volumen paramirum*, P I, 1, 166–72.

71. For a sympathetic interpretation of Hippocrates on *virtus*, *Opus Paramirum*, P I, 9, 227–8.

72. *Astronomia magna*, P I, 12, 148, 190; *Zwei bücher von der pestilenz*, P I, 8, 372; *Labyrinthus medicorum errantium*, P I, 11, 208; *Sieben defensiones*, P I, 11, 125–6, 159–60.

73. The patriarchs feature at the bottom, to the immediate left of the central tree. Their modern academic dress emphasizes that they are the analogues of the Wittenberg reformers. Moses bears the scriptural tablets that look more book-like than in other presentations, suggesting their analogy to the New Testament. Immediately to the side of the patriarchs are the two figures representing death and the Devil, the latter prominently sporting a cardinal's hat and showing its cords, all indicating that the Roman church decisively belongs on the side of the discredited *ancien régime*.

74. *Erklärung der ganzen astronomie*, P I, 12, 148, 190.

75. *De vera influentia rerum*, P I, 14, 214.

76. *Sieben defensiones*, P I, 11, 131–6.

77. *Septem punctis*, P II, 3, 5–6.

78. Stayer, *Anabaptists and the Sword*, 128–9, representing the views of the Swiss Brethren and Michael Sattler.

79. For more extended discussion of the links of Paracelsus with the radical movement and relevant secondary sources, see Chapter VI.

80. *De coena domini*, Sudhoff, *Versuch*, II, 315, 318. For a similar sentiment, see quotation at the head of this chapter.

81. Hamm, 'Laienthologie zwischen Luther und Zwingli', 236.

82. *Septem punctis*, P II, 3, 6.

83. Commentary on Matthew 1–5, Sudhoff, *Versuch*, II, 239.

84. Utz Rychsner, *Eine schöne Unterweisung daß wir in Christo alle Brüder und Schwester sind* (Augsburg: H. Steiner, 1524), in Laube, et al. (eds), *Flugschriften der frühen Reformationsbewegung*, vol. 1, 422–39, at 427.

85. Johannes Spörl, 'Das Alte und das Neue im Mittelalter', *Historisches Jahrbuch*, 50 (1930), 297–341, 498–542.

86. Judas Nazarei, *Vom alten und nüen Gott, Glauben und Ler* (Basel, 1521), discussed by Hofacker, '*Vom alten und nüen Gott, Glauben und Ler*', in Nolte, Tompert and Windhorst, *Kontinuität und Umbruch*, 145–77. Judas Nazarei's old/new distinction was taken up by Heinrich von Kettenbach, *Ein gespräch mit einem frommen altmütterlein* (1522), and by Urbanus Rhegius, *Novae doctrinae ad veterem collatio* (1526). The latter was translated by William Turner, the English botanist, as *A Comparison betwene the Olde Learnynge & the Newe* (London, 1537).

87. Hofacker, '*Vom alten und nüen Gott, Glauben und Ler*', in Nolte, Tompert and Windhorst, *Kontinuität und Umbruch*, 145–77, 150.

88. *Von allen offenen schäden*, P I, 6, 210; *Spital-Buch*, P I, 7, 391; *Sieben defensiones*, P I, 11, 135.

89. *Herbarius*, P I, 2, 33–4.

90. *Septem punctis*, P II, 7.

91. *De causis morborum invisibilium*, P I, 9, 260–4; *De peste libri tres*, P I, 9, 602–3; *Astronomia magna*, P I, 12, 15–18, 31–51.

92. Franck included heathen luminaries in this pantheon and therefore sided more with the *prisca sapientia* tradition than was acceptable to Paracelsus.

93. *Astronomia magna*, P I, 12, 306–20; *De virtute humana*, P II, 2, 98; *De genealogia Christi*, P II, 3, 71–3, 132–3; *De limbo aeterno I*, Sudhoff, *Versuch*, II, 273–4; *Prologus in vitam beatam*, Matthießen, 80–1, Goldammer, *RSSchr*, 5.
94. Commentary on Psalm 91 (92), P II, 4, 246.
95. Commentary on Psalm 146 (147), P II, 7, 90–3.
96. The tented encampment in the upper left relates to Numbers 21: 9, where Moses quietens his mutinous followers by erecting a brazen serpent on a pole, which duly cures their diseases.
97. Commentary on Psalm 91 (92), P II, 4, 244–5; *Sieben defensiones*, P I, 11, 123–31.
98. *Astronomia magna*, P I, 12, 25–31, 273, Cor. 5: 8 for *sauerteig*, Matt. 10: 14, etc. for dust (*staub, kleit*).
99. *De generatione stultorum*, fragment, P I, 14, 94.
100. *Labyrinthus medicorum errantium*, P I, 11, 172–3.
101. John 3: 8, a rendition shared with Eckhart and Luther. Paracelsus adds, in an abbreviated form, the relevant expression *frei und niemands eigen sey*, free and nobody's servant. This was used in legal testimonies of the time and is also found in articles of grievance against abuses connected with serfdom. It also connects with the quotation attached to the famous AH portrait, *alterius non sit qui suus esse potest*, let nobody belong to another who can belong to himself. For full discussion of the sources of this quotation, but without making the connection with this passage from the *Labyrinthus*, Robert-Henri Blaser, 'Die Quelle des paracelsischen "Alterius non sit"', in Blaser, *Paracelsus in Basel*, 9–19. For a representative German rendition, *Keines anderen Knecht sei, wer seine eigener Herr sein kann*, see Benzenhöfer, *Paracelsus*, 106. It is quite likely that the direct source for Paracelsus was Heinrich Steinhöwel/ Sebastian Brant, *Esopi appologi sive mythologi* (Basel, 1501), 69–70. Paracelsus also cited *der Geist geistet* ... to attack the dogmatism of the Aristotelians. Their attitude, he maintained, was contrary to the instinct of the human spirit to explore all alternatives, *Liber meteororum*, P I, 13, 156. For employment of *der Geist geistet* ... in an apocalyptic context, *Astronomia magna*, P I, 12, 137. It is generally assumed that the AH portrait and associated motto were produced in connection with the projected publication of the *Labyrinthus* and related writings. But it is also possible that there was a link with the contemporaneous *Astronomia magna*. It is worth noting that the latter contains the aphorism *ein ietlicher tut das sein, also ich auch das mein*, which is cognate with *alterius non sit* ..., P I, 12, 403. For further amplification concerning this proverb, *De felici liberalitate*, P II, 2, 6.
102. 2 Cor. 5: 17, Col. 3: 9, etc. See quotation at head of this chapter and related notes.
103. Matt. 7: 6. In his *Herbarius*, Paracelsus attacked the medical humoralists for failing to exploit the magnalia of nature and for turning *sophia* into sophistry. As a consequence, they had crushed the pearls of nature out of existence and failed to impede the course of diseases. The pearls of nature could not be thrown to such humoralist pigs, P I, 2, 25. Similarly in *Von den natürlichen dingen*, physicians were censured for allowing the sick to suffer rather than admitting their own ignorance of the pearls of nature, P I, 2, 137. In *Astronomia magna* he used the example of the sow to warn humans against reversion to animal nature and neglect of the gospel message, P I, 10, 305–6, 318. In *De nymphis* he used the pearls quotation to support his call for attention to the spirit world, P I, 14, 117.
104. Matt. 7: 7, 8; Luke 11: 9, echoing Jer. 29: 13. This quotation was repeated three times in this short section of the *Labyrinthus medicorum errantium*, and it was cited elsewhere at important points in the argument, for instance *De causis morborum invisibilium*, P I, 9, 255, and regularly in other tracts, for instance *Astronomia magna*, P I, 12, 24, 29–30, 279, 303–5, 380, 400; *Prologus in vitam beatam*, Matthießen, 80,

Goldammer, *RSSchr*, 4. In *De natura rerum*, the injunctions to ask, seek and knock were elevated into three high principles that constituted the whole basis for the magical and kabbalistic arts, P I, 11, 394; see also *De inventione artium*, P I, 14, 265, 269, 272, 273, 274–5.

105. Rom. 7: 6, 2 Cor. 3: 6. For reference to these passages in the early religious writings of Paracelsus, see Chapter III.

106. 1 Cor. 2: 1, 6–7.

107. Eccles. 1: 7, 16–17.

108. Matt. 7:9–11, James 1: 17.

109. For two convenient surveys, Howard Clark Kee, 'Magic and Messiah', and Susan R. Garrett, 'Light on a Dark Subject ... Magic and Magicians in the New Testament', in Jacob Neusner, Ernest S. Frerichs and Paul V. MC. Flescher (eds), *Religion, Science and Magic. In Concert and In Conflict* (New York, etc: Oxford University Press, 1987), 121–41, 142–65.

110. See for instance 2 Cor. 12: 12.

111. *Von den miraceln und zeichen des brotts und weins Christi*, Sudhoff, *Versuch*, II, 290–1.

112. *Prologus in vitam beatam*, Matthießen, 78, Goldammer, *RSSchr*, 4, *darumb geistet der [heiligen] geist nit in vilen.*

113. Gen. 3: 19. *Liber meteororum*, P I, 13, 155.

114. *De virtute humana*, P II, 2, 98.

115. Matt. 25: 1–13. *De decem virginibus*, P II, 2, 121–5.

116. *De generatione hominum*, P I, 1, 298–301; *De causis morborum invisibilium*, P I, 9, 255–6; *Speculum, sive lumen naturale*, Sudhoff, *Versuch*, II, 546–7.

117. A particularly impressive example is the broadsheet on the theme of God's lamentation for his vineyard (*c.* 1532), with woodcuts by Erhard Schön and long verses by Hans Sachs. Scribner, *For the Sake of Simple Folk*, 190–3; Roland Belgrave et al, *Prints as Propaganda. The German Reformation* (London: History of Art Dept. UCL, 1999), 86–7, 98–9.

118. For the fruitful and barren tree, Matt. 7: 17, 12: 33; for the barren tree, Isa. 56: 3, 57: 5. *BdE*, 22–3, 26; *Labyrinthus medicorum errantium*, P I, 11, 190–5.

119. *Prologus in vitam beatam*, Matthießen, 81–2, Goldammer, *RSSchr*, 5.

120. Commentary on Psalm 91 (92), P II, 4, 249–51.

121. For fruitfulness in the eschatological context, see also Commentary on Daniel, P II, 7, 355.

122. Commentary on Psalm 147 (148), P II, 7, 293.

123. *Astronomia magna*, P I, 12, 319. McGinn, *The Mystical Thought of Meister Eckhart*, 71–113.

124. Paul Wyser, 'Taulers Terminologie von Seelengrund', in Ruh, *Altdeutsche und altniederländische Mystik*, 324–52, esp. 349–50.

125. Commentary on Psalm 103 (104), P II, 5, 1–18.

126. *De vera influentia rerum*, P I, 14, 215; *Labyrinthus medicorum errantium*, P I, 11, 169–73. Commentary on Psalm 103 (104), P II, 5, 1–6.

127. *Astronomia magna*, P I, 12, 316–17.

Chapter V: Matter and Magic

1. *De genealogia Christi*, P II, 3, 65. 'Nature is similar to the Trinity in its symmetry and mode of action ... all proceeds according to the order and monarchy of the godhead, in the same way that the image of man proceeds from God.'

2. Gen. 1: 28; Ps. 8: 6.

3. *Paragranum*, P I, 8, 45–50.

4. Ibid., P I, 8, 56–7, 137–9.
5. Garin, *De hominis dignitate*, 146, Section 35, *novam afferre velle philosophiam*. At the opening of Section 36 Pico announced a specific new philosophy employing numbers, conceding that it originated among ancient theologians, especially Pythagoras. Paracelsus accepted similar debts to the most ancient past.
6. Woodcut, verso of title-page, Heinrich Seuse, *Horologium eterne sapientie* (Cologne: Cornelius von Zieriksee, 1503).
7. For fuller discussion, Pagel, *Das medizinische Weltbild des Paracelsus. Seine Zusammenhänge mit Neuplatonismus und Gnosis*; idem, 'The Prime Matter of Paracelsus'; Pagel with Winder, 'The Higher Elements and Prime Matter in Renaissance Naturalism and in Paracelsus'. For a recent and challenging reinterpretation, Daniel, 'Invisible Wombs'.
8. The late-medieval defence of the Neoplatonist position relied heavily on Proclus's *Elements of Theology*, P.O. Kristeller, 'Proclus as a Reader of Plato and Plotinus', in J. Pépin and H.D. Saffrey (eds), *Proclus: Lecteur et interprète des anciens* (Paris: CNRS, 1987), 191–211; Alain de Libera, *La Mystique Rhénane*, 25–33.
9. See especially Pagel, *Paracelsus*, 104–17 and passim; idem, *Das medizinische Weltbild des Paracelsus*; Pagel with Winder, 'The Higher Elements and Prime Matter'.
10. For a recent discussion of the tension between four and seven symbolism in early Christian sources, J.A. Whitlark and M.C. Parsons, ' "The Seven Last Words": A Numerical Motivation for the Insertion of Luke 23.34a', *New Testament Studies*, 52 (2006), 188–204. Illustration 2 provides a reminder of the varied applications of four symbolism.
11. *Liber meteororum*, P I, 13, 134. Paracelsus may well also have been thinking of the difference between white lead and the quartz-like ore from which it derived.
12. *Philosophia de generationibus et fructibus quatuor elementorum*, P I, 13, 15. Here it is specifically stated that the Creator opted for four rather than eight iliastri and elements. Pagel highlights the use of eight symbolism by Paracelsus, particularly with respect to the eightness of Adam, but the sources for this idea lie mainly outside the genuine writings: Pagel and Winder, 'The Eightness of Adam and Related "Gnostic" Ideas in the Paracelsian Corpus'; Pagel, 'Das Rätsel der "Acht Muetter" im Paracelsischen Corpus'. More relevant to Paracelsus was the kabbalistic trinitarian bias, indicated, for instance, by the importance attached to the association of the three 'mother' letters and the three elements, fire, air and water.
13. *Liber de sancta trinitate*, P II, 3, 239. Further examples of the unity–trinity nexus, *Liber meteororum*, P I, 13, 134–9; *Prognostikation*, P I, 10, 581.
14. Aegidius Sadeler, engraved title-page to Oswald Croll, *Basilica chymica* (Frankfurt am Main: Claudius Marnius & Heredes Joahnnis Aubrii, 1609). For discussion, Owen Hannaway, *The Chemists and the Word. The Didactic Origins of Chemistry* (Baltimore, MD: Johns Hopkins University Press, 1975), Wilhelm Kühlmann and Joachim Telle (eds and trans.), *Oswald Croll, De signaturis internis rerum* (Stuttgart: Franz Steiner, 1996).
15. The tripartite approach to theory has been located in medieval alchemy, see Wilhelm Ganzenmüller, 'Das Buch der heiligen Dreifaltigkeit', *Archiv für Kulturgeschichte*, 29 (1939), 93–146. Although authorities such as Keil and Pagel assume that this source influenced Paracelsus, the evidence is not convincing. As a presentation, this type of alchemical work was unlikely to appeal to Paracelsus. See below, note 38.
16. *Paragranum*, P I, 8, 145. In his final plan for this book, with the inclusion of medicine, the three pillars became four (see also *Grosse Wundarznei, II*, P I, 10, 322).
17. *De vita longa*, P I, 3, 262; *Elf tractat*, P I, 1, 3–4.
18. *Liber meteororum*, P I, 13, 134.

19. Ibid., P I, 13, 136.
20. Ibid., P I, 13, 142.
21. Hartmut Rudolph, 'Kosmosspekulation und Trinitätslehre'.
22. *De genealogia Christi*, P II, 3, 63–7.
23. Ibid., P II, 3, 66–7.
24. Ibid., P II, 3, 65–6. Gen. 1: 26. The same image was developed at greater length in *Astronomia magna*, although here the special importance of humans was emphasized on account of their possession of the quintessence. Humans were described as being like the work of a goldsmith. P I, 12, 36–43.
25. *Liber meteororum*, P I, 13, 134–6. For a full discussion of these terms and the wider terminology of Paracelsus, see Michael Kuhn, *De nomine et vocabulo*.
26. *Opus paramirum*, P I, 9, 46–7.
27. See Chapter IV, note 23.
28. *Opus paramirum*, P I, 9, 41–3. For the mystic background, Gnädinger, *Johannes Tauler*, 250–1.
29. Ibid., P I, 9, 90.
30. *Labyrinthus errantium medicorum*, P I, 11, 180. *Opus paramirum*, P I, 9, 51 lists *resina, gummi, botin, axungia, pinguedo, butyrum, oleum, vinum ardens* as synonyms for suphur.
31. For instance, *De vita longa* ascribes the balsamic property to sulphur, P I, 3, 262. The same is implied in *Von den natürlichen dingen*, on account of linking balsam with *harz* and *resin*, P I, 2, 61.
32. *Von den ersten dreien essentiis*, P I, 3, 3.
33. *Von des bades Pfäfers*, P I, 1, 142
34. *Von den natürlichen dingen*, P I, 2, 99.
35. *De mineralibus*, P I, 2, 43.
36. *Opus paramirum*, P I, 9, 46–7, 92.
37. *Grosse Wundarznei, III*, P I, 10, 478–9.
38. *Herbarius*, P I, 2, 26–30. The following section concurs with Kuhn, *De nomine et vocabulo*, 114–15, while rejecting the view of Keil and others that the tripartite theory of matter derived from the St Gallen period and was dependent on Paracelsus's acquaintance with the *Buch der heilige Dreifaltigkeit* at that date. See Keil in Volker Zimmermann (ed.), *Paracelsus* (Stuttgart: Franz Steiner, 1995), 33–6.
39. *De podagricis*, P I, 1, 311–44.
40. *Volumen paramirum*, P I, 1, 185–6, 198–9.
41. *Elf tractat*, P I, 1, 66–7, 148–9.
42. *Von den natürlichen dingen*, P I, 2, 98–9: *alles das do ist, das selbig ist in die drei stük gesetzt und weder in mer noch in minder.* 'Every single thing that exists is constituted from three parts, and not more or less.'
43. *Von den natürlichen dingen*, P I, 2, 126–38.
44. Pagel, *Paracelsus*, 152–65.
45. *Von der bergsucht*, P I, 9, 467–8, which Rosner ascribes to an early date. For further discussion, Pagel, *Paracelsus*, 153–61.
46. *De podagricis*, P I, 1, 334–8.
47. Fragment on colours, P I, 13, 259–60.
48. Fragment on winds, P I, 13, 259.
49. Rudolf Allers, 'Microcosmus: From Anaximandros to Paracelsus', *Traditio*, 2 (1944), 319–407, schematically comprehensive but deeply disappointing with respect to Paracelsus; G.P. Conger, *Theories of Macrocosms and Microcosms in the History of Philosophy* (New York: Columbia University Press, 1922); Adolf Meyer, *Wesen und Geschichte der Theorie vom Mikro- und Makrokosmos* (Berner Studien, 25), (Bern: Sturzenegger, 1900).

50. Rom. 15: 7. For a summary of Ficino's analogy between macrocosm and microcosm, with a survey of its influence, Panofsky, *Studies in Iconology*, 129–69.
51. Gen. 1: 27.
52. *Paragranum*, P I, 9, 94. Gen. 2: 7, '*Deus hominem de limo terrae*.' In an early work of Paracelsus, limbus is also used as approximately equivalent to *materia prima*. The term was in use to denote the foreground of hell. Ingenuity has been expended to connect Paracelsus with this usage. But the term also denoted the zodiac, which would seem to relate better to the macrocosm–microcosm aspect of limbus in both the senses applied by Paracelsus. Kurt Goldammer, 'Bemerkungen zur Struktur des Kosmos und der Materie bei Paracelsus' (1971), *Paracelsus in neuen Horizonten*, 263–87, especially 282–3, note 34; Daniel, 'Paracelsus' Declaratio on the Lord's Supper. A Summary with Remarks on the Term Limbus'; Rudolph, 'Hohenheim's Anthropology in the Light of his Writings on the Eucharist', 193–7.
53. *Paragranum*, P I, 9, 95–6.
54. McGinn, *The Mystical Thought of Meister Eckhart*, 71–113.
55. *De mineralibus*, P I, 3, 39–40.
56. Ibid., P I, 3, 42–3.
57. *De felici liberalitate*, P II, 2, 8.
58. *De mineralibus*, P I, 3, 49–51. Paracelsus was the first western author to give prominence to these 'new' metals and their compounds, and the first to provide tolerably clear descriptions of their properties.
59. *Paragranum*, P I, 9, 96–7.
60. *De mineralibus*, P I, 3, 50.
61. *Von der bergsucht*, P I, 9, 476. For a full discussion of mutual enmity in the animal kingdom, with two magnificent woodcut illustrations by the Petrarca Meister, see Eckhard Keßler (ed.) and Rudolf Schottlaender (trans. and comment.), *Petrarca, Heilmittel gegen Glück und Unglück* (Munich: Wilhelm Fink Verlag, 1988), 152–85, 254–6.
62. *Paragranum*, P I, 9, 89–90.
63. Ibid., P I, 9, 101–13.
64. Ibid., P I, 9, 113–17.
65. For a summary of late-medieval humoral theory, Maclean, *Logic, Signs and Nature*, 241–2; Siraisi, *Medieval & Early Renaissance Medicine*, 104–9.
66. Fragment from *Paramirum*, P I, 9, 236; in similar terms, *Von den ersten dreien essentiis*, P I, 3, 6; *De morbis ex tartaro*, P I, 5, 16; *Paragranum*, P I, 8, 87–9. For Pagel's summary of the homoeopathic argument, *Paracelsus*, 146–8.
67. Giovanni Pico della Mirandola, *Oratio* (generally called Oration On the Dignity of Man), Section 38; Garin, *De hominis dignitate*, 152. For the same idea in Pico's *Apologia*, *Opera* (Basel, 1572), 121. Perhaps the form of these texts most accessible to Paracelsus was the 1504 Strasbourg edition.
68. *De occulta philosophia*, I, 37. V. Perrone Campagni (ed.), *Cornelius Agrippa De occulta philosophia libri tres* (Leiden: Brill, 1992), 154. Agrippa's Book I was not published until 1531 and the entire work in 1533.
69. For Jean Gerson's use of alchemical imagery, suggesting that the *unio mystica* is furthered by separating out and purifying the part of the spirit that has the greatest similitude with God, Ozment, *Homo spiritualis*, 73–9, and for parallel ideas in Tauler, idem, 40–6. Illustration 2 provides a reminder of the finest German expression of the *Amores* theme. It is even possible that the wreath in this illustration, at its top right and left, contains reference to the legendary sympathy between the vine and the elm. This also features in Pico's *Oratio*, Section 38, a few lines after the citation in note 67. The classical precedents for this amity between vine and elm are numerous.
70. Dionysius, *Divine Names*, 4: 20–21.

71. *Von der bergsucht*, P I, 9, 476–7.
72. Ibid., P I, 9, 477–8.
73. Ibid., P I, 9, 481.
74. *Opus paramirum*, P I, 9, 227, with respect to the falling sickness in women.
75. *Sieben defensiones*, P I, 11, 136–41.
76. Ibid., P I, 11, 138: *alle ding sind gift und nichts on gift; alein die dosis macht das ein ding kein gift ist.*
77. W.B. Deichmann, D. Henschler, B. Holmstedt and G. Keil, 'Review of "What is there that is not Poison?" A Study of the *Third Defense* by Paracelsus', *Archives of Toxicology*, 58 (1986), 207–13, includes the relevant texts and helpful information, reaching positive conclusions on the dose–response question.
78. *Von den natürlichen dingen*, P I, 2, 137–9.
79. *Herbarius*, P I, 2, 49–57, 137–9; *Von den natürlichen dingen*, P I, 2, 122–3, which fails to execute the expected revision.
80. Bianchi, *Signatura rerum*, 31–86.
81. Pagel, *Paracelsus*, 55–6, 101.
82. *Von dem fleisch und mumia*, P I, 13, 343–9.
83. *Von der corporum und spirituum*, P I, 13, 350–1.
84. *Von den natürlichen dingen*, P I, 2, 61–72. Just as the inner mumia was the best cure for wounds, the highest of all medicines was the balsam mumiae, which was capable of curing the plague, *Zwei bücher von der pestilenz*, P I, 8, 393.
85. *Paragranum*, P I, 9, 92–3; *De morbis somnii*, P I, 9, 359.
86. *De causis morborum invisibilis*, P I, 9, 249–68. For further discussion, Heinz Schott, 'Invisible Diseases – Imagination and Magnetism: Paracelsus and the Consequences', in Grell (ed.), *Paracelsus*, 309–22.
87. *De generatione hominis*, P I, 1, 295; *Zwei bücher von der pestilenz*, P I, 8, 391–3.
88. *Zwei bücher von der pestilenz*, P I, 8, 383–4; *De peste libri tres*, P I, 9, 573–4. For just a few of the representative uses of basilisk imagery in the social and theological context, *De virtute humana*, P II, 2, 100–1; Commentary on Psalm 90 (91), P II, 4, 237–41; Commentary on Daniel, P II, 7, 326.
89. *De causis morborum invisibilis*, P I, 9, 295, 301, where the poisonous nature of the glance of the basilisk is ascribed to the strength of its imagination.
90. *Von der bergsucht*, P I, 9, 476.
91. *De podagricis*, P I, 1, 327.
92. For representative statements on the Book of Nature from *Sieben defensiones* and *Labyrinthus medicorum errantium*, P I, 11, 145–6, 164, 175–8.
93. Goldammer, 'Der Beitrag des Paracelsus zur neuen wissenschaftlichen Methodologie und zur Erkenntnislehre' (1966), in *Paracelsus in neuen Horizonten*, 229–49; idem, *Der Göttliche Magier und die Magierin Natur*, 53–6; Ernst Robert Curtius, *Europäische Literatur und lateinisches Mittelalter* (Bern: A. Franke AG Verlag, 1948), 321–7; Pagel, *Paracelsus*, 356–7.
94. Representative of relevant recent literature, Werner Beierwaltes, 'Die Metaphysik des Lichtes in der Philosophie Plotins', *Zeitschrift für philosophische Forschung*, 15 (1961), 334–62; Kurt Goldammer, 'Lichtsymbolik in philosophischer Weltanschauung, Mystik und Theosophie vom 15. zum 17. Jahrhundert', *Studium Generale*, 13 (1960), 670–82; Klaus Hedwig, *Sphaera Lucis* (Münster: Aschendorff, 1980); Hans H. Malmede, *Die Lichtsymbolik im Neuen Testament* (Wiesbaden: Harrassowitz, 1986). For sources more specifically relating to the medieval German mystics, see Chapter VI, note 183.
95. Pagel, *Das medizinische Weltbild*, 120–6.
96. *Practica in scientiam divinationis*, P I, 12, 488.
97. *Liber de sancta trinitate*, P II, 3, 261–4.
98. *De podagricis*, P I, 1, 319.

99. *Prognostikation auf 24 jahre*, P I, 10, 582. Paracelsus intentionally selected 32 figures as the basis for his apocalyptic predictions, which coincided with the 32 paths of Kabbalistic wisdom, a number based on the 10 *sefirot* and 22 elemental letters of the Hebrew alphabet: Reuchlin, *On the Art of the Kabballah*, 255–61.

100. *De generatione hominis*, P I, 1, 9, 298–303.

101. *De podagricis*, P I, 1, 338–9.

102. Ibid., P I, 1, 317.

103. *De morbis somnii*, P I, 9, 259–62. I Pet. 3: 18, '*Christus … ist getötet nach dem Fleisch, aber lebendig gemacht nach dem geist.*'

104. *De nymphis*, P I, 14, 115–17.

105. *Von der bergsucht*, P I, 9, 492.

106. Kurt Goldammer, 'Magie bei Paracelsus', *Studia Liebnitiana*, 7 (1978), 30–51; idem, *Göttliche Magier und die Magierin Natur*, 27–51; Pagel, *Paracelsus*, 62–5; Will-Erich Peuckert, 'Paracelsische Zauberei', *Nova Acta Paracelsica*, 8 (1957), 71–93; Heinrich Schipperges, 'Magia et Scientia bei Paracelsus', *Sudhoffs Archiv*, 60 (1976), 76–92.

107. Pre-empting the critics, at the opening of the section on magic in his Oration, Pico pleaded that he was solely concerned with the form of magic that represented the true perfection of natural philosophy, whereas he completely eschewed the demonic aspect of magic that he conceded was aborrent and monstrous: Garin, *De hominis dignitate*, 152.

108. Clark, *Thinking with Demons*, 214–32; Daxelmüller, *Zauberpraktiken*, 218–47.

109. Clark, *Thinking with Demons*, 215–50.

110. Garin, *De hominis dignitate*, 152–60.

111. Ibid., 154–60; J.H. Lupton (ed.), *Ioannes Coletus super opera dionysii* (London: Bell and Daldy, 1869), 109–11. For recent commentary, Stephen A. Farmer, *Syncretism in the West*; Brian P. Copenhaver, 'The Secret of Pico's Oration: Cabala and Renaissance Philosophy', in Peter A. French, Howard K. Wettstein and Bruce Silver (eds), *Renaissance and Early Modern Philosophy* (Midwest Studies in Philosophy, 26), (Boston: Blackwell, 2002), 56–81; idem, 'Number, Shape, and Meaning in Pico's Christian Cabala: The Upright Tsade, the Closed Mem, and the Gaping Jaws of Azazel', in Anthony Grafton and Nancy Siraisi (eds), *Natural Particulars: Nature and Disciplines in Renaissance Europe* (Cambridge, MA: MIT Press, 1999), 25–76; Moshe Idel, 'The Magical and Neoplatonic Interpretations of the Kabbalah in the Renaissance', in Bernard Dov Cooperman (ed.), *Jewish Thought in the Sixteenth Century* (Cambridge, MA: Harvard University Press, 1983), 186–242.

112. John Donne, *Essays in Divinity*, ed. E.M. Simpson (Oxford: Clarendon Press, 1952), 48.

113. Chaim Wirszubski, *Pico della Mirandola's Encounter with Jewish Mysticism* (Jerusalem: The Israel Academy of Sciences and Humanities, 1989), 194–200.

114. Ibid., 196.

115. Johann Reuchlin, *On the Art of the Kabbalah*, trans. and ed. Martin and Sarah Goodman (Lincoln, NE: University of Nebraska Press, 1993), 117–25.

116. For an insight into the perceived danger represented by these itinerant practitioners, Jeffrey Hamburger, 'Bosch's "Conjuror": An Attack on Magic and Sacramental Heresy', *Simiolus: Netherlands Quarterly for the History of Art*, 14 (1984), 4–23.

117. *Herbarius*, P I, 2, 59.

118. Representative of the more recent literature, Baxandall, *Limewood Sculptors of Renaissance Germany*, 50–93; Peter Blickle et al. (eds), *Macht und Ohnmacht der Bilder. Reformatorischer Bildersturm im Kontext der europäischen Geschichte* (Munich: R. Oldenbourg, 2002); C.M.N. Eire, *War against Idols. The Reformation of Worship from Erasmus to Calvin* (Cambridge: Cambridge University Press, 1986); Robert

Scribner (ed.), *Bilder und Bildersturm im Spätmittelalter und in der frühen Neuzeit* (Wiesbaden, Harrassowitz, 1990); Klaus Schreiner (ed.), *Laienfrömmigkeit im späten Mittelalter* (Munich: R. Oldenbourg, 1992); Margarete Stirm, *Die Bilderfrage in der Reformation* (Gütersloh: Gütersloher Verlagshaus Gerd Mohn, 1977); Webster, 'Paracelsus Confronts the Saints: Miracles, Healing and the Secularization of Magic', *Social History of Medicine*, 8 (1995), 403–21.

119. Baxandall, *Limewood Sculptors of Renaissance Germany*, 252–4. The exhibition, Manfred Mohr, *Der heilige Wolfgang in Geschichte, Kunst und Kult. Ausstellungs des Landes Oberösterreich* (Linz: Amt der Oberösterreichen Landesregierung, Kulturabteilung, 1976) indicates the importance of the Wolfgang cult in generating demand for locally manufactured amulets, talismans and other lucrative healing objects.

120. Johann Eberlin von Günzburg, 'Mich wundert, dass kein Geld im Land ist', in Ludwig Enders (ed.), *Johann Eberlin von Günzburg, Ausgewählte Schriften*, 3 vols (Halle: Max Niemeyer, 1896–1902), vol. 3, 147–81, 175–8.

121. Karlstadt, *Von Abtuung der Bilder* (1522), in Laube, et al. (eds), *Flugschriften der frühen Reformationsbewegung*, vol. 1, 107–8, 115–19; Kettenbach, *Ein Gespräch mit einen frommen Altmütterlein* (1522), in Laube, et al. (eds), *Flugschriften der frühen Reformationsbewegung*, vol. 1, 202–5; Sebastian Lotzer, *Eine heilsame Ermahnung* (1523), ibid., 256; Ludwig Hätzer, *Ein Urteil Gottes* (1523), ibid., 279–80; Utz Rychsner, *Eine schöne Unterweisung* (1524), ibid., 427–9. Most of the relevant *Flugschriften* critics include Einsiedeln among their specific targets of criticism; Kettenbach also mentions St Wolfgang (205). For fabrications, Erasmus and Franck, see Baxandall, *Limewood Sculptors of Renaissance Germany*, 55–60.

122. Craig Harbison, 'Dürer and the Reformation Problem of the Re-dating of the St Philip Engraving', *The Art Bulletin*, 58 (1976), 368–73.

123. J.J. de Manlius, P. Melanchthon and S. Sulcer (eds), *Locorum communium collectanea* (1562), cited from O. Clemen, 'Zur Lebensgeschichte Heinrich Stromers von Auerbach', *Neues Archiv für Sächsische Geschichte und Altertumskunde*, 24 (1903), 107–8.

124. *De felici liberalitate*, P II, 2, 15. *De imaginibus* goes even further in acknowledging the wonder-working powers of images, P I, 13, 361–86.

125. *Von der messe*, Sudhoff, *Versuch*, II, 290.

126. Fragment from *De causis morborum invisibilis*, P I, 9, 361–2.

127. *Von den natürlichen dingen*, P I, 2, 138; *Paragranum* draft, P I, 8, 47.

128. *Zwei bücher von der pestilenz*, P I, 8, 385–6.

129. For a survey of Paracelsus on the falling sickness, Temkin, *The Falling Sickness*, 169–77, but without specific comment on the *Elf tractat*.

130. Temkin, *The Falling Sickness*, 138–44.

131. *Elf tractat*, P I, 1, 143–8.

132. *Zwei bücher von der pestilenz*, P I, 8, 378–80.

133. *De peste libri tres*, P I, 9, 567.

134. *Zwei bücher von der pestilenz*, P I, 8, 378–80.

135. Ibid., P I, 8, 382–5.

136. Ibid., P I, 8, 391–3.

137. For Paracelsus, Kämmerer, *Das Leib–Seele–Geist Problem*; for the late medieval and Renaissance perspective on this important subject, M. Fattori and M.L. Bianchi (eds), *Spiritus. IV Colloquio internazionale* (Rome: Edizioni dell-Ateneo, 1984); C. Vasoli, 'La ratio nella filosofia di Marsilio Ficino', in M. Fattori and M.L. Bianchi (eds), *Ratio. VII Colloquio internazionale* (Florence: Olscki, 1994), 219–37; Katherine Park, 'The Organic Soul', in Charles B. Schmitt et al. (eds), *Cambridge History of Renaissance Philosophy*, 464–84; D.P. Walker, 'The Astral Body in Renaissance

Medicine', *Journal of the Warburg and Courtauld Institutes*, 21 (1958), 119–33; idem, *Spiritual and Demonic Magic from Ficino to Campanella* (London: Warburg Institute, 1958), 38–48 and passim (Ficino); idem, *The Ancient Theology* (London: Duckworth, 1972), 110–22 (Servetus).

138. *De generatione hominis*, P I, 1, 305–6, citing in Latin, but not coinciding with the Vulgate, John 10: 16, *ich habe noch andere Schafe, die sind nicht aus diesem Stalle ... sie werden meine Stimme hören, und wird eine Herde und ein Hirte werden. Von dem underscheit der corporum und spirituum*, P I, 13, 350–1. In the latter text Paracelsus named the spirits of fire *salamander*, of air *sylvani*, of water *nymphae*, and earth *sylphes, pygmaei, schrötlin, büzlin*, and *bergmannlein*. In *De nymphis* he used similar names and also alternatives, for fire *vulcani*, air *sylvestres*, water *undina*, and earth *bergleuten*, P I, 14, 124. For further discussion, Webster, 'Paracelsus and Demons: Science as a Synthesis of Popular Belief', 15 for further variant terminology on spirit beings.

139. *Von dem schlaf und wachen der leiber und geister*, P I, 13, 352–3. For Enoch and the Enochdienses, P I, 2, 281, 286, 289; 13, 358, 383; 14, 185, 192, 552, 581, 637. This corner of Gnostic influence is not much considered by Pagel, but for relevant context, see Ithamar Gruenwald, *Apocalyptic and Merkavah Mysticism* (Leiden: Brill, 1980).

140. *De mineralibus*, P I, 3, 44. Job 37: 14–16, Ps. 72: 18, Ps. 86: 10, Ps. 119: 19, 27, Ps. 145: 5.

Chapter VI: Radical Reform

1. *Septem punctis*, P II, 3, 51. 'The way to salvation requires tranquillity; shrillness is to no avail; [salvation] must flow from the innermost recesses of the heart to the outside and not by cleaving to outer things.'

2. The old cemetery associated with the new church building of St Sebastian in Salzburg was traditionally reserved for the poor.

3. *De secretis secretorum theologiae*, P II, 3, 167–231.

4. Commentary on Matthew 24, in *De secretis secretorum theologiae*, P II, 3, 212–31, 230.

5. Joannes Baptista Montanus, *In nonum librum Rhasis ad Regem Almansorem lectiones* (Basel: Petrus Perna, 1562), quoted by Gilly, 'Theophrastica Sancta', 431. Exchanges between Gessner and Crato are discussed by Gilly, 'Zwischen Erfahrung und Spekulation', and Webster, 'Conrad Gessner and the Infidelity of Paracelsus'.

6. Johann Schelhammer, *Widerlegung der vermeynten Postill Valentini Weigelij* (Leipzig/ Hamburg: Rauscher/Frobenius, 1621), 7, 40f.

7. Webster, *From Paracelsus to Newton*, 1–14.

8. Heinrich Bornkamm, 'Paracelsus' (1929), in *Das Jahrhundert der Reformation. Gestalten und Kräfte* (Göttingen: Vandenhoeck & Ruprecht, 1961), 162–77; Rufus M. Jones, *Spiritual Reformers of the 16th and 17th Centuries* (London: Macmillan, 1914); Alexandre Koyré, 'Paracelse' (1933), in *Mystiques, spirituels, alchimistes du XVIe siècle allemand* (Paris: Gallimard, 1971), 75–129; Gustav Adolf Benrath, 'Die Lehre der Spiritualisten', in Carl Andresen (ed.), *Handbuch der Dogmen- und Theologiegeschichte*, vol. 2 (Göttingen: Vandenhoeck & Ruprecht, 1980), 611–58.

9. George Hunston Williams, *The Radical Reformation*, 195–8, 325–7. In various of his short studies Rudolph detects links with the radicals, but also points of difference, often explained with reference to the Neoplatonic background of Paracelsus, 'Theophrast von Hohenheim (Paracelsus): Arzt und Apostel der

neuen Kreatur'; idem, 'Paracelsus' Laientheologie in traditionsgeschichtlicher Sicht'.

10. Goertz, *Pfaffenhaß und groß Geschrei*; idem, 'Die Radikalität reformatorischer Bewegungen'; Laube, 'Die Reformation als soziale Bewegung'; idem, 'Radicalism as a Research Problem in the History of the Early Reformation'; Stayer, 'The Radical Reformation'; Stayer, Packull and Deppermann, 'From Monogenesis to Polygenesis'.

11. For helpful modern assessments, Biegger, *Paracelsus und die Marienverehrung*, 49–56; Gause, *Paracelsus*, 285–9; idem, 'Paracelsus und Jesus Christus'.

12. Haas, *Der Kampf um den Heilige-Geist. Luther und die Schwärmer*. Luther, *Dass eine Christliche versammlung* (1523), WA 11, 408–16; Luther, *Von den Schleichern und Winkelpredigern* (1532), WA 30, *Abteilung III*, 518–27.

13. Osiander, 'Schlußrede auf dem Religionsgespräch', *Osiander Gesamtausgabe*, vol. 1, 1975, 549; Osiander, 'Gutachten zur Verteidigung der Visitation', *Osiander Gesamtausgabe*, vol. 3, 1979, 277–82. Seebaß, 'An sint persequendi haeretici'. For Karlstadt's reservations about *winkelprediger*, Hans-Peter Hasse, 'Beobachtungen zum Selbstverständnis des Karlstadt', in Bubenheimer and Oehmig, *Querdenker*, 49–73, 59.

14. Dopsch, 'Bauernkrieg und Glaubensspaltung', in Dopsch and Spatzenegger (eds), *Geschichte Salzburgs. Stadt und Land. II, 1*, 11–83; Florey, 'Sozialrevolution und Reformation im Erzstift Salzburg', in Barton (ed.), *Sozialrevolution und Reformation*, 42–61.

15. The first notable Lutheran offender was Stephan Kastenbauer (Agricola), who was pursued from 1520 to 1524, when he left the archdiocese: Sallaberger, *Kardinal Matthäus Lang*, 269–78.

16. Barton, *Geschichte der Evangelischen*, 183–4; Rogge, *Jakob Strauß*, 16–19; Rummel, *The Confessionalization of Humanism*, 105–11; Zschoch, *Reformatorische Existenz und konfessionelle Identität*, 44–93.

17. Hans-Jürgen Goertz, 'Brüderlichkeit', in Schmidt, Holenstein and Würgler (eds), *Gemeinde, Reformation und Widerstand*, 161–78, 166–7.

18. Sallaberger, *Kardinal Matthäus Lang*, 302–17.

19. Ibid., 326, 333; Dopsch, 'Bauernkrieg und Glaubensspaltung', 36–7.

20. Sallaberger, *Kardinal Matthäus Lang*, 337; Dopsch, 'Bauernkrieg und Glaubensspaltung', 39–40.

21. Barton, *Geschichte der Evangelischen*, 185; Wiswedel, 'Die alten Täufergemeinden und ihr missionarisches Wirken', *Archiv für Reformationsgeschichte*, 41 (1948), 115–32, 124 for the out of the way places selected for Anabaptist gatherings.

22. Packull, *Hutterite Beginnings*; Klaus Rischar, 'The Martyrdom of the Salzburg Anabaptists in 1527', *Mennonite Quarterly Review*, 43 (1969), 322–7.

23. Vadian, *Deutsch Historische Schriften*, ed. Ernst Götzinger, vol. 3 (St Gallen: Zollikofer, 1879), 458–9.

24. Packull, *Hutterite Beginnings*, 179.

25. Franz, *Der Deutsche Bauernkrieg*, vol. 2, *Aktenband*, 335–7.

26. Packull, *Hutterite Beginnings*, 240–1.

27. Grete Mecenseffy, *Österreich, III*, 241, 258–61 (Sterzing, June/July, 1534), 262–3 (Wölfl, Wölflin).

28. *Septem punctis*, P II, 3, 3–10, 14. Jer. 7: 11, Matt. 21: 13 (*spelunca latronum*).

29. *In Esaiam prophetam philosophia*, P II, 7, 256.

30. *De secretis secretorum theologiae*, P II, 3, 199–201.

31. Ibid., P II, 3, 204.

32. Goldammer, *SSSchr*, 85, 90.

33. A typical example is provided by the friendship circle of Martin Luther in Erfurt. Most went along with Luther, but Hutten died under the protection of Zwingli;

Konrad Mutian opposed the break-up of the Catholic church, while Johann Crotus was first a fervent Lutheran, but later reverted to an attractive Catholic archepiscopal post.

34. Goeters, 'Die Vorgeschichte des Täufertums'; Stayer, 'Die Anfänge der schweizerischen Täufertums'. For the wider constitutional context, Blickle, *Die Revolution von 1525, Die Reformation im Reich* and *Gemeindereformation*. For a short overview, Goertz, *Pfaffenhaß*, 235–50. For a critique of all of these points of view, Strübind, *Eifriger als Zwingli*, 19–47, 79–119.

35. For a reconstruction of the preaching of Vischer and Wölfl, Packull, *Hutterite Beginnings*, 176–81. For Castelberger, Strübind, *Eifriger als Zwingli*, 129–47.

36. Hamm, 'Geistbegabte gegen Geistlose', 416–29, identifies this group as spiritualists, the third out of four groups in his pneumatological typology. With respect to Nuremberg, Hans Greiffenberger is discussed with reference to the influence of Denck and Karlstadt. See also Goertz, 'Clerical Anticlericalism', 506–7, for Jakob Strauß and associated thinkers.

37. Hans-Peter Hasse, 'Beobachtungen zum Selbstverständnis des Karlstadt', in Bubenheimer and Oehmig (eds), *Querdenker*, 49–73, 61–8.

38. *De genealogia Christi*, P II, 3, 160.

39. *Septem punctis*, P II, 3, 4–10.

40. Ibid., P II, 3, 11, 17; *De genealogia Christi*, P II, 3, 160.

41. *Septem punctis*, P II, 3, 20.

42. *Sermones in similitudines et parabolis Christi*, cited from Goldammer, *SSSchr*, 90.

43. Matthew Commentary, cited from from Goldammer, *SSSchr*, 90–91; *De secretis secretorum theologiae*, P II, 3, 189, 195.

44. Commentary on Psalm 139 (140), P II, 7, 25–38.

45. *Außlegung des brauchs des nachtmahls*, Sudhoff, *Versuch*, II, 278. See also *De usu coenae domini*, Sudhoff, *Versuch*, II, 288.

46. Commentary on Matthew 1–5, Chapter 3, Sudhoff, *Versuch*, II, 242.

47. *De sacramento corporis Christi*, Sudhoff, *Versuch*, II, 354–5.

48. Deppermann, *Melchior Hoffman*, 233–5, proposed a rigid four-level hierarchy, which severely restricted the rights of the laity.

49. *De modo missae*, Sudhoff, *Versuch*, II, 289–90.

50. *De coena domini*, Sudhoff, *Versuch*, II, 314.

51. Matt. 18: 3. Fragment from *De morbis ex incantationibus*, P I, 9, 355.

52. *Buch der Erkanntnis*, *BdE*, 52–3. Relevant to this theme is Illustration 2 where Cranach shows the small response to the challenging teaching of Christ.

53. Matt. 20: 16, 22: 14.

54. Matt. 7: 14.

55. Matt. 9: 37, Luke 10: 2.

56. *Buch außlegung aus S. Paulo*, Sudhoff, *Versuch*, II, 275.

57. *De genealogia Christi*, P II, 3, 150–1. For Hoffman's similar use of the bridegroom metaphor, Deppermann, *Melchior Hoffman*, 202–3.

58. *De martyrio Christi*, Matthießen, 194–5, Goldammer, *RSSchr*, 55, Sudhoff, *Versuch*, II, 256–7. For the *selige leben*, Fussler, *Les Idées éthiques, sociales et politiques de Paracelse*; Goldammer, *Paracelsus, Sozialethische und sozialpolitische Schriften*; idem, *Paracelsus. Natur und Offenbarung*; idem, *Paracelsus. Religiöse und sozialphilosophische Schriften*.

59. Friesen, *Erasmus, the Anabaptists, and the Great Commission*.

60. Paola Zambelli, 'Magic and Radical Reformation in Agrippa of Nettesheim', *Journal of the Warburg and Courtauld Institutes*, 39 (1976), 69–103.

61. Packull, *Mysticism and the Early South German-Austrian Anabaptist Movement*; idem, *Hutterite Beginnings*.

62. *De causis morborum invisibilium*, P I, 9, 280–1, 337, 350. Goldammer, *Paracelsus*

in neuen Horizonten, 178–85 (1958); Midelfort, *Madness in Sixteenth-Century Germany*, 123.

63. *De causis morborum invisibilium*, P I, 9, 350; Commentary on Psalm 147 (148), P II, 7, 104.
64. Rosner, 'Studien zum Leben und Wirken des Paracelsus in St Gallen'.
65. Biegger, *Paracelsus und die Marienverehrung*, 55–6; Gause, *Paracelsus*, 58–9, 173–6, 179–82; Goldammer, *SSSchr*, 69–93; Goldammer, *Paracelsus in neuen Horizonten*, 27, 89–90, 144.
66. Bonorand, 'Joachim Vadian und die Täufer'.
67. Vadian, *Deutsch Historische Schriften*, vol. 3, 468. Similarly Paracelsus declared that the Old Testament was the way to death and the New Testament the means to eternal life: Sudhoff, *Versuch*, II, 274.
68. For a recent exhaustive consideration of the background to this situation, concentrating on events before 1528, Strübind, *Eifriger als Zwingli*, 471–546.
69. Bonorand, 'Joachim Vadian und die Täufer', 49–50. The Vadian and Anabaptist angles are not included in the otherwise compendious treatment of this epidemic by John L. Flood in *Renaissance Studies*, 17 (2003), 147–76.
70. Paracelsus travelled to Nördlingen in 1529 and Sterzing in 1534 specifically to confront plague epidemics. For full discussion, Heinrich Dormeier, 'Die Flucht vor der Pest als religiöses Problem', in Klaus Schreiner, *Laienfrömmigkeit im späten Mittelalter* (Schriften des Historischen Kollegs, Kolloquien, 20), (Munich: Oldenbourg, 1992), 331–97.
71. Bonorand, 'Joachim Vadian und die Täufer', 64–72. Vadian, *Deutsch Historische Schriften*, vol. 3, 458–502.
72. Fussler, *Les Idées éthiques, sociales et politiques de Paracelse*, for the most recent full discussion.
73. For an early commitment, see *Septem punctis* (1525) where Theophrastus insists on compliance with Matt. 19: 21 concerning the selling of all goods and distribution of the proceeds to the poor, P II, 3, 15. The community of goods is usually raised in the context of the idealization of poverty. Goldammer, 'Eschatologie II' (1952) lists half a dozen relevant tracts, *Paracelsus in neuen Horizonten*, 134.
74. The strictures on tithes and rents in *Septem punctis* aligned Paracelsus with the Anabaptists and with common demands in petitions associated with the German Peasants' War. As seen above, especially in Chapters III and IV, his complaints about unjust taxes were frequent. For a general critique of unfair taxation, 'Sermo "Date Caesari quae sunt Caesaris"', Goldammer, *RSSchr*, 153–65. See also *Auslegung über die zehen gebott gottes*, P II, 7, 181–90, 216–24, and *De secretis secretorum theologiae*, P II, 3, 198–202.
75. For early opposition to the death penalty, Commentary on Matthew 1–5, Chapter 5 (1525), Sudhoff, *Versuch*, II, 244. For further comment, see *Auslegung über die zehen gebott gottes*, P II, 7, 153–68. See also *De magnificis et superbis*, P II, 2, 132–3.
76. Religious and civil oaths were frequently attacked and were the subject of his *De votis alienis*, P I, 14, 276–98; see also Commentary on Psalm 75 (76), P II, 4, 1–13; *Auslegung über die zehen gebott gottes*, P II, 7, 130–6; *Lamentationes*, P II, 7, 236–7; and *De secretis secretorum theologiae*, P II, 3, 198–200.
77. For representative discussions of peace and war, *Auslegung über die zehen gebott gottes*, P II, 7, 153–68; Commentary on Psalm 139 (140), P II, 7, 25–38; *De secretis secretorum theologiae*, P II, 3, 205–6, 216–17. For context, Goldammer, *SSSchr*, 51–5; idem, 'Friedensidee und Toleranzgedanke bei Paracelsus' (1955), in *Paracelsus in Neuen Horizonten*, 153–76. Paracelsus was more of a pacifist than Müntzer, Hubmaier and Hut. Grebel and Mantz came round to a pacifist position after their earlier support for Zwingli's acceptance of coercion on matters of faith: Stayer, *Anabaptists and the Sword*.

78. For further discussion of issues raised in the above paragraph, Fussler, *Les Idées éthiques, sociales et politiques de Paracelse*.
79. Kautz, *Sieben Artikel* (1527), in Laube et al. (eds), *Flugschriften vom Bauernkrieg*, vol.2, 702–7.
80. Benjamin W. Farley, *John Calvin Treatises against the Anabaptists and Against the Libertines* (Grand Rapids, MI: Baker Book House, 1982); Willem Balke, *Calvijn en de Doperse Radikalen* (Amsterdam: Uitgeverij Ton Bolland, 1973), 37–70, 97–124. For Paracelsus on soul sleep, especially *De animabus hominum post mortem apparentibus*, P I, 14, 299–304, Commentary on Psalm 95 (96), P II, 4, 290. Briefly discussed in Goldammer, 'Eschatologie II' (1952), in *Paracelsus in neuen Horizonten*, 129–31. See also note 84.
81. Haugk, *Ain christlich ordenung* (composed about 1524, but first published 1526), in Laube et al. (eds), *Flugschriften vom Bauernkrieg*, vol.2, 667–86.
82. Hut, *Von dem geheimnus der tauf*, in Müller (ed.), *Glaubenszeugnisse*, 12–28. This general statement of the ideas of Hut derives from the period 1525–27; it was still in draft at Hut's death in 1527.
83. Hut, *Von dem geheimnus der tauf*, in Müller (ed.), *Glaubenszeugnisse*, 14.
84. For these subjects, Williams, *The Radical Reformation*, 20–4, 104–6, 580–92; Jürgen Kaiser, *Ruhe der Seele und Siegel der Hoffnung*, 183–218 for Anabaptists, but without reference to Paracelsus; Michael Klein, 'Geschichtsdenken und Ständekritik in apokalyptischer Perspektive', 191–4, for Paracelsus.
85. Wolfgang Schäufele, *Die missionarische Bewußtsein und Wirken der Taufer*.
86. Mark 16: 15–18. Also Matt. 28: 19, teach and baptize.
87. Matt. 24: 18; Dan. 7: 14.
88. Schäufele, *Die missionarische Bewußtsein und Wirken der Taufer*, 75–7.
89. For the need for believers to risk sacrificing their lives for their faith, Commentary on Psalm 96 (97), P II, 4, 295; Commentary on Psalm 97 (98), P II, 4, 298. As already noted, Paracelsus was opposed to any gratuitous sacrifice of life, which was regarded as avoidance of the obligation to fulfil a useful calling.
90. Mark 16: 15, with the pronoun as dative singular.
91. Mark 16: 15, with the pronoun as genitive singular. Romans 16: 20; Col. 1: 16, 23.
92. Haugk, *Christliche Ordnung*, in Laube et al. (eds), *Flugschriften vom Bauernkrieg*, vol.2, 669–70, 779; Hut, *Von dem geheimnus der tauf*, in Müller (ed.), *Glaubenszeugnisse*, 16–17; see also Hut, *Christliche Unterrichtung*, in Laube et al. (eds), *Flugschriften vom Bauernkrieg*, vol.2, 691. For representative recent discussions on the much-debated gospel of creatures, Mau, 'Gott und Schöpfung bei Thomas Müntzer'; Packull, *Mysticism and the Early South German-Austrian Anabaptist Movement*, 68–71; Seebaß, *Müntzers Erbe*, 400–12.
93. An important background influence was Aquinas, for whom see studies by Norman Kretzmann. At the popular level, Raimond Sebond was important. For representative studies, Claude Blum (ed.), *Montaigne 'Apologie de Raimond Sebond'. De la 'Theologia' à la 'Théologie'* (Paris: Champion, 1990); Jaume de Puig i Oliver, *Les Sources de la pensée philosophique de Raimond Sebond (Ramon Sibiuda)* (Paris: Champion, 1994); idem, *La filosofia de Ramón Sibiuda* (Barcelona: Institut d'Estudis Catalans, 1997); C.C.J. Webb, *Studies in the History of Natural Theology* (Oxford: Clarendon Press, 1915), 233–312. The *Theologia naturalis* of Sebond was available in print from 1480 onwards, and was mentioned by Agrippa von Nettesheim.
94. In his *Horologium sapientiae*, Book I, 3, Seuse cites as one of his main supports Romans 1: 20, which was also the standard reference point for the justification of natural theology.
95. *De genealogia Christi*, P II, 3, 155.
96. With pronoun in dative plural. *De genealogia Christi*, P II, 3, 161; *Vom tauf der Christen*, Goldammer, *RSSchr*, 117.

97. For many examples of metaphors from mythology and nature, *Auff das licht der natur* and *Irrdischen weissagungen nach innehalt der magnalia gottes*, Sudhoff, *Versuch*, II, 276–7; *De coena domini ex lumine naturae*, Sudhoff, *Versuch*, II, 355–6.
98. *De fundamento scientiarum*, P I, 13, 312–24.
99. *De felici liberalitate*, P II, 2, 12.
100. For a characteristic synopsis, *De inventione artium*, P I, 14, 266–72.
101. *Prologus in vitam beatam*, Matthießen, 72–5, Goldammer, *RSSchr*, 2–3. Similarly, Tauler ascribed lack of inner faith to the dominance of '*hündischer Mensch*', Vetter, *Die Predigten Taulers*, No. 45, 199: 8–21.
102. *Liber de lunaticis, II 'De allegoriis ex Christo'*, P I, 14, 50–7.
103. *Astronomia magna*, P I, 12, 58, 68.
104. *Von der widergeburt dess menschen*, Sudhoff, *Versuch*, II, 324–5; *Astronomia magna*, P I, 10, 306.
105. *De inventione artium*, P I, 14, 266–71.
106. *De natura rerum*, P I, 11, 377–80. Commentary on Psalm 146 (147a), P II, 7, 94–5.
107. *Von den natürlichen dingen*, P I, 2, 165.
108. The radical perspective on the *ordo rerum* was developed by Müntzer: Bubenheimer, *Thomas Müntzer*, 210–16 and idem, 'Thomas Müntzer und der Humanismus', on the importance of Tertullian as a source; Goertz, *Inner und äussere Ordnung*, 39–45; Schwarz, *Die apokalyptische Theologie Thomas Müntzers*, 115–26; Seebaß, *Müntzers Erbe*, 383–9.
109. *De inventione artium*, P I, 14, 263–5, 270–5; Commentary on Psalm 91 (92), P II, 4, 246–9.
110. Seuse, *Horologium sapientiae*, II, 4; see note 187 for Tauler on the seven sacraments.
111. *Quod sanguis et caro Christi*, Sudhoff, *Versuch*, II, 326–7, where Paracelsus summarizes the issues of controversy.
112. Recent studies by Daniel and Rudolph accept that the dissertations by Török and Bunners, dating from 1946 and 1961 respectively, are not entirely superseded. Daniel, 'Paracelsus – die Sakramentenlehre'; idem, 'Paracelsus' *Declaratio* on the Lord's Supper'; idem, 'Paracelsus on the Lord's Supper'; idem, 'Paracelsus on Baptism and the Acquiring of the Eternal Body'; Rudolph, 'Hohenheim's Anthropology in the Light of his Writings on the Eucharist'. Both Daniel and Rudolph concentrate on exposition of the relevant primary sources. With respect to the alignments of Paracelsus, Daniel briefly mentions parallels with Franck and Karlstadt, while Rudolph concentrates on the Italian Neoplatonists.
113. *Außlegung etlicher spruech*, Sudhoff, *Versuch*, II, 275.
114. *Quae ex S. Paulo de coena domini*, Sudhoff, *Versuch*, II, 281. '*Hagarisch*' refers to the Agarenes, customarily identified with the Saracen or Ottoman Turkish menace, usually at this date with apocalyptic overtones. Under his magical interpretation in his Lichtenberger commentary, Paracelsus identified the Agarenes as the false Christians, who were the oppressors of the community of saints, P I, 7, 526–7.
115. *De genealogia Christi*, P II, 3, 133.
116. For representative characterizations of John the Baptist, *De genealogia Christi*, P II, 3, 118–21, 156.
117. John 1: 23, 'I am a voice of one crying in the wilderness'. Luther has '*stimme eines predigers in der wüste*', which is less portentous than Paracelsus. Commentary on Matthew (1525), cited by Gause, *Paracelsus*, 178 and Sudhoff, *Versuch*, II, 241; *De genealogia Christi*, P II, 3, 146.
118. Commentary on Matthew 1–5, Chapter 3, Sudhoff, *Versuch*, II, 241–2.
119. Commentary on Matthew 1–5, Chapter 3, quoted by Gause, *Paracelsus*, 178.

120. *Vom tauf der Christen, libellus de baptismate Christiano,* Matthießen, 317–59; P II, 2, 327–78; Goldammer, *RSSchr,* 113–23; Karant-Nunn, *The Reformation of Ritual,* 43–61.
121. Commentary on Matthew 1–5, Chapter 3, Sudhoff, *Versuch,* II, 241–2.
122. *Von der widergeburt dess menschen,* Sudhoff, *Versuch,* II, 324–5; Commentary on Psalm 115 (116b), P II, 5, 216–17.
123. Gause, *Paracelsus,* 142, 180.
124. Stephens, *Theology of Zwingli,* 194, 207–8, 217.
125. Gause, *Paracelsus,* 180.
126. *De genealogia Christi,* P II, 3, 128–32; *Astronomia magna,* P I, 12, 308–18.
127. John 3: 31, *der von oben her kommt, ist über alle.*
128. John 3: 4–6.
129. *Astronomia magna,* P I, 12, 310, *alein es sei dan sach, das ir widergeboren, neugeboren werdet;* Commentary on Psalm 115 (116b), P II, 5, 216.
130. *Astronomia magna,* P I, 12, 310, *auf irem glauben als dan sollen sie getauft werden und auf iren unglauben nicht getauft.*
131. *Astronomia magna,* P I, 12, 310, *was aber nit getauft wird und vom heiligen geist incarnirt, das selbig gehet in die verdamnus.*
132. *Astronomia magna,* P I, 12, 310–11, 316–17.
133. Commentary on Psalm 115 (116b), P II, 5, 216–17. The exclusive concern of this baptismal text with adults is reinforced by citations from the same verses with respect to the Lord's Supper, which of course was itself limited to adults, Sudhoff, *Versuch,* II, 276.
134. *De genealogia Christi,* P II, 3, 128, *darumb soll der glaub gepredigt werden in der ganzen welt allen creturen, damit die erwöhlten zum glauben und zum tauf komben.*
135. Stephens, *Theology of Zwingli,* 196–7.
136. Commentary on Psalm 116 (117), P II, 5, 225.
137. *De genealogia Christi,* P II, 3, 156.
138. Ibid., P II, 3, 154–7.
139. *I. Liber de limbo aeterno,* Sudhoff, *Versuch,* II, 274. *De modo missae,* Sudhoff, *Versuch,* II, 290, accepts that those with mental disease are eligible to accept the baptism of believers.
140. *Auslegung über die zehen gebott gottes,* P II, 7, 194. The editorial suggestion that the intention of Paracelsus was to criticize Anabaptists for willingness to dispense with baptism cannot be accepted. Anabaptists would have agreed with Paracelsus in his insistence that living according to the natural order was insufficient to earn salvation.
141. Karant-Nunn, *The Reformation of Ritual,* 107–18.
142. *Buch außlegung aus S. Paulo,* Sudhoff, *Versuch,* II, 275; *De modo missae,* Sudhoff, *Versuch,* II, 289–90.
143. *II. Buch ex Joanne evangelista: Außlegung etlicher spruech,* Sudhoff, *Versuch,* II, 274–5; *De modo missae,* Sudhoff, *Versuch,* II, 290.
144. *Buch ex Joanne evangelista,* Sudhoff, *Versuch,* II, 274; *De modo missae,* Sudhoff, *Versuch,* II, 290.
145. For a recent review of the Eucharistic debate, but only from the perspective of the Lutheran, Reformed and the Catholic churches, Lee Palmer Wandel, *The Eucharist in the Reformation: Incarnation and Liturgy* (Cambridge: Cambridge University Press, 2006).
146. Ernest Evans, *Tertullian's Treatise on the Incarnation* (London: SPCK, 1956).
147. For sources, see note 80.
148. Gause, *Paracelsus,* discussing both Docetic and monophysite tendencies, 33–9, 285–6 and passim; Biegger, *Paracelsus und die Marienverehrung,* 53–4, 248–53. The (Eutychian) monophysite position suggested that at the birth of Christ there

occurred a union in which the divine absorbed the physical nature, which resulted in a single divine nature.

149. See particularly the collection of short chapters headed *Libri VII, De coena domini ad Clementem VII papam*, Sudhoff, *Versuch*, II, 271–8, 331–2. See also the important text edited and discussed by Daniel, 'Paracelsus' *Declaratio* on the Lord's Supper'; idem, 'Paracelsus on the Lord's Supper' for this text; and see also Sudhoff, *Versuch*, II, 308–10.

150. *De genealogia Christi*, P II, 3, 62–3, 96–7, 131–3.

151. *Ex divo Paulo 1 Cor. 15*, Sudhoff, *Versuch*, II, 280; *Quae ex S. Paulo de coena domini*, Sudhoff, *Versuch*, II, 281.

152. *De usu coenae domini*, Sudhoff, *Versuch*, II, 288.

153. *Ex textibus trium Evangelistarum*, Sudhoff, *Versuch*, II, 274.

154. Gause, *Paracelsus*, 26–42 shows full awareness of these parallels. See also Deppermann, *Melchior Hoffman*, 186–90, 197–202; McLaughlin, 'Schwenckfeld and the South German Eucharistic Controversy, 1526–1529'; idem, 'The Schwenckfeld–Vadian Debate'; idem, *Caspar Schwenckfeld*, 62–76, 85–90, 202–24; Schoeps, *Von himmlischen Fleisch Christi*; Schantz, *Crautwald and Erasmus*, 101–32; Williams, *Radical Reformation*, 326–37.

155. Mark 16: 15 was bypassed, but 2 Cor. 3: 6 was subject to frequent and lengthy discussion in Franck's *Paradoxa*: Wollgast (ed.), *Paradoxa*, 104, 203, 286–91, 349, 423, 427.

156. The roots of the Marian theology of Paracelsus are explored by Gause, *Paracelsus*, and especially by Biegger, *Paracelsus und die Marienverehrung*. For context, Baxandall, *Limewood Sculptors of Renaissance Germany*, 56–8, 164–72; Stephan Beissel, *Geschichte der Verehrung Marias*; Klaus Schreiner, *'Maria'. Jungfrau, Mutter, Herrscherin* (Munich: G. Hanser, 1994). Schwenckfeld disagreed with Hoffman over the status of the Virgin Mary. Hoffman sided with Karlstadt and Sattler about the imperfection of Mary, while Ziegler and Schwenckfeld broadly coincided with Paracelsus over her reputation for spotlessness, Deppermann, *Melchior Hoffmann*, 157–8, 189–91. At the end of his *Christlicher Unterrichtung* Hut cited Mary as an ideal for believers to follow Müller (ed.), *Glaubenszeugnisse*, 33. For a similar expression by Hans Schwalb, *Beklagung eines laien*, in Laube et al. (eds), *Flugschriften der frühen Reformationsbewegung*, vol.1, 63.

157. Hans-Jürgen Goertz, 'Brüderlichkeit'.

158. C. Arnold Snyder, *Anabaptist History and Theology*, 47–8.

159. The *Horologium sapientiae* edition featured in Illustration 6 was first printed in Cologne in 1480; four more editions appeared in Cologne before 1540, and others were produced in three other publishing centres.

160. Bräuer and Junghans, *Der Theologe Thomas Müntzer*; Goertz, *Innere und äussere Ordnung*; Hasse, *Karlstadt und Tauler*; Ozment, *Homo spiritualis*; Packull, *Mysticism*, 17–34. Otto Langer, 'Inneres Wort und inwohnender Christus. Zum mystischen Spiritualismus Sebastian Francks und seinen Implikationen', in Müller (ed.), *Sebastian Franck*, 55–69. The sermons of Tauler and *Theologia Deutsch* were among the most commonly cited sources in the *Paradoxa* of Franck, each accounting for about twenty references, see Wollgast (ed.), *Paradoxa*, index.

161. Goldammer, *Paracelsus. Natur und Offenbarung*, 95.

162. Ozment, *Homo spiritualis*, 13–48; Gnädinger, *Johannes Tauler*, 241–51. For *grunt*, see also McGinn, *The Mystical Thought of Meister Eckhart*, 37–52. For an example of striking use of *gemuete* and its variants by Paracelsus, *De genealogia Christi*, P II, 3, 67, 74, 106, 114, 145 (where the term is used on three occasions in one line of text, and on many other instances in adjacent lines). For a review of *gelassenheit*, Ludwig Völker, '"Gelassenheit". Zur Enstehung des Wortes in der Sprache Meister Eckharts und seiner Überlieferung in der nacheckhartischen Mystik bis Jakob

Böhme', in Franz Hundsnurscher and Ulrich Müller (eds), *'Getempert und gemischet' für Wolfgang Mohr zum 65. Geburtstag* (Göppingen: Verlag Alfred Kümmerle, 1972), 281–312; for Tauler, 288–93.

163. As for instance indicated by Luther's marginal annotations on Tauler, Steven E. Ozment, 'An Aid to Luther's Marginal Comments on Johannes Tauler's Sermons', *The Harvard Theological Review*, 63 (1970), 305–11.

164. Use of the verb *kleben* and its compounds was favoured particularly by Tauler, Egerding, *Die Metaphorik*, 344–5.

165. Typically, to achieve liberation, dispense with all earthly possession and become an empty or free (*lärer, freien*) spirit, *De felici liberalitate*, P II, 2, 6. For Tauler on the requirement for emptying of obligations, Vetter, *Die Predigten Taulers*, No. 1, 9–10, No. 60e, 305–6; following the example of Christ in humbling himself, Phil. 2: 7–8.

166. *Astronomia magna*, P I, 12, 7–9. For further examples of elimination of intermediaries, see *De virtute humana*, P II, 2, 99; Commentary on Psalm 118 (119), P II, 6, 16, 50–1, 89–90, 103. The *ohne mittel* theme was taken up by Tauler from Eckhart and often expressed, Vetter, *Die Predigten Taulers*, No. 6, 24, No. 20, 84, No. 22, 91, No. 39, 154, No. 57, 267, No. 60b, 290, No. 62, 336, 340–1. For emphasis on *ohne mittel*: by Denck, *Von gesetz Gottes*, Entfelder, *Von den mannigfalten zerspaltungen*, both in Laube et al., *Flugschriften vom Bauernkrieg, vol. 2*, 638, 950–1; Franck, discussed by Müller, 'Buchstabe, Geist, Subjekt …', 658, 665.

167. *Astronomia magna*, P I, 12, 316–20; Commentary on Psalm 75 (76), P II, 4, 3–8, deriving from James 1: 17, … *alle vollkommene Gabe kommt von oben herab*; see also Col. 3: 2. The same text was the basis for the sermon *Omne datum optimum* by Eckhart: Steer, Sturlese, Gottschall (eds), *Lectura Eckhardi I*, 2–9. For Sebastian Franck on this theme, Müller, 'Buchstabe, Geist, Subjekt …', 658–9.

168. *Volgen die irrdischen weissagungen nach innehalt der magnalia Gottes*, Sudhoff, *Versuch*, II, 277; Commentary on Psalm 75 (76), P II, 4, 3–8.

169. Commentary on Psalm 91 (92), P II, 4, 245–6. Goertz, *Innere und äussere Ordnung*, 39–45, for Tauler on the *ordo rerum*. Ozment concludes his discussion of Tauler by quoting his view that spiritual perfection lay in the utterly inward, hidden and deepest ground of the soul *in dem allerinnigesten, in dem allerverborgensten tieffesten grunde der selen, do sú daz in dem grunde …*, Vetter, *Die Predigten Taulers*, No. 60d, 300, 17f., which Ozment in turn links with the German writings of Eckhart, *Homo spiritualis*, 25–6.

170. For *grunt*, Egerding, *Metaphorik*, 279–309; for *tief*, Egerding, *Metaphorik*, 539–52.

171. For *stille*, Egerding, *Metaphorik*, 552–6.

172. Commentary on Psalm 91 (92), P II, 4, 250. Similarly, Commentary on Daniel, P II, 7, 355.

173. For *fliessen* and its compounds, Egerding, *Metaphorik*, 624–58.

174. *Auß dem closter lauffen*, Sudhoff, *Versuch*, I, 523–4.

175. *De virtute humana*, P II, 2, 99.

176. *Paragranum*, P I, 8, 41–2. Indicative of the appeal to Paracelsus of *grünen* imagery in the Psalms commentary, P II, 4, 51, 65, 217, 246, 249, 320, 342. The related *viriditas* symbolism was closely identified with Hildegard of Bingen. Egerding, *Metaphorik*, 109–25.

177. McGinn, *The Mystical Thought of Meister Eckhart*, 48.

178. Cited from Appendix to Matthew Commentary 1525–26, from Gause, *Paracelsus*, 230–1. For *smelzen* and *versmelzung*, Egerding, *Die Metaphorik*, 523–8, noting that Tauler was particularly attached to the use of *versmelzung*, 525–6.

179. Friesen, *Thomas Muentzer*, 10–32, 32.

180. McGinn, *The Mystical Thought of Eckhart*, 38–52. Gnädinger, *Johannes Tauler*, 241–51. See also Paul Wyser, 'Taulers Terminologie von Seelengrund'.

181. Ibid., 37. Like Eckhart and Tauler, Paracelsus used *grunt* in a variety of senses ranging from the more literal 'basis' or 'reason' to the mystic expression for the innermost depth of the soul and nearest point of identity with God.

182. Werner Beierwaltes, '*Primum est dives per se*: Meister Eckhart und der "*Liber de causis*"', in E.P. Bos and P.A. Meijer (eds), *Proclus and his Influence in Medieval Philosophy* (Leiden: Brill, 1992), 141–69; Josef Koch, 'Augustinischer und dionysischer Neuplatonismus im Mittelalter', in Beierwaltes (ed.), *Platonismus in der Philosophie des Mittelalters*, 317–42; Kurt Ruh, 'Neuplatonische Quellen Meister Eckhart', in Claudia Brinker et al. (eds), *Contemplata aliis tradere: Studien zum Verhältnis von Literatur und Spiritualität* (Frankfurt am Main: Peter Lang, 1995), 317–52.

183. Gnädinger, *Johannes Tauler*, 129–35; Alois M. Haas, '*Nim din selbes war.*' *Studien zur Lehre von der Selbsterkenntnis bei Meister Eckhart, Johannes Tauler und Heinrich Susso* (Freiburg/Schweiz: Universitätsverlag, 1971), 76–153; idem, *Sermo mysticus. Studien zu Theologie und Sprache der deutschen Mystik* (Freiburg/Schweiz: Universitätsverlag, 1979); Alain de Libera, *Eckhart, Suso, Tauler, ou la divinisation de l'homme* (Paris: Bayard Editions, 1996); Loris Sturlese, 'Tauler im Kontext: Die philosophischen Voraussetzungen des "Seelengrund" in der Lehre des deutschen Neuplatonikers Berthold von Moosburg', *Beiträge zur Geschichte der deutschen Sprache und Literatur*, 109 (1987), 390–426.

184. Haas, *Sermo mysticus*, 52–5; Josef Koch, 'Über die Lichtsymbolik im Bereich der Philosophie und der Mystik im Mittelalter', *Studium Generale*, 13 (1960), 653–70; Egerding, *Metaphorik*, 359–410; Weiß, *Die deutschen Mystikerinnen*, vol. 1, 285–347 and also the sections on *herrlichkeit* and *klarheit*, 213–85.

185. The dichotomous and trichotomous anthropologies were weighed up as alternatives by Erasmus in his *Enchiridion*; he was perhaps reflecting Gabriel Biel. For commitment of Erasmus to this idea, M.A. Screech, *Erasmus. Ecstacy and the Praise of Folly* (London: Duckworth, 1980), 96–112. The idea was also prominent in Tauler, who represented a trail of thinking going back through Eckhart to Origen. Like Erasmus, Paracelsus made use of both the trichotomous and dichotomous alternatives, Kämmerer, *Das Leib–Seele–Geist–Problem*; Midelfort, 'The Anthropological Roots of Paracelsus' Psychiatry', in Dilg-Frank, *Kreatur und Kosmos*, 67–77; idem, *Madness in Sixteenth-Century Germany*, 108–38, especially 113–16. For the earlier history, Henri Crouzel, 'L'Anthropologie d'Origène', in Ugo Bianchi and Henri Crouzel (eds), *Arché e Telos. L'antropologia di Origene e di Gregorio di Nissa* (Studia patristica Mediolanensia, 12), (Milan: Vita e Pensiero, 1981), 36–49; Paul Wyser, 'Taulers Terminologie von Seelengrund'. The trichotomous approach was rejected by Luther but adopted by Denck, Hubmaier and Hoffman: Deppermann, *Melchior Hoffman*, 197–202; Joest, *Ontologie der Person bei Luther*, 137–62, 196–210, 265–9; Windhorst, *Täuferisches Taufverständnis*, 205–8.

186. Vetter, *Die Predigten Taulers*, No. 20, 81.

187. Isa. 11: 1–3, interpreted by Christians as the seven gifts of the Holy Spirit. Vetter, *Die Predigten Taulers*, No. 26, 103–10.

188. For the support for Isaiah of New Testament sources, J.A. Whitlark and M.C. Parsons, ' "The Seven Last Words": A Numerical Motivation for the Insertion of Luke 23.34a', *New Testament Studies*, 52 (2006), 188–204.

189. Laube et al. (eds), *Flugschriften vom Bauernkrieg*, vol. 2, 682. For a parallel on the Sabbath from Paracelsus, Commentary on Psalm 117 (118), P II, 5, 252–4. Kaiser, *Ruhe der Seele und Siegel der Hoffnung*, 215–18.

Chapter VII: Endzeit

1. *Prologus in vitam beatam*, Matthießen, 82, Goldammer, *RSSchr*, 5. 'The age of philosophy has come to its end; the winter of my sufferings is over. The summer time is here, and so also is arrived the time appointed for the blissful and eternal existence.'

2. For Paracelsus on prophecy and eschatology from various angles, Goldammer, 'Paracelsische Eschatologie' (1949 and 1952), in *Paracelsus in neuen Horizonten*, 87–152; Webster, *From Paracelsus to Newton*, 15–28. For general context, many classics, including Norman Cohn, *Pursuit of the Millennium* (London: Secker & Warburg, 1957), Ernest Lee Tuveson, *Millennium and Utopia* (Berkeley: The University of California Press, 1949), and especially Peuckert, *Die Grosse Wende*. For the more recent literature, apart from other titles cited in other notes, which are necessarily selective and confined to recent titles from a vast literature: Robin Bruce Barnes, *Prophecy and Gnosis: Apocalypticism in the Wake of the Lutheran Reformation* (Stanford, CA: Stanford University Press, 1988); Klaus Bergdolt and Walther Ludwig, *Zukunftsvoraussagen in der Renaissance*; Kate Cooper and Jeremy Gregory (eds), *Signs, Wonders, Miracles. Representations of Divine Power in the Life of the Church* (Woodbridge, Suffolk: Boydell Press, 2005); Bernard McGinn (ed.), *The Encyclopedia of Apocalypticism. Volume 2, Apocalypticism in Western History and Culture* (New York: Continuum, 1998); Andrew Cunningham and Ole Peter Grell, *The Four Horsemen of the Apocalypse. Religion, War, Famine and Death in Reformation Europe* (Cambridge: Cambridge University Press, 2000); Manfred Jakubowski-Tiessen, Hartmut Lehmann, Johannes Schilling and Reinhart Staats (eds), *Jahrhundertwenden, Endzeit- und Zukunftsvorstellungen vom 15. bis zum 20. Jahrhundert* (Göttingen: Vandenhoeck & Ruprecht, 1999); Manfred Jakubowski-Tiessen and Hartmut Lehmann (eds), *Um Himmels Willen. Religion in Katastrophenzeiten* (Göttingen: Vandenhoeck & Ruprecht, 2003).

3. *Prognostikation auf 24 zukünftige jahre*, P I, 10, 582: ... *die zeichen verkünt, die dan nun den anfang geben. Aber in der operation ist noch kein end, waren nur anfang. Est ist aber iez die zeit ... das sie zum end gehen werden.*

4. Ps. 1: 1, Vulgate: *cathedra pestilentiae*, Luther: *noch sitzt, da die spotter sitzen.*

5. *De secretis secretorum theologiae*, P I, 3, 223. Mark 3: 29.

6. Hut, *Von dem geheimnus der tauf*, in Müller, *Glaubenszeugnisse*, 13: *Dieweil die letzt und allergferlichest zeit diser welt itzt auf uns gelanget.* See Illustration 7(a), for an Old Testament prophet, and 7(b), for the representation insired by a text of Paracelsus of the prophetic figure at the end of time. 7(a) Hans Holbein d.J., woodcut illustration to Jonah 4: 5–6, from *Historia veteris testamenti icones* (Lyons: Trechsel & Frellon partners, 1538). 7(b), woodcut, Figure XXXII, from *Die Prognostikation auf 24 zukünftige jahre* (1536), H, vol.10, Appendix, 224.

7. *Philosophia de generationibus quatuor elementorum*, P I, 13, 27.

8. *Opus paramirum*, P I, 9, 99.

9. *De ente astrale*, P I, 1, 237; *Volumen paramirum*, P I, 1, 225–33.

10. *Opus paramirum*, P I, 9, 99–100.

11. *Von ursprung der franzosen*, P I, 7, 185–6.

12. *Sieben defensiones*, P I, 11, 135–6.

13. *De peste libri tres*, P I, 9, 587–8.

14. Ibid., P I, 9, 593.

15. Ibid., P I, 9, 588–90. For the *potentia ordinata/absoluta* distinction in astrology, see Laura A. Smoller, *History, Prophecy, and the Stars* (Princeton, NJ: Princeton University Press, 1994), 122–30.

16. Ibid., P I, 9, 590–1.

17. *Elf tractat*, P I, 1, 25–6.

18. *Auslegung aphorismorum Hippocratis*, P I, 4, 495–6.
19. A relevant reference to sharpness occurs in Illustration 2, where immediately in front of Philosophia is an obelisk, the mysterious needle-shaped stone, upon which are inscribed the Greek symbols for the seven liberal arts, also two Greek letters at the base and summit, perhaps indicating the rising scale from the world of nature to the province of God. Robert, *Konrad Celtis und das Projekt*, 123–6.
20. *Paragranum*, P I, 8, 41–50.
21. Matt. 21: 18–20, Mark 11: 12–14, 20–1.
22. Matt. 3: 10, Luke 3: 9.
23. Matt. 24: 32–3, Mark 13: 28–9, Luke 21: 29–31.
24. Paracelsus evidently assumed that the inhabitants of Nineveh were punished, whereas after token contrition involving sackcloth and ashes they were forgiven. Jonah 3.
25. Luke 21: 25, *super terram pressura gentium prae confusione*. For the same expression in Paracelsus, see sources cited in note 29.
26. Luke 21: 24, ... *donec impleantur tempora nationum*. See also *Prognostikation auf 24 zukünftige jahre*, P I, 10, 582, *es ist aber iez die zeit (tempora nationum) das ist zum end gehen werden*.
27. *Grosse Wundarznei, III*, P I, 10, 451–4; *Sieben defensiones*, P I, 11, 41–50. Mark 13: 14–27; Luke 21: 5–36.
28. *Astronomia magna*, P I, 12, 364–5.
29. *Grosse Wundarznei, III*, P I, 10, 454; *Sieben defensiones* P I, 11, 136; *Astronomia magna*, P I, 12, 403; *Erklärung der ganzen astronomie*, P I, 12, 476–7.
30. Commentary on Psalm 91 (92), P II, 4, 249–50.
31. Ibid., P II, 4, 246–7.
32. Ibid., P II, 4, 26; *In Esaiam prophetam philosophia*, P II, 7, 258.
33. *In Esaiam prophetam philosophia*, P II, 7, 258.
34. Matt. 7: 14; Matt. 9: 37, Luke 10: 2, Matt. 20: 16, 22: 14.
35. *Astronomia magna*, P I, 12, 403–6.
36. Klaassen, *Living at the End of the Ages*, 19–32.
37. Wolfgang Hübner, 'Astrologie in der Renaissance', in Bergdolt and Ludwig, *Zukunftsvoraussagen in der Renaissance*, 241–80; Kurze, 'Popular Astrology and Prophecy in the Fifteenth and Sixteenth Centuries'.
38. McGinn (ed.), *The Encyclopedia of Apocalypticism. Volume 2*, 74–466; Rau, *Das Bild des Antichrist im Mittelalter*.
39. Reeves, *The Influence of Prophecy in the Later Middle Ages*.
40. This was perhaps the first German vernacular alchemical work. For its apocalyptic bias, Barbara Obrist, *Les Débuts de l'imagerie alchemique (XIVe–XVe siècles)* (Paris: Le Sycomore, 1982), 126–40.
41. Robert E. Lerner, 'Refreshment of the Saints: The Time after Antichrist as a Station for Earthly Progress in Medieval Thought', *Traditio*, 32 (1976), 97–144; idem, 'The Medieval Return to the Thousand-Year Sabbath', in Richard K. Emmerson and Bernard McGinn (eds), *The Apocalypse in the Middle Ages* (Ithaca etc: Cornell University Press, 1992), 51–71. Smoller, *History, Prophecy, and the Stars*, 85–101.
42. Besides others mentioned in the text, among the many medical professionals contributing to prophecy and astrology from various political angles between 1500 and 1540 were Lorenz Fries, Joseph Grünpeck, Alexander Seitz, Georg Tannstetter, Theodericus Ulsenius and Johann Virdung. For the importance of a humanist medical scholar as a collector of prophetic manuscripts, see Robert E. Lerner, 'Prophetic Manuscripts of the "Renaissance Magus" Pierleone of Spoleto', in Gian Luca Potestà (ed.), *Il profetismo gioachimita tra Quattrocento e Cinquecento* (Genoa: Marietti, 1991), 97–116.

43. Bernhard Töpfer, *Das kommende Reich des Friedens: zur Entwicklung chiliastischer Zukunftshoffnungen im Hochmittelalter* (Berlin: Akademie-Verlag, 1964).
44. Klaus H. Lauterbach, 'Der "oberrheinische Revolutionär" – der Theoretiker aufständischer Bauern?', in Peter Blickle and Thomas Adam (eds), *Bundschuh: Untergrombach 1502, das unruhige Reich und die Revolutionierbarkeit Europas* (Stuttgart: Franz Steiner Verlag, 2004), 140–79.
45. Kurze, *Johannes Lichtenberger. Eine Studie zur Geschichte der Prophetie und Astrologie*; Sarah Slattery, 'Wunderzeichen und Propaganda'; Heike Talkenberger, *Sintflut: Prophetie und Zeitgeschehen*, 56–119.
46. Reflecting the positive associations of Saturn for the Jews, the conjunction was interpreted by R. Yohanan Alemanno as an encouragement to his nation and its prophets: Idel, *Absorbing Perfections*, 149–50. Alemanno's friend, Giovanni Pico, was also caught up in the apocalyptic frenzy.
47. Tilman Struve, 'Utopie und gesellschaftliche Wirklichkeit. Zur Bedeutung des Friedenskaisers im späten Mittelalter', *Historische Zeitschrift*, 225 (1977), 65–95.
48. Panofsky, *Life and Art of Dürer*, 51–9.
49. Luther, *Das Evangelium am Tage der heyligen drey Künige*, WA 10, *Erste Abteilung, 1 Hälfte*, 571.
50. Barnes, *Prophecy and Gnosis*, 87–91, 96–9, 104–12, 143–51 and *passim*; Stefano Caroti, 'Comete, portenti, causalità naturale e escatologia in Filippo Melantone', in Zambelli, *Scienza, credenze occulte*, 393–426; Talkenberger, *Sintflut*, 368–78, 285–300.
51. Talkenberger, *Sintflut*, 58–61. Ten editions of Lichtenberger were produced in Germany between 1526 and 1528: Kurze, 'Popular Astrology', 189. In Germany no editions of Lichtenberger were produced between 1497 and 1526.
52. *Osiander, Gesamtausgabe*, vol. 2, 421–2.
53. Lerner, *The Power of Prophecy*, 157–74; F. U. Prietz, 'Geschichte und Reformation. Die deutsche Chronica des Johannes Carion als Erziehungsbuch und Fürstenspiegel', in Oliver Auge and Cora Dietl (eds), *Universitas. Die mittelalterliche und frühneuzeitliche Universität im Schnittpunkt wissenschaftlicher Disziplinen. Festschrift für Georg Wieland zum 70. Geburtstag* (Tübingen: Francke Verlag 2007), 153–65.
54. Lerner, The Power of Prophecy, 16.
55. Manfred Schulze, 'Onus ecclesiae: Last der Kirche – Reformation der Kirche', in Dykema and Oberman (eds), *Anticlericalism*, 318–42. Berthold was Bishop of Chiemsee, but his duties were performed in Salzburg.
56. Lerner, 'Medieval Prophecy and Religious Dissent', 17.
57. Gengenbach, *Der Nollart. Dies sind die prophetien sancti Methodii und Nollardi* (Basel: P. Gegenbach, 1517). Kurze, 'Prophecy and History', 67; Talkenberger, *Sintflut*, 173–7, 302–6. See also note 93.
58. Dietrich Kurze, 'Nationale Regungen in der spätmittelalterlichen Prophetie', 16–17.
59. Martin Borrhaus (Cellarius), *De operibus dei* (Strasbourg, 1527). Irena Backus, *Martin Borrhaus* (Bibliotheca Dissidentium, 2), (Baden-Baden: Valentin Koerner, 1981); Lucia Felici, *Tra riforma ed eresia. La giovinezza di Martin Borrhaus (1499–1528)* (Florence: Olschki, 1995); Seifert, 'Reformation und Chiliasmus'.
60. Klaassen, *Living at the End of the Ages*, 26–7; Packull, *Mysticism and the Early South German–Austrian Anabaptist Movement*, 78–87, 110–12; Seebaß, *Müntzers Erbe*, 349–65.
61. Klaassen, *Living at the End of the Ages*, 84–5; Sondheim, *Thomas Murner als Astrolog*, 98–100.
62. Hoffman, *Auslegung der heimlichen Offenbarung des Apostels und Evangelisten Johannes*, in Laube et al. (eds), *Flugschriften vom Bauernkrieg*, vol. 1, 492–500.
63. Deppermann, *Melchior Hoffman*, 305–14; Klaassen, *Living at the End of the Ages*, 27–9.

64. Otto Brunfels, *Almanach ewig werend* (Strasbourg: J. Schott, 1526), briefly discussed by Ginsberg, *Il nicodemismo*, 29–30; more fully by Talkenberg, *Sintflut*, 357–9.
65. Benzing, *Bibliographie Lorenz Fries*, Talkenberg, *Sintflut*, 257–9, 286–7.
66. Benzing, No. 1; Scribner, *For the Sake of Simple Folk*, 127.
67. Benzing, Nos 7 and 8; Talkenberger, *Sintflut*, 300–1.
68. Osiander, Foreword to Letter of Argula von Grumbach to the Rector of the University of Ingolstadt, 1523, *Osiander Gesamtausgabe*, vol. 1, 91–2.
69. *St Hildegardten Weissagung* (Nuremberg, 1527); Gottfried Seebaß, *Bibliographica Osiandrica* (Nieuwkoop: B. De Graaf, 1971), No. 121.1–3. For the edition by Hans-Ulrich Hofmann, Osiander Gesamtausgabe, vol. 2, 485–501.
70. Sachs, 'Disputation zwischen einem Chorherren und Schuchmacher' (1524), in Seufert, *Die Wittenbergisch Nachtigall*, 45–71.
71. Benzing, Nos 18–26. Fries began publishing on syphilis before 1518 and completed his last work on this subject just before his death in 1532.
72. Sudhoff, *Versuch*, I, No. 2.
73. P I, 7, 48–9. The Wellcome Library, London, contains a variant of the 1529 edition unrecorded by Sudhoff, showing good demand for this initial publication. A copy of this variant was also recently in the stock of Jonathan A. Hill, Bookseller of New York.
74. Sudhoff, *Versuch*, I, 4–36.
75. *Prognostikation auf 24 zukünftige jahre*, P I, 10, 582–3.
76. *Auslegung über etliche figuren J. Lichtenbergers*, P I, 7, 477–530. Internal evidence suggests that Paracelsus worked on this text until 1530.
77. *Ein wunderliche Weissagung von dem Babstumb* (Nuremberg, 1527); Seebaß, *Bibliographica Osiandrica*, No. 11.1–4. The success of the Papal Prophecies is suggested by its issue in Wittenberg, Zwickau and Oppenheim, also in 1527. For *Ein wunderliche Weissagung*, edited by Hans-Ulrich Hofmann, Osiander Gesamtausgabe, vol. 2, introduction 403–18 (414–16 for dissemination); for text and illustrations, 421–84. The Osiander series was an amalgam of two sets of images, each of fifteen figures, both dating from the first half of the fourteenth century. Osiander claimed to base his edition on two different manuscripts from Nuremberg, but quite possibly his source was one of the recent Italian editions.
78. *Auslegung der papstbilder*, P I, 12, 511–85. Sudhoff, *Versuch*, I, No. 106, 1569 (German), No. 115, 1570 (Latin). Reeves, *The Influence of Prophecy*, 454 mistakenly dates the first Latin edition from 1530; also it is not correct that the Latin edition preceded a German 'translation' of 1532. As indicated in note 95, circumstantial evidence suggests that Paracelsus took Osiander's edition as the source for his images.
79. Hans-Ulrich Hofmann, in Osiander Gesamtausgabe, vol. 2, 411–14.
80. *Prognostikation auf 24 zukünftige jahre*, Sudhoff, *Versuch*, I, No. 17; P I, 10, 580–620. For a brief exposition of contemporary marginal notes, very much supportive of Paracelsus and even more radical in its sentiments, Bernhard Milt, 'Prognostikation auf 24 zukünftige Jahre von Theophrastus Paracelsus und eine zeitgenössischer Deutungsversuch', *Gesnerus*, 8 (1951), 38–53.
81. Indicative of the hostile context, the publisher was criticized for including a letter from a radical ally of Paracelsus in the first edition of the *Großen Wundartznei*. Hans-Jörg Künast, '*Getruckt zu Augspurg*', 206.
82. Milt, 'Prognostikation'.
83. *Aus der philosophia super Esaiam prophetam*, P I, 12, 506.
84. For the lively world of prophets, visions and dreams, Deppermann, *Melchior Hoffman*, 178–86; Hoyer, 'Die Zwickauer Storchianer'; Seebaß, *Müntzers Erbe*, 379–400.
85. *Practica in scientiam divinationis*, P I, 12, 488–9.
86. Ibid., P I, 12, 492.

87. Ibid., P I, 12, 492–3.
88. Matt. 24: 30, Mark 13: 4, Luke 21: 11, 25.
89. *Aus der philosophia super Esaiam prophetam*, P I, 12, 506–7.
90. *De divinatione*, P I, 12, 506–7.
91. De *martyrio Christi*, Matthießen, 177–95, Goldammer, *RSSchr*, 49–55, Sudhoff, *Versuch*, II, 256–7.
92. *Auslegung Lichtenbergers*, P I, 7, 507–9.
93. Ibid., P I, 7, 510–30. *Nollbrüder*, like *nollhart* or *lollhart*, indicated a low-level, often dire, putable or even heretical monastic attendant, as in the case of Gengenbach (see above, n. 57).
94. Ibid., P I, 7, 525–7. Jeremiah 7, 26 and 31. For the Agarenes, Baruch 3: 23. Klein, 'Geschichtsdenken und Ständkritik in apokalyptischer Perspektive', 191–4 for Paracelsus. For Sattler, Thieleman J. van Braght (ed.), *Martyrs Mirror* (Scottdale, PA: Herald Press, 1987), 416. See also John W. Bohnstedt, 'The Turkish Menace as seen by German Pamphleteers of the Reformation Era', *Transactions of the American Philosophical Society*, 58 Part 9 (1968); Keith Moxey, *Peasants, Warriors and Wives. Popular Imagery in the Reformation* (Chicago: Chicago University Press, 1989), 67–100.
95. *Ein wunderliche Weissagung, Osiander Gesamtausgabe*, vol. 2, 468–70; *Auslegung der papstbilder*, P I, 12, 560–2, 569–72, ninth, thirteenth and twentieth figures. Chipps Smith, *Nuremberg*, 167, No. 65. For an interesting discussion of the twentieth image, indicating Osiander's residual hope for rapprochement between the Lutherans and Charles V, David Heffner, '*Regnum vs Sacerdotum* in a Reformation Pamphlet', *Sixteenth Century Journal*, 20 (1989), 617–30. Heffner also provides helpful insight into the fire-iron symbol, which was adapted from the capital 'B' that appears in medieval manuscripts and in the Italian editions. Since the fire-iron also occurs in Paracelsus, it is evident that the source for his illustrations was the Osiander edition.
96. *Auslegung der papstbilder*, P I, 12, 558–9, nineteenth figure.
97. Ibid., P I, 12, 536, 556, eleventh and eighteenth figures.
98. Ibid., P I, 12, 550, sixteenth figure.
99. Ibid., P I, 12, 577–82, twenty-seventh to twenty-ninth figures.
100. Ibid., P I, 12, 583–5, thirtieth figure and conclusions.
101. *Prognostikation auf 24 zukünftige jahre*, P I, 10, 581.
102. Milt, 'Prognostikation'.
103. Paul of Middelburg to Marsilio Ficino, 1492: Ficino, *Opera omina* (Basel, 1576), vol. 1, 944.
104. Idel, *Absorbing Perfections*, 149–50.
105. Particularly aptly described by Farmer in his *Syncretism in the West*, 41–5.
106. Baron, 'The "Querelle" of the Ancients and Moderns as a Problem for Renaissance Scholarship'; Buck, *Die Rezeption der Antike in den romanischen Literaturen der Renaissance*, 228–36.
107. Kaiser, *Ruhe der Seele und Siegel der Hoffnung*, 183–235; Lerner, 'Refreshment of the Saints: The Time after Antichrist as a Station for Earthly Progress'; Seebaß, *Müntzers Erbe*, 346–8.
108. *Prologus in vitam beatam*, Goldammer, *RSSchr*, 1 (no equivalent at this point in the Matthießen edition).
109. *Prologus in vitam beatam*, Matthießen, 77, Goldammer, *RSSchr*, 3.
110. *Prologus in vitam beatam*, Matthießen, 80, Goldammer, *RSSchr*, 4–5.
111. In language and concept, the call for immediate and radical change, and the objection to compromise or to sparing the counterfeit work of the establishment, are all reminiscent of the objections to proceeding slowly with reform by Karlstadt in his *Ob man gemach faren, und des ergernüssen der schwachen verschonen soll* (Basel 1524); and similarly Grebel, in Harder, *Sources of Swiss Anabaptism*, vol. 2, 671, 677.

112. *Prologus in vitam beatam*, Matthießen, 82, Goldammer, *RSSchr*, 5.
113. Ibid.
114. Commentary on Psalm 103 (104), P II, 5, 15–16.
115. Ibid., P II, 5, 13, 18–20.
116. Commentary on Psalm 146 (147a), P II, 7, 92.
117. Commentary on Psalm 103 (104), P II, 5, 16–18.
118. Commentary on Psalm 79 (80), P II, 4, 93; ibid., P II, 4, 107; Commentary on Psalm 89 (90), P II, 4, 211; Commentary on Psalm 144 (145), P II, 7, 69.
119. Matt. 24: 36, *Von dem Tage aber und von der Stunde weiß niemand, auch die Engel nicht im Himmel sondern allein mein Vater. Außlegung etlicher spruech*, Sudhoff, *Versuch*, II, 275.
120. *De secretis secretorum theologiae*, P II, 3, 212–31.
121. *De natura rerum*, P I, 11, 272–3. Although this work is generally treated as a genuine writing, there is an element of doubt, especially about the Preface. But it is also accepted that for the most part *De natura rerum* reflects the genuine ideas of Paracelsus, for which parallels exist elsewhere in his writings. My own view is that this is a case of a competent distillation based on authentic Paracelsus sources, akin to *De occulta philosophia*, *De pestilitate*, and the well-known summaries of his ethical and religious writings.
122. Matt. 24: 30 says no more than the 'power and glory' of Christ's appearance; Matt. 25: 31 has 'throne of his glory', and Rev. 20: 11 'great white throne'. Rom. 14: 10 and 2 Cor. 5: 10, like Paracelsus, keep to the simple judgement seat. Also, like Paracelsus, such texts create ambiguity over the respective roles of the Father and Christ in dispensing judgement. Consistent with other New Testament texts, Paracelsus gives the impression that Christ undertook the judging on the Father's behalf, John 5: 22, 27, Acts 10: 42, 1 Cor. 15: 20–8.
123. Matt. 25: 31 and Mark 8: 38 have the accompaniment of angels.
124. Matt. 24: 31, which says that the trumpets were directed to the four winds and throughout the heavens. See 1 Thess. 4: 13–18 for the arrival of the dead.
125. John 5: 25, 1 Thess. 4: 16.
126. Matt. 19: 28. Paracelsus bypasses 1 Cor. 6: 2, which gives the saints a role in the judgement of the world.
127. Matt. 25: 31–3 which in German reads sheep and rams/goats, but Paracelsus is more specific about innocent and offensive animals.
128. Commentary on Psalm 103 (104), P II, 5, 18 for smoke as symbol of the majesty of God.
129. 1 Thess. 4: 17 has ascent into the clouds. Matt. 25: 41 has everlasting fire for those on the left, something reserved for Satan and his party by Paracelsus.
130. 2 Peter 3: 7. Also Rev. 20: 10 for the final fate of Satan and his last defeated allies.
131. Matt. 25: 35–40, 42–4.
132. Matt. 25: 46, John 5: 29, Rom. 2: 7.
133. John 14: 2.
134. 2 Peter 3: 10,12,13.
135. Commentary on Psalm 146 (147a), P II, 7, 90–6; Commentary on Psalm 147 (148), P II, 7, 97–105.
136. Commentary on Psalm 146 (147a), P II, 7, 90–1.
137. Commentary on Psalm 147 (148), P II, 7, 97–9.
138. Commentary on Psalm 146 (147a), P II, 7, 90–3; *Astronomia magna*, P I, 12, 135.
139. Dan. 11: 33, 35, 12: 3–4, 10.
140. Dan. 12: 3, *fulgebunt quasi splendor firmamenti; et qui ad iustitiam erudiunt multos, quasi stellae in perpetuas aeternitates.*
141. In Commentary on Daniel, P I, 7, 354–5, referring to Daniel 12: 3, Paracelsus points out that the *heiligen* of Daniel would confound the higher priesthood and

the monarchs, who would be consigned to damnation. For the early Christian period, F.F. Bruce, 'The Book of Daniel and the Qumran Community', in E.E. Ellis and M. Wilcox (eds), *Neotestamentica et Semitica* (Edinburgh, T. and T.Clark, 1969), 221–35; E. Earle Ellis, 'The Role of the Christian Prophet in Acts', in W. Ward Gasque and Ralph P. Martin (eds), *Apostolic History and the Gospel* (Exeter: Paternoster Press, 1970), 55–67.

142. Dan. 12: 4. Commentary on Daniel, P I, 7, 354–5, where Paracelsus identified Daniel's *'zeit der erkantnis'* as *'der zeit Christi'*. For the impact made by this verse on the reformists of the English Revolution, Charles Webster, *The Great Instauration, Science Medicine and Reform, 1626–1660* (London: Duckworth, 1975).

143. Commentary on Daniel, P I, 7, 355.

144. Acts 5: 12, 14: 3.

145. For a representative synopsis indicating fusion of all of these ideas, see the sixth chapter of the first book of the *Astronomia magna*. In the concluding paragraphs Paracelsus pointed to the example of the physician and the magus, who between them were granted the capacity to exploit the full powers intrinsic to the heavens and earth, with respect to both natural and supernatural phenomena. At their most effective they fulfilled the promise of the prophet that humans would gain mastery over the whole of nature (Ps. 8: 6–8, depending on Gen. 1: 26, 28) (*und was die natur vermag, das muß under dem menschen sein*). Such achievement was possible only by reference to the teaching and example of Christ, which meant rejecting books and their dead print, which should be burnt or torn up. Instead, the aspiring magi would turn to the Light of Nature, the living Word that needed to be read with the help of the fiery tongue and the Holy Spirit. Theses were mysterious sources, but nevertheless secure (*der geist geistet*, etc., John 3: 8). Such enlightenment would enable humans to capture all the powers and wisdom from the heavens, so that they would become themselves like stars or comets (*wir das gestirn selbs seient*). Indeed he speculated that such powers were inborn, so that the Magi might in themselves be regarded as the *mysteria* or *magnalia* of God (*diser mensch wird geborn als ein comet*). Such magi would glorify God by their exposition of His wonders and they would help to bring about complete harmony with the Creator. By becoming companions of God, they were equipped with eternal truths and thereby would be able to lead all others to the truth. P I, 12, 135–7.

Conclusions

1. *Liber meteororum*, P I, 13, 153: 'the works of God are divided into two parts, into the works of nature that are the province of philosophy, and the works of Christ that are the concern of theology. We should dedicate the time allotted to us on earth to both of these avocations, so that we may die in contentment.' The same sentiments are expressed in the opening paragraph of his exposition of the fifth commandment, P II, 7, 153–4.

2. See Illustration 8, Emblem from the title-page of Menasseh ben Israel, *Conciliador o de la conviniencia de los lugares de la S. Escriptura, que repugnantes entre si parecen*, Part 2 (Amsterdam: Nicolaes van Ravensteyn, 1641). Although this is taken from a seventeenth-century source, the pilgrimage ideal for the scholar was well established, for instance among the medieval mystics. Paracelsus believed that pilgrimage, laying emphasis on a wandering existence, free from all material constraints, represented the model laid down by Christ as appropriate for those accepting his mission objectives, *BdE*, 52–3; *De felici liberalitate*, P II, 2, 6; *De genealogia Christi*, P II, 3, 102.

SELECT BIBLIOGRAPHY

I. Editions of the Writings of Paracelsus

Abbreviations for these editions used in the Notes are given in brackets at the end of each item. The major editions are cited in chronological order, followed by more specialized collections, texts and digests in a logical order.

Huser, Johannes (ed.), *Erster [-zehender] Theil der Bücher und Schrifften des Edlen ... Philosophi und Medici Philippi Theophrasti Bombast von Hohenheim, Paracelsi genannt, jetzt ... an Tag geben durch Johannem Huserum Brisgoium*, 10 vols (Basel: Conrad Waldkirch, 1589–90). (Huser)

Sudhoff, Karl (ed.), *Theophrast von Hohenheim/ Paracelsus. Sämtliche Werke I. Abteilung. Medizinische, naturwissenschaftliche und philosophische Schriften*, 14 vols (Munich/ Berlin: R. Oldenbourg Verlag, 1922–33). (P I)

Sudhoff, Karl and Wilhelm Matthießen (eds), *Theophrast von Hohenheim/ Paracelsus. Sämtliche Werke II. Abteilung. Die theologischen und religionsphilosophischen Schriften, Erster Band* (Munich: Otto Wilhelm Barth, 1923). (Matthießen)

Goldammer, Kurt (ed.), *Theophrast von Hohenheim/ Paracelsus. Sämtliche Werke II. Abteilung. Theologische und religionsphilosophische Schriften*, vols 2–7 (Wiesbaden: Franz Steiner Verlag, 1955–86). (P II)

Goldammer, Kurt (ed.), *Theophrast von Hohenheim/ Paracelsus. Sämtliche Werke. Theologische und religionsphilosophische Schriften. Supplement. Religiöse und sozial-philosophische Schriften in Kurzfassungen* (Wiesbaden: Franz Steiner Verlag, 1973). (Goldammer, *RSSchr*)

Goldammer, Kurt (ed.), *Paracelsus, Sozialethische und sozialpolitische Schriften. Aus dem theologisch-religionsphilosophischen Werk ausgewält, eingeleitet und mit erklärenden Anmerkungen* (Tübingen: J.C.B. Mohr (Paul Siebeck), 1952). (Goldammer, *SSSchr*)

Karl Sudhoff, *Versuch einer Kritik der Echtheit der Paracelsischen Schriften*, 2 vols (Berlin: Georg Reimer Verlag, 1894–99). (Sudhoff, *Versuch*, I&II)

Goldammer, Kurt (ed.), *Das Buch der Erkanntnus des Theophrast von Hohenheim gen. Paracelsus* (Texte des späten Mittelalters und der frühen Neuzeit, 18) (Berlin: Erich Schmidt Verlag, 1964). (*BdE*)

II. Other Sources

Abramowski, Luise and J.F. Gerhard Goeters (eds), *Studien zur Geschichte und Theologie der Reformation. Festschrift für Ernst Bizer* (Neukirchen-Vluyn: Neukirchener Verlag, 1969).

Andersson, Christiane, 'Popular Imagery in German Reformation Broadsheets', in Tyson and Wagonheim, *Print and Culture in the Renaissance*, 120–50.

Armour, Rollin S., *Anabaptist Baptism. A Representative Study* (Scottdale, PA: Herald Press, 1966).

Arnold, Martin, *Handwerker als theologische Schriftsteller. Studien zu Flugschriften der frühen Reformation (1523–1525)* (Göttingen: Vanderhoeck & Ruprecht, 1990).

Backus, Irena, ' "Corpus-anima-spiritus". Spiritual Renewal in the Theology of Hubmaier and Borrhaus', in Rott and Verheus, *Anabaptistes et dissidents au XVIe siècle*, 121–30.

Baron, Hans, 'The "Querelle" of the Ancients and Moderns as a Problem for Renaissance Scholarship', *Journal of the History of Ideas*, 20 (1959), 3–22.

Barton, Peter Friedrich (ed.), *Sozialrevolution und Reformation. Aufsätze zur Vorreformation, Reformation und zu den 'Bauernkrieg' in Südmitteleuropa* (Studien und Texte zur Kirchengeschichte und Geschichte, 2) (Vienna etc: Böhlau, 1975).

—— *Die Geschichte der Evangelischen in Österreiche* (Jahrbuch für die Geschichte des Protestantismus in Österreiche, 101), (Vienna: Evangelischer Pressverband in Österreiche, 1985).

Baxandall, Michael, *The Limewood Sculptors of Renaissance Germany* (New Haven/ London: Yale University Press, 1981).

Baylor, Michael G., 'Andreas Bodenstein von Karlstadt und der gemeine Mann', in Bubenheimer/Oehmig (eds), *Querdenker*, 251–64.

Baylor, Michael G. (ed.), *The Radical Reformation* (Cambridge: Cambridge University Press, 1991).

Beierwaltes, Werner, 'Neuplatonisches Denken als Substanz der Renaissance', in *Studia Leibnitiana. Sonderheft 7, Magia Naturalis und die Entstehung der Modernen Naturwissenschaften* (Wiesbaden, Franz Steiner Verlag, 1978), 1–16.

—— (ed.), *Platonismus in der Philosophie des Mittelalters* (Darmstadt: Wissenschaftliche Buchhandlung, 1969).

Beissel, Stephan, *Geschichte der Verehrung Marias in Deutschland während des Mittelalters* (Freiburg/ Breisgau: Herdersche Verlagshandlung, 1909).

Benzenhöfer, Udo, 'Zum Brief des Johannes Oporinus über Paracelsus. Die bislang älteste bekannte Briefüberlieferung in einer "Oratio" von Gervasius Marstaller', *Sudhoffs Archiv*, 73 (1989), 55–63.

—— *Paracelsus* (Reinbek, Hamburg: Rowohlt, 1997).

Benzing, Josef, 'Bibliographie der Schriften des Colmarer Arztes Lorenz Fries', *Philobiblion*, 6 (1962), 121–40.

Bergdolt, Klaus, *Arzt, Krankheit und Therapie bei Petrarca* (Weinheim: VCH Verlaggesellschaft, 1992).

—— and Walther Ludwig (eds), *Zukunftsvoraussagen in der Renaissance* (Wiesbaden: Harrassowitz Verlag, 2005).

Bianchi, Massimo Luigi, *Signatura rerum. Segni, magia e conoscenza da Paracelso a Leibniz* (Rome: Edizioni dell'Ateneo, 1987).

Biegger, Katharina, *'De invocatione beatae Mariae virginis'. Paracelsus und die Marienverehrung* (Stuttgart: Franz Steiner Verlag, 1990).

Bittel, Karl, 'Die Elsässer Zeit des Paracelsus. Hohenheims Wirken in Straßburg und Kolmar, sowie seine Beziehungen zu Lorenz Fries', *Elsasser-Lothringisches Jahrbuch*, 21 (1943–44), 157–86.

Blanke, Fritz, 'Reformation und Alkoholismus', *Zwingliana*, 9 (1949), 75–89.

Blaser, Robert-Henri, *Paracelsus in Basel* (St Arbogast: Verlag Muttenz, 1979).
Blickle, Peter, *Gemeindereformation. Die Menschen des 16. Jahrhunderts auf dem Weg zum Heil. Studienausgabe* (Munich: R. Oldenbourg, 1985).
—— *Die Revolution von 1525*, 4th edn (Munich: R. Oldenbourg, 2004).
—— *Die Reformation im Reich*, 3rd edn (Stuttgart: UTB, 2000).
Bonorand, Conradin, 'Joachim Vadian und die Täufer', *Schweizer Beiträge zur Allgemeinen Geschichte*, 11 (1953), 43–72.
Brady, Thomas A. Jr. and Elisabeth Müller-Luckner (eds), *Die deutsche Reformation zwischen Spätmittelalter und Früher Neuzeit* (Munich: R. Oldenbourg, 2001).
Brady, Thomas A. Jr., Heiko A. Oberman, and James D. Tracy (eds), *Handbook of European History 1400–1600*, 2 vols (Leiden: Brill, 1995).
Bräuer, Siegfried and Helmar Junghans (eds), *Der Theologe Thomas Müntzer. Untersuchungen zu seiner Entwicklung und Lehre* (Göttingen: Vandenhoeck & Ruprecht, 1989).
Brecht, Martin, 'Die Predigt des Simon Haferitz zum Fest der heiligen drei Könige 1524 in Allstedt' (1991), in Martin Brecht, *Ausgewälte Aufsätze*, vol. 1 (Stuttgart: Calwer Verlag, 1995), 300–11.
Brunner, Walter, 'Aufrührer wider Willen. Beiträge zur Geschichte der Aufstandsbewegung des Jahres 1525 in oberen Murtal', *Mitteilungen des steiermarkisches Landesarchiv*, 48 (1998), 143–236.
Bubenheimer, Ulrich, *Thomas Müntzer. Herkunft und Bildung* (Leiden: Brill, 1989).
—— 'Thomas Müntzer und der Humanismus', in Bräuer and Junghans, *Der Theologe Thomas Müntzer*, 302–28.
—— and Stefan Oehmig (eds), *Querdenker der Reformation – Andreas Bodenstein von Karlstadt und seine frühe Wirkung* (Würzburg: Religion und Kultur Verlag, 2001).
Buck, August, *Die Rezeption der Antike in den romanischen Literaturen der Renaissance* (Berlin: Erich Schmidt Verlag, 1976).
Bücking, Jürgen, *Michael Gaismair, Reformer, Sozialrebell und Revolutionär* (Stuttgart: Klett-Cotta, 1978).
Chrisman, Miriam U., *Lay Culture, Learned Culture. Books and Social Change in Strasbourg 1480–1599* (New Haven, CT: Yale University Press, 1982).
—— *Conflicting Visions of Reform. German Lay Propaganda Pamphlets, 1519–1530* (Atlantic Highlands, NJ: Humanities Press, 1996).
Clasen, Claus-Peter, *Anabaptism. A Social History, (1525–1618)* (Ithaca, NY: Cornell University Press).
Cornette, James C. Jr., *Proverbs and Proverbial Expressions in the German Works of Martin Luther*, ed. Wolfgang Mieder and Dorothee Racette (Berne: Peter Lang, 1997).
Cranefield, P.F. and W. Federn, 'The Begetting of Fools. An Annotated Translation of Paracelsus, *De generatione stultorum*', *Bulletin of the History of Medicine*, 41 (1967), 56–74, 161–74.
Dan, Joseph (ed.), *The Christian Kabbalah: Jewish Mystical Books and their Christian Interpreters* (Cambridge, MA: Harvard College Library, Harvard University Press, 1997).
Daniel, Dane Thor, 'Paracelsus – die Sakramentenlehre und das Verhältnis von Religion und Naturwissenschaften in der wissenschaftlichen Revolution', *Manuskripte, Thesen, Informationen der Deutschen Bombastus-Gesellschaft*, 16 (2000), 17–26.
—— 'Paracelsus' *Declaratio* on the Lord's Supper. A Summary with Remarks on the Term Limbus', *Nova Acta Paracelsica*, N.F. 16 (2002), 141–62.
—— 'Paracelsus on the Lord's Supper: *Coena Dominj Nostrj Jhesu Christj Declaratio*. A Transcription of the Leiden Codex Voss.Chym. fol. 24, f.12r–29v', *Nova Acta Paracelsica*, N.F. 16 (2002), 107–39.
—— 'Paracelsus on Baptism and the Acquiring of the Eternal Body', in Williams and Gunnoe, *Paracelsian Moments*, 117–34.

—— 'Invisible Wombs: Rethinking Paracelsus's Concept of Body and Matter', *Ambix*, 53 (2006), 129–42.

Deppermann, Klaus, *Melchior Hoffman. Soziale Unruhen und apocalyptische Visionen im Zeitalter der Reformation* (Göttingen: Vandenhoeck & Ruprecht, 1979).

Dilg, Peter and Hartmut Rudolph (eds), *Resultate und Desiderata der Paracelsus-Forschung* (Sudhoffs Archiv, Beiheft 31), (Stuttgart: Franz Steiner Verlag, 1993).

Dilg-Frank, Rosemarie (ed.), *Kreatur und Kosmos. Internationale Beiträge zur Paracelsus-forschung* (*Medizinhistorisches Journal*, 16 (1981), Heft 1/2), (Stuttgart: Gustav Fischer, 1981).

Dopsch, Heinz, 'Bauernkrieg und Glaubensspaltung', in Dopsch and Hans Spatzenegger, *Geschichte Salzburgs. Stadt und Land. II, 1* (Salzburg: Universitätsverlag Anton Pustet, 1988), 11–83.

—— and Peter F. Kramml (eds), *Paracelsus und Salzburg. Vorträge bei den Internationalen Kongressen in Salzburg und Badgastein anläßlich des Paracelsus-Jahres 1993* (Mitteilungen der Gesellschaft für Salzburger Landeskunde, 14), (Salzburg: Gesellschaft für Salzburger Landeskunde, 1994).

Dykema, Peter A. and Heiko A. Oberman (eds), *Anticlericalism in Late Medieval and Early Modern Europe* (Leiden: Brill, 1993).

Edwards, Marc U. Jr., *Printing, Propaganda, and Martin Luther* (Berkeley, CA: California University Press, 1994).

Egerding, Michael, *Die Metaphorik der Spätmittelalterlichen Mystik.Bd.II* (Paderborn etc: Ferdinand Schöningh, 1997).

Enders, Ludwig (ed.), *Johann Eberlin von Günzburg, Ausgewählte Schriften*, 3 vols, (Halle: Max Niemeyer, 1896–1902).

Erb, Peter C., *Schwenckfeld and Early Schwenckfeldianism* (Pennsburg, PA: Schwenckfelder Library, 1986).

Farmer, Stephen Alan, *Syncretism in the West: Pico's 900 Theses (1486). The Evolution of Traditional Religious and Philosophical Systems* (Tempe, AZ: Medieval & Renaissance Texts & Studies, 1998).

Felici, Lucia, *Tra riforma ed eresia. La giovinezza di Martin Borrhaus (1499–1526)* (Florence: Olschki, 1995).

Florey, Gerhard, 'Sozialrevolution und Reformation im Erzstift Salzburg', in Barton, *Sozialrevolution und Reformation*, 42–61.

Franz, Adolf, *Die kirchlichen Benediktionen im Mittelalter* (Freiburg/Breisgau: Herdersche Verlagshandlung, 1909).

Franz, Günther, *Der Deutsche Bauernkrieg*, 2 vols (Munich: R. Oldenbourg, 1935).

—— (ed.), *Quellen zur Geschichte des Bauernkrieges* (Munich: R. Oldenbourg, 1963.

—— (ed.), *Thomas Müntzer. Schriften und Briefe. Kritische Gesamtausgabe* (Gütersloh: Gütersloher Verlagshaus Gerd Mohn, 1968).

Friedmann, Robert, 'The Nicolsburg Articles: A Problem of Early Anabaptist History', *Church History*, 36 (1967), 391–409.

Friesen, Abraham, *Thomas Muentzer, a Destroyer of the Godless. The Making of a Sixteenth Century Religious Revolutionary* (Berkeley etc., CA: University of California Press, 1990).

—— *Erasmus, the Anabaptists, and the Great Commission* (Grand Rapids, MI: Eerdmans Publishing, 1998).

Furcha, Edward J. (ed.), *The Essential Carlstadt* (Waterloo, Ontario/ Scottdale, PA: Herald Press, 1995).

Fussler, Jean-Pierre, *Les Idées éthiques, sociales et politiques de Paracelse (1493–1541) et leur fondement* (Strasbourg: Association des Publications près les Universités de Strasbourg, 1986).

Ganzenmüller, Wilhelm, 'Das Buch der heiligen Dreifaltigkeit', *Archiv für Kulturgeschichte*, 29 (1939), 93–146.

—— 'Paracelsus und die Alchemie des Mittelalters', *Ausgewandte Chemie*, 54 (1941), 427–31.

Garin, Eugenio (ed.), *G. Pico della Mirandola. De hominis dignitate, Heptaplus, De Ente et Uno* (Florence: Vallecchi Editore, 1942).

Gause, Ute, 'Zum Frauenbild im Frühwerk des Paracelsus', in Telle, *Parerga Paracelsica*, 45–56.

—— *Paracelsus (1493–1541). Genese und Entfaltung seiner frühen Theologie* (Tübingen: J.C.B. Mohr (Paul Siebeck), 1993).

—— 'Aspekte der theologischen Anthropologie des Paracelsus', in Peter Dilg and Rudolph, *Neue Beiträge zur Paracelsus-Forschung Hartmut* (Stuttgart: Akademie der Diözese Rottenburg/Stuttgart, 1995), 59–70.

—— 'Paracelsische Erkenntnistheorie in den frühen Theologica und in der "Astronomia Magna"', *Salzburger Vorträge 1996* (Salzburger Beiträge zur Paracelsusforschung, 30) (Vienna: Verband der wissenshaftlichen Gesellschaften Österreichs, 1997), 99–115.

—— 'On Paracelsus' Epistemology in his Early Theological Writings and in his "Astronomia Magna"', in Grell, *Paracelsus*, 207–21.

—— 'Paracelsus und Jesus Christus. Paracelsus als theologischer Denker zwischen Reformation und radikalem Individualismus', *Manuskripte, Thesen, Informationen. Herausgegeben von der Deutschen Bombastus-Gesellschaft*, 15 (2000), 4–15.

—— 'Einleitung zu Paracelsus, Die sieben Punkte des christlichen Götzendienstes', in Theodor Strohm and Michael Klein (eds), *Die Entstehung einer sozialen Ordnung Europas, Bd. 1: Historische Studien und exemplarische Beiträge zur Sozialreform im 16. Jahrhundert* (Heidelberg: Universitätsverlag Carl Winter, 2004), 256–65.

Gensthaler, Gerhard, *Das Medizinalwesen in der Freien Reichstadt Augsburg bis zum 16 Jahrhundert* (Augsburg: H. Mühlburger, 1973).

Gilly, Carlos, 'Zwischen Erfahrung und Spekulation. Theodor Zwinger und die religiöse und kulturelle Krise seiner Zeit', *Basler Zeitschrift für Geschichte und Altertumskunde*, Part I, 77 (1977), 57–137; Part II, 79 (1979), 125–223.

—— 'Das Sprichwort "Die gelehrten die verkehrten" oder der Verrat der Intellektuellen im Zeitalter der Glaubensspaltung', in Rotondò, *Forme e destinazione del messaggio religioso*, 229–375.

—— ' "Theophrastia Sancta". Der Paracelsismus als Religion im Streit mit den offiziellen Kirchen', in Telle, *Analecta Paracelsica*, 426–88.

Gilmont, Jean-François (ed.), *The Reformation and the Book* (Aldershot: Ashgate, 1998).

Ginsberg, Carlo, *Il nicodemismo. Simulazione e dissimulazione religiosa nel Europa del '500* (Turin: Einaudi, 1970).

Gnädinger, Louise, *Johannes Tauler Lebenswelt und mystische Lehre* (Munich: C.H. Beck, 1993).

Goertz, Hans-Jürgen, *Innere und äussere Ordnung in der Theologie Thomas Müntzers* (Leiden: Brill, 1967).

—— *Pfaffenhaß und groß Geschrei. Die reformatorischen Bewegungen in Deutschland 1517–1529* (Munich: C.H. Beck, 1987).

—— *Die Täufer. Geschichte und Deutung*, 2nd edn (Munich: C.H. Beck, 1988).

—— '"What a tangled and tenuous mess the clergy is!" Clerical Anticlericalism in the Reformation Period', in Dykema and Oberman, *Anticlericalism*, 499–519.

—— 'Brüderlichkeit – Provokation, Maxime, Utopie. Ansätze einer fraternitären Gesellschaft in der Reformationszeit', in Schmidt, Holenstein and Würgler, *Gemeinde, Reformation und Widerstand*, 161–78.

—— '"A Common Future Conversation": A Revisionist Interpretation of the September 1524 Grebbel Letters to Thomas Müntzer', in Packull and Dipple, *Radical Reformation Studies*, 73–90.

—— 'Die Radikalität reformatorischer Bewegungen. Plädoyer für ein kulturgeschichtliches Konzept', in Goertz and Stayer, *Radikalität und Dissent*, 29–42.

—— (ed.), *Umstrittenes Täufertum: 1525–1975. Neue Forschungen* (Göttingen: Vandenhoeck & Ruprecht, 1975).

—— (ed.), *Radikale Reformatoren. 21 biographische Skizzen von Thomas Müntzer bis Paracelsus* (Munich: C.H. Beck, 1978).

—— and James M. Stayer (eds), *Radikalität und Dissent im 16. Jahrhundert/Radicalism and Dissent in the Sixteenth Century* (Berlin: Duncker & Humblot, 2002).

Goeters, J.F. Gerhard, 'Die Vorgeschichte des Täufertums in Zürich', in Abramowski and Goeters, *Studien zur Geschichte und Theologie der Reformation*, 239–81.

Götze, Alfred and Hans Volz (eds), *Frühneuhochdeutsche Lesebuch*, 5th edn (Göttingen: Vandenhoeck & Ruprecht, 1968).

Goldammer, Kurt, *Paracelsus. Natur und Offenbarung* (Hannover-Kirchrode: Theodor Oppermann Verlag, 1953).

—— *Paracelsus in neuen Horizonten. Gesammelte Aufsätze* (Salzburger Beiträge zur Paracelsusforschung, 24) (Vienna: Verband der wissenshaftlichen Gesellschaften Österreichs, 1986).

—— *Der Göttliche Magier und die Magierin Natur. Religion, Naturmagie und die Anfänge der Naturwissenschaft vom Spätmittelalter bis zur Renaissance. Mit Beiträgen zum Magie-Verständnis des Paracelsus* (Kosmosophie. Forschungen und Texte zur Geschichte des Weltbildes etc., 5), (Stuttgart: Franz Steiner Verlag, 1991).

Grell, Ole Peter (ed.), *Paracelsus. The Man and his Reputation, his Ideas and their Transformation* (Studies in the History of Christian Thought, 85) (Leiden: Brill, 1998).

Haas, Alois M., *Der Kampf um den Heilige-Geist. Luther und die Schwärmer* (Freiburg/Schweiz: Universitäts Verlag, 1997).

Habermann, Mechthild, *Deutsche Fachtexte der frühen Neuzeit. Naturkundlich-medizinische Wissensvermittlung im Spannungsfeld von Latein und Volkssprache* (Berlin, etc.: Walter de Gruyter, 2001).

Hamm, Berndt, 'Laienthologie zwischen Luther und Zwingli', in Nolte, Tompert and Windhorst, *Kontinuität und Umbruck*, 222–332.

—— 'Geistbegabte gegen Geistlose: Typen des pneumatologischen Antiklerikalismus – zur Vielfalt der Luther-Rezeption in der frühen Reformationsbewegung (vor 1525)', in Dykema and Oberman, *Anticlericalism*, 379–440.

—— Bernd Moeller and Dorothea Wendebourg, *Reformationstheorien. Ein kirchenhistorischer Disput über Einheit und Vielfalt der Reformation* (Göttingen: Vandenhoeck & Ruprecht, 1995).

Harder, Leland (ed.), *The Sources of Swiss Anabaptism. The Grebel Letters and Related Documents* (Scottdale, PA: Herald Press, 1985).

Harmening, Dieter, *Superstitio. Überlieferungs- und theoriegeschichtliche Untersuchungen zur kirchlich-theologischen Aberglaubensliteratur des Mittelalters* (Berlin: Erich Schmitt Verlag, 1979).

Hasse, Hans-Peter, *Karlstadt und Tauler.Untersuchungen zur Kreuzestheologie* (Gütersloh: Gütersloher Verlagshaus Gerd Mohn, 1993).

—— '"Von mir selbs nicht halden". Beobachtungen zum Selbstverständnis des Andreas Bodenstein von Karlstadt', in Bubenheimer and Oehmig, *Querdenker*, 49–73.

Helm, Jürgen, 'Protestant and Catholic Medicine in the Sixteenth Century? The Case of Ingolstadt Anatomy', *Medical History*, 45 (2001), 83–96.

Helmrath, Johannes, Ulrich Muhlack and Gerrit Walther (eds), *Diffusion des Humanismus. Studien zur nationalen Geschichtsschreibung europäischer Humanisten* (Göttingen: Walstein Verlag, 2002).

Hertzsch, Erich (ed.), *Karlstadts Schriften aus den Jahren 1523–1525*, 2 vols (Halle: Max Niemeyer, 1956–57).

Hess, Günter, *Deutsch-lateinische Narrenzunft. Studien zum Verhältnis von Volkssprache und Latinität in der satirischen Literatur des 16 Jahrhunderts* (Münchener Texte und Untersuchungen zur deutschen Literatur des Mittelalters, 41) Munich: C.H. Beck, 1971.

Hillerbrand, Hans J. (ed.), *Radical Tendencies in the Reformation* (Kirksville, MO: Sixteenth Century Journal Publishers, 1988).

Hofacker, Hans-Georg, '*Vom alten und nüen Gott, Glauben und Ler*. Untersuchungen zum Geschichtsverständnis und Epochenbewußtsein einer anonymen reformatorischen Flugschrift', in Nolte, Tompert and Windhorst, *Kontinuität und Umbruch*, 145–77.

Hohenberger, Thomas, *Lutherische Rechtfertigungslehre in den reformatorischen Flugschriften der Jahre 1521–22* (Tübingen: J.C.B. Mohr (Paul Siebeck), 1996).

Hoyer, Siegfried, 'Die Zwickauer Storchianer–Vorläufer der Täufer?', in Rott and Verheus, *Anabaptistes et dissidents au XVIe siècle*, 65–84.

—— 'Lay Preaching and Radicalism in the Early Reformation', in Hillerbrand (ed.), *Radical Tendencies*, 85–98.

Idel, Moshe, 'The Magical and Neoplatonic Interpretations of the Kabbalah in the Renaissance', in Bernard Dov Cooperman, *Jewish Thought in the Sixteenth Century* (Cambridge, MA: Harvard University Press, 1983), 186–242.

—— 'Jewish Magic from the Renaissance Period to Early Hasidism', in Jacob Neusner, Ernest A. Frerichs, and Paul V. McC. Flesher, *Religion, Science and Magic. In Concert and in Conflict* (New York, etc.: Oxford University Press, 1987), 82–117.

—— *Absorbing Perfections. Kabbalah and Interpretation* (New Haven, CT: Yale University Press, 2002).

Joest, Wilfried, *Ontologie der Person bei Luther* (Göttingen: Vandenhoeck & Ruprecht, 1967).

Kaiser, Jürgen, *Ruhe der Seele und Siegel der Hoffnung. Die Deutungen des Sabbats in der Reformation* (Göttingen: Vandenhoeck & Ruprecht, 1996).

Kämmerer, Ernst Wilhlem, *Das Leib–Seele–Geist–Problem dei Paracelsus und einigen Autoren des 17. Jahrhunderts* (Kosmosophie. Forschungen und Texte zur Geschichte des Weltbildes etc., 3), (Wiesbaden: Franz Steiner Verlag, 1971).

Karant-Nunn, Susan C., *The Reformation of Ritual. An Interpretation of Early Modern Germany* (London: Routledge, 1997).

Klaassen, Walter, *Living at the End of the Ages. Apocalyptic Expectation in the Radical Reformation* (Lanham: University Press of America, 1992).

Klein, Michael, 'Geschichtsdenken und Ständekritik in apokalyptischer Perspektive. Martin Luthers Meinungs- und Wissensbildung zur "Türkenfrage"', doctoral dissertation, FernUniversität Hagen, 2004.

Koch, Josef, 'Augustinische und dionysischer Neuplatonismus im Mittelalter', in Beierwaltes, *Platonismus in der Philosophie des Mittelalters*, 317–42.

Koepplin, Dieter and Tilman Falk, *Lukas Cranach. Gemälde, Zeichnungen, Druckgraphik* (Basel/Stuttgart: Birkhäuser Verlag, 1976).

Köhler, Hans-Joachim (ed.), *Flugschriften als Massenmedium der Reformationszeit* (Stuttgart: Klett-Cotta, 1981).

—— Hildegard Hebenstreit-Wilfert and Christoph Weismann, *Flugschriften des frühen 16. Jahrhunderts* (Zug/Schweiz: IDC, 1978–87).

Könneker, Barbara, *Wesen und Wandlung der Narrenidee im Zeitalter des Humanismus. Brant-Murner-Erasmus* (Wiesbaden: Franz Steiner Verlag, 1966).

Krause, Armin, *Zur Sprache des Reformators Andreas Bodenstein von Karlstadt. Untersuchungen zum Einfluß von Verstehens- und Sprachtraditionen auf die Ausprägung individuellen Sprach- und Schriftverständnisses, Sprachverhaltens und die Bedeutung ausgewählter Schlüsselwörter der Reformationszeit* (Stuttgarter Arbeiten zur Germanistik, 236) (Stuttgart: H-D. Heinz, 1990).

Kroon, Marrijn de and Friedhelm Krüger (eds), *Bucer und seine Zeit* (Wiesbaden: Franz Steiner Verlag, 1976).

Kühlmann, Wilhelm and Joachim Telle (eds), *Der Frühparacelsismus. Erster Teil* (Tübingen: Max Niemeyer Verlag, 2001).

Kuhn, Michael, *De nomine et vocabulo. Der Begriff der medizinischen Fachsprache und die Krankheitsnamen bei Paracelsus (1493–1541)* (Heidelberg: Universitätsverlag C. Winter, 1996).

Künast, Hans-Jörg, *'Getruckt zu Augspurg'. Buchdruck und Buchhandel in Augsburg zwischen 1468 und 1555* (Tübingen: Max Niemeyer Verlag, 1997).

Kurze, Dietrich, 'Prophecy and History. Lichtenberger's Forecasts of Events to Come … their Reception and Diffusion', *Journal of the Warburg and Courtauld Institutes*, 21 (1958), 63–85.

—— 'Nationale Regungen in der spätmittelalterlichen Prophetie', *Historische Zeitschrift*, 202 (1966), 1–23.

—— 'Popular Astrology and Prophecy in the Fifteenth and Sixteenth Centuries', in Zambelli, *'Astrologi hallucinati'*, 177–93.

—— *Johannes Lichtenberger. Eine Studie zur Geschichte der Prophetie und Astrologie* (Historische Studien, Heft 379) (Lübeck, etc.: Matthiesen, 1960).

Laube, Adolf, 'Die Reformation als soziale Bewegung', *Zeitschrift für Geschichtswissenschaft*, 33 (1985), 421–41.

—— 'Radicalism as a Research Problem in the History of the Early Reformation', in Hillerbrand, *Radical Tendencies in the Reformation*, 9–24.

—— Annerose Schneider and Sigrid Looß (eds), *Flugschriften der frühen Reformationsbewegung (1518–1524)*, 2 vols (Vaduz, Liechtenstein/Berlin: Topos/Akademie Verlag, 1983).

—— Annerose Schneider and Ulman Weiß (eds), *Flugschriften vom Bauernkrieg zum Täuferreich (1526–1535)* (Berlin: Akademie-Verlag, 1992).

—— and Hans Werner Seiffert (eds), *Flugschriften der Bauernkriegszeit* (Berlin: Akademie-Verlag, 1975).

Lerner, Robert E., 'Medieval Prophecy and Religious Dissent', *Past and Present*, 72 (1976), 3–24.

—— 'Refreshment of the Saints: The Time after Antichrist as a Station for Earthly Progress in Medieval Thought', *Traditio*, 32 (1976), 97–144.

—— *The Power of Prophecy. The Cedar of Lebanon Vision from the Mongol Onslaught to the Dawn of the Enlightenment* (Berkeley, CA: University of California Press, 1983).

—— 'The Medieval Return to the Thousand-Year Sabbath', in Richard K. Emmerson and Bernard McGinn (eds), *The Apocalypse in the Middle Ages* (Ithaca, etc., NY: Cornell University Press, 1992), 51–71.

Libera, Alain de, *La Mystique Rhénane d'Albert le Grand à Maître Eckhart* (Paris: Éditions du Seuil, 1994).

—— *Eckhart, Suso, Tauler, ou la divinisation de l'homme* (Paris: Éditions Bayard, 1996).

Lienhard, Marc, 'La Percée du mouvement évangélique à Strasbourg: Le rôle et la figure de Mathieu Zell (1477–1548)', in Livet and Rapp, *Strasbourg au Coeur Religieux*, 85–98.

—— and Jean Rott, 'Die Anfänge der evangelischen Predigt in Strassburg und ihr erstes Manifest', in Kroon and Krüger (eds), *Bucer und seine Zeit*, 54–73.

List, Günther, *Chiliastische Utopie und Radikale Reformation. Die Erneuerung der Idee vom tausende-jährigen Reich im 16. Jahrhundert* (Munich: Wilhelm Fink Verlag, 1973).

Livet, Georges and Francis Rapp (eds), *Strasbourg au coeur religieux du XVIe siècle. Hommage à Lucien Febvre* (Strasbourg: Librairie Istra, 1977).

Looß, Sigrid, 'Reformatorische Ideologie und Praxis im Dienst des Rates und der Bürgerschaft Straßburgs', *Jahrbuch für Geschichte des Feudalismus*, 5 (1981), 255–90.

Luh, Peter, *Kaiser Maximilian gewidmet. Die unvollendete Werkausgabe des Conrad Celtis und ihre Holzschnitte* (Bern, etc.: Peter Lang, 2001).

Maclean, Ian, *Logic, Signs and Nature in the Renaissance. The Case of Learned Medicine* (Cambridge: Cambridge University Press, 2002).

McGinn, Bernard, *The Mystical Thought of Meister Eckhart* (New York: The Crossroad Publishing Company, 2001).

McLaughlin, R. Emmet, 'Schwenckfeld and the South German Eucharistic Controversy, 1526–1529', in Erb, *Schwenckfeld and Early Schwenckfeldianism*, 181–210.

—— 'The Schwenckfeld–Vadian Debate', in Erb, *Schwenckfeld and Early Schwenckfeldianism*, 237–58.

—— *Caspar Schwenckfeld. Reluctant Radical. His Life to 1540* (New Haven, CT: Yale University Press, 1986).

Matheson, Peter (ed.), *The Collected Works of Thomas Müntzer* (Edinburgh: T. and T. Clark, 1988).

Mau, Rudolph, 'Gott und Schöpfung bei Thomas Müntzer', in Bräuer and Junghans, *Der Theologe Thomas Müntzer*, 11–32.

Mecenseffy, Grete, *Österreich, III* (Quellen zur Geschichte der Täufer, XIV) (Gütersloh: Gütersloher Verlagshaus Gerd Mohn, 1968).

Meier, Pirmin, *Paracelsus. Arzt und Prophet*, 3rd edn (Zürich: Amman Verlag, 1993).

Midelfort, Erik H.C., 'The Anthropological Roots of Paracelsus' Psychiatry', in Dilg-Frank, *Kreatur und Kosmos*, 67–77.

—— *A History of Madness in Sixteenth-Century Germany* (Stanford, CA: Stanford University Press, 1999).

Miller-Guinsberg, Arlene, 'Paracelsian Magic and Theology. A Case Study of the Matthew Commentaries', in Dilg-Frank, *Kreatur und Kosmos*, 125–39.

Müller, Jan-Dirk, 'Buchstabe, Geist, Subjekt: Zu einer frühneuzeitlichen Problemfigur bei Sebastian Franck', *MLN*, 106 (1991), 648–74.

—— (ed.), *Sebastian Franck (1499–1542)* (Wolfenbütteler Forschungen, 56), (Wiesbaden: Harrassowitz Verlag, 1993).

Müller, Lydia (ed.), *Glaubenszeugnisse oberdeutscher Taufgesinnter, I.* (Quellen und Forschungen zur Reformationsgeschichte, 20) (Leipzig: M. Heinsius Nachfolger, 1938).

Müller-Jahncke, Wolf-Dieter, *Astrologisch-magische Theorie und Praxis in der Heilkunde der frühen Neuzeit* (Sudhoffs Archiv, Beiheft 25) (Stuttgart: Franz Steiner Verlag, 1985).

Nolte, Josef, Hella Tompert and Christof Windhorst (eds), *Kontinuität und Umbruch. Theologie und Frömmigkeit in Flugschriften und Kleinliteratur an der Wende vom 15. zum 16. Jahrhundert* (Stuttgart: Klett-Cotta, 1978).

Overfeld, James H., *Humanism and Scholasticism in Late Medieval Germany* (Princeton, NJ: Princeton University Press, 1984).

Ozment, Steven E., *Homo spiritualis. A Comparative Study of the Anthropology of [Tauler, Gerson and Luther] in the Context of their Theological Thought* (Leiden: Brill, 1969).

—— *Mysticism and Dissent. Religious Ideology and Social Protest in the Sixteenth Century* (New Haven, CT: Yale University Press, 1973).

—— *The Reformation in the Cities* (New Haven, CT: Yale University Press, 1980).

Packull, Werner O., *Mysticism and the Early South German–Austrian Anabaptist Movement 1525–1531* (Scottdale, PA: Herald Press, 1977).

—— 'Die Anfäng des Schweizer Täufertums im Gefüge der Reformation des Gemeinen Mannes', in Rott and Verheus, *Anabaptistes et dissidents au XVIe siècle*, 53–64.

—— *Hutterite Beginnings. Communitarian Experiments during the Reformation* (Baltimore, MD: Johns Hopkins University Press, 1995).

—— 'In Search of the "Common Man" in Early German Anabaptist Ideology', *Sixteenth Century Journal*, 17 (1986), 51–67.

—— and Geoffrey L. Dipple (eds), *Radical Reformation Studies. Essays Presented to James M. Stayer* (Aldershot: Ashgate, 1999).

Pagel, Walter, *Paracelsus. An Introduction to Philosophical Medicine in the Era of the Renaissance* (Basel: Karger, 1958); second revised edn (Basel: Karger, 1982).

—— 'Paracelsus and Techellus the Jew', *Bulletin of the History of Medicine*, 34 (1960), 274–7.

—— 'Paracelsus and the Neoplatonic and Gnostic Tradition', *Ambix*, 8 (1960), 125–66.

—— 'The Prime Matter of Paracelsus', *Ambix*, 9 (1961), 117–35.

—— *Das medizinische Weltbild des Paracelsus. Seine Zusammenhäng mit Neuplatonismus und Gnosis* (Kosmosophie. Forschungen und Texte zur Geschichte des Weltbildes, etc., 1) (Wiesbaden: Franz Steiner Verlag, 1962).

—— 'Paracelsus' äetheränliche Substanzen und ihre pharmakologische Auswertung an Hühnern. Sprachgebauch (*Henbane*) und Konrad von Megenbergs *Buch der Natur* als mögliche Quellen', *Gesnerus*, 21 (1964), 113–25.

—— 'Das Rätsel der "Acht Mütter" im Paracelsischen Corpus', *Sudhoffs Archiv*, 59 (1975), 254–66.

—— 'The Paracelsian Elias Artista and the Alchemical Tradition', *Medizinhistorisches Journal*, 16 (1981), 6–19.

—— and Marianne Winder, 'Gnostisches bei Paracelsus und Konrad von Megenburg', in *Fachliteratur des Mittelalters. Festschrift für Gerard Eis* (Stuttgart: Metzler, 1968), 359–71.

—— 'The Eightness of Adam and Related "Gnostic" Ideas in the Paracelsian Corpus', *Ambix*, 16 (1969), 119–39.

—— 'The Higher Elements and Prime Matter in Renaissance Naturalism and in Paracelsus', *Ambix*, 21 (1974), 93–127.

Panofsky, Erwin, *Studies in Iconology. Humanistic Themes in the Art of the Renaissance* (New York: Oxford University Press, 1939).

—— *The Life and Art of Albrecht Dürer*, 4th edn (Princeton, NJ: Princeton University Press, 1955).

Pelling, Margaret, *Medical Conflicts in Early Modern London. Patronage, Physicians, and Irregular Practitioners, 1550–1640* (Oxford: Clarendon Press, 2003).

Peuckert, Will-Erich, *Die grosse Wende. Das apocalyptische Saeculum und Luther. Geistgeschichte und Volkskunde* (Hamburg: Claasen & Goverts, 1948).

Rau, Horst Dieter, *Das Bild des Antichrist im Mittelalter. Von Tyconius zum deutschen Symbolismus* (Münster: Aschendorff, 1973).

Reeves, Marjorie, *The Influence of Prophecy in the Later Middle Ages* (Oxford: Clarendon Press, 1969).

Reuchlin, Johann, *On the Art of the Kabbalah*, trans. and ed. Martin and Sarah Goodman (Lincoln, NE: University of Nebraska Press, 1993).

Rhein, Stefan, 'Vergil oder die "Königskerze": War Paracelsus ein Humanist?', *Nova Acta Paracelsica*, NF 7 (1993), 45–71.

Robert, Jörg, *Konrad Celtis und das Projekt der deutschen Dichtung. Studien zur humanistischen Konstitution von Poetik, Philosophie, Nation und Ich* (Tübingen: Max Niemeyer Verlag, 2003).

Rogge, Joachim, *Der Beitrag des Predigers Jakob Strauß zur frühen Reformationsgeschichte* (Berlin: Evangelische Verlagsanstalt, 1957).

Rosner, Edwin, 'Hohenheims Bergsuchtmonographie', in Dilg-Frank, *Kreatur und Kosmos*, 20–52.

—— 'Studien zum Leben und Wirken des Paracelsus in St Gallen', *Nova Acta Paracelsica*, N.F. 3 (1988), 32–54.

Rotondò, Antonio (ed.), *Forme e destinazione del messaggio religioso. Aspetti della propaganda religiosa nel cinquecento* (Florence: Olschki, 1991).

Rott, Jean-Georges and Simon L. Verheus (eds), *Anabaptistes et dissidents au XVIe siècle* (Baden-Baden: Valentin Koerner, 1987).

Rublack, Ulinka, *Reformation Europe* (Cambridge: Cambridge University Press, 2005).

Rudolph, Hartmut, 'Theophrast von Hohenheim (Paracelsus): Arzt und Apostel der neuen Kreatur', in Goertz, *Radikale Reformatoren*, 231–42.

—— 'Kosmosspekulation und Trinitätslehre. Ein Beitrag zur Beziehung zwischen Weltbild und Praxis in der Heilkunde der frühen Neuzeit', in *Paracelsus in der Tradition* (Salzburger Beiträge zur Paracelsusforschung, 21) (Vienna: Verband der wissenschaftlichen Gesellschaften Österrreich, 1980), 32–47.

—— 'Einige Gesichtspunkte zum Thema "Paracelsus und Luther"', *Archiv für Reformationsgeschichte*, 78 (1981), 34–53.

—— 'Schriftauslegung und Schriftverständnis bei Paracelsus', in Dilg-Frank, *Kreatur und Kosmos*, 101–24.

—— 'Individuum und Obrigkeit bei Paracelsus', *Nova Acta Paracelsica*, NF 3 (1988), 69–76.

—— 'Paracelsus' Laientheologie in traditionsgeschichtlicher Sicht und in ihrer Zuordnung zu Reformation und katholischer Reform', in Dilg and Rudolph, *Resultate und Desiderata*, 79–98.

—— 'Hohenheim's Anthropology in the Light of his Writings on the Eucharist', in Grell, *Paracelsus*, 187–206.

Ruh, Kurt, *Geschichte der abendländischen Mystik*, vol. 3 (Munich: Verlag C.H. Beck, 1996).

—— (ed.), *Altdeutsche und altniederländische Mystik* (Darmstadt: Wissenshaftliche Buchgesellschaft, 1964).

Rummel, Erika, *The Confessionalization of Humanism in Reformation Germany* (Oxford, etc.: Oxford University Press, 2000).

Sallaberger, Johann, *Kardinal Matthäus Lang von Wellenburg (1468–1540)* (Salzburg, etc.: Anton Pustet, 1997).

Schantz, Douglas H., *Crautwald and Erasmus. A Study in Humanism and Radical Reform in Sixteenth Century Silesia* (Baden-Baden: Valentin Koerner, 1992).

Schäufele, Wolfgang, *Die missionarische Bewußtsein und Wirken der Täufer* (Neukirchen-Vluyn: Neukirchener Verlag, 1966).

Schmidt, Heinrich Richard, André Holenstein and Andreas Würgler (eds), *Gemeinde, Reformation und Widerstand. Festschrift für Peter Blickle zum 60. Geburtstag* (Tübingen: Bibliotheca Academica Verlag, 1998).

Schmitt, Charles B. et al., *The Cambridge History of Renaissance Philosophy* (Cambridge: Cambridge University Press, 1988).

Schoeps, Hans-Joachim, *Vom himmlischen Fleisch Christi. Eine dogmengeschichtliche Untersuchung* (Tübingen: J.C.B. Mohr (Paul Siebeck), 1951).

Schott, Heinz, 'Invisible Diseases – Imagination and Magnetism: Paracelsus and the Consequences', in Grell, *Paracelsus*, 309–22.

Schulze, Manfred, '*Onus ecclesiae*: Last der Kirche – Reformation der Kirche', in Dykema and Oberman, *Anticlericalism*, 318–42.

Schütze, Ingo, 'Zur Ficino-Rezeption bei Paracelsus', in Telle, *Parerga Paracelsica*, 39–44.

Schwarz, Reinhard, *Die apokalyptische Theologie Thomas Müntzers und die Taboriten* (Tübingen: J.C.B. Mohr (Paul Siebeck), 1977).

Schwitalla, Johannes, *Deutsche Flugschriften 1460–1525. Textsortengeschichtliche Studien* (Reihe Germanistische Linguistik, 45), (Tübingen: M. Niemeyer, 1983).

Scott, Tom, 'The Reformation and Modern Political Economy: Luther and Gaismair Compared', in Brady and Müller-Luckner, *Die deutsche Reformation*, 173–202.

Scribner, Robert W., *Popular Culture and Popular Movements in Reformation Germany* (London: Ronceverte, 1987).

—— *For the Sake of Simple Folk. Popular Propaganda for the German Reformation*, 2nd edn (Oxford: Clarendon Press, 1994).

Seebaß Gottfried, *Das reformatorische Werk des Andreas Osiander* (Nuremberg: Vereins für Bayerischen Kirchengeschichte, 1967).

—— '*An sint persequendi haeretici*: Die Stellung des Johannes Brenz und Bestrafung der Täufer', *Blätter für württembergische Kirchengeschichte*, 70 (1970), 40–99.

—— 'Das Zeichen der Erwählten: Zum Verständnis der Taufe bei Hans Hut', in Goertz, *Umstrittenes Täufertum*, 138–64.

—— *Artikelbrief, Bundesordnung und Verfassungsentwurf. Studien zu drei zentralen Dokumenten des südwestdeutschen Bauernkrieges* (Heidelberg: Carl Winter, 1988).

—— *Müntzers Erbe. Werk, Leben und Theologie des Hans Hut* (Gütersloh: Gütersloher Verlagshaus Gerd Mohn, 2002).

Seifert, Arno, 'Reformation und Chiliasmus: Die Role des Martin Cellarius (Borrhaus)', *Archiv für Reformationsgeschichte*, 77 (1986), 226–64.

Seufert, Gerald H. (ed.), *Die Wittenbergisch Nachtigall. Spruchgedicht, vier Reformationsdialoge und das Meisterlied 'Das Walt Got'* (Stuttgart: Philipp Reclam, 1974).

Sider, Ronald J., *Andreas Bodenstein von Karlstadt. The Development of his Thought 1517–1525* (Leiden: Brill, 1974).

Slattery, Sarah, 'Astrologie, Wunderzeichen und Propaganda. Die Flugschriften des Humanisten Joseph Grünpeck', in Bergdolt and Ludwig, *Zukunftsvoraussagen in der Renaissance*, 329–48.

Snyder, C. Arnold, *Anabaptist History and Theology: An Introduction* (Kitchener, Ontario: Pandora Press, 1995).

Snyder, C. Arnold (ed.), *Sources of South German/Austrian Anabaptism*, trans. Walter Klaassen, Frank Friesen and Werner O. Packull (Kitchener, Ontario: Pandora Press/ Herald Press, 2001).

Sondheim, Moriz, *Thomas Murner als Astrolog* (Strasbourg: Elsass-Lothringische Wissenschaftliche Gesellschaft, 1938).

Spörl, J., 'Das Alte und das Neue im Mittelalter', *Historisches Jahrbuch*, 50 (1930), 297–341, 498–542.

Stafford, William S., *Domesticating the Clergy. The Inception of the Reformation in Strasbourg 1522–1524* (Missoula, MT: Scholars Press, 1976).

Stauber, Reinhard, 'Hartmann Schedel, der Nürnberger Humanistenkreis und die "Erwieterung der deutschen Nation"', in Johannes Helmrath, Ulrich Muhlack and Gerrit Walther (eds), *Diffusion des Humanismus. Studien zur nationalen Geschichtsschreibung europäischer Humanisten* (Göttingen: Walstein Verlag, 2002), 159–85.

Stayer, James M., *Anabaptists and the Sword* (Lawrence, KS: Coronada Press, 1972).

—— 'Die Anfänge der schweizerischen Täufertums im reformierte Kongregationalismus', in Goertz, *Umstrittenes Täufertum*, 19–49.

—— *The German Peasants' War and Anabaptist Community of Goods* (Montreal, etc.: McGill-Queen's University Press, 1991).

—— 'The Radical Reformation', in Brady, Oberman, and Tracy, *Handbook of European History*, vol. 2, 249–82.

—— Werner O. Packull and Klaus Deppermann, 'From Monogenesis to Polygenesis: The Historical Discussion of Anabaptist Origins', *Mennonite Quarterly Review*, 49 (1975), 83–121.

Steer, Georg, Loris Sturlese and Dagmar Gottschall (eds), *Lectura Eckhardi I* (Stuttgart, etc.: W. Kohlhammer, 1998).

Steinmetz, David C., 'The Baptism of John the Baptist and the Baptism of Jesus in Huldrych Zwingli, Balthasar Hubmaier and late Medieval Theology', in F. Forrester Church and Timothy George, *Continuity and Discontinuity in Church History. Essays presented to George Hunston Williams on the Occasion of his 65th Birthday* (Leiden: Brill, 1979), 169–81.

Stephens, W.P., *The Theology of Huldrych Zwingli* (Oxford: Clarendon Press, 1986).

Strauss, Gerald, *Law, Resistance, and the State. The Opposition to Roman Law in Reformation Germany* (Princeton, NJ: Princeton University Press, 1986).

Strübind, Andrea, *Eifriger als Zwingli. Die frühe Täuferbewegung in der Schweiz* (Berlin: Duncker & Humblot, 2001).

Struve, Tilman, 'Utopie und gesellschaftliche Wirklichkeit: zur Bedeutung des Friedenskaisers im späten Mittelalter', *Historische Zeitschrift*, 225 (1977), 65–95.

Talkenberger, Heike, *Sintflut: Prophetie und Zeitgeschehen in Texten und Holzschnitten astrologischer Flugschriften 1488–1528* (Tübingen: Niemeyer, 1990).

Telle, Joachim, 'Wolfgang Talhauser. Zu Leben und Werk eines Augsburger Stadtarztes und seinen Beziehungen zu Paracelsus und Schwenckfeld', *Medizinhistorisches Journal*, 7 (1972), 1–30.

—— 'Wissenschaft und Öffentlichkeit im Spiegel der deutschen Arzneibuchliteratur. Zum deutsch-lateinischen Sprachenstreit in der Medizin des 16. und 17. Jahrhunderts', *Medizinhistorisches Journal*, 14 (1979), 35–52.

—— 'Paracelsus als Alchemiker', in Dopsch and Kramml, *Paracelsus und Salzburg*, 157–72.

—— (ed.) *Pharmazie und der gemeine Mann. Hausarznei und Apotheke in deutschen Schriften der frühen Neuzeit* (Ausstellungskataloge der Herzog August Bibliothek, 36) (Wolfenbüttel: Herzog August Bibl. 1982); 2nd edn (Weinheim, etc.: VCH Verlaggesellschaft, 1988).

—— (ed.), *Parerga Paracelsica. Paracelsus in Vergangenheit und Gegenwart* (Heidelberger Studien zur Naturkunde der frühen Neuzeit, 3) (Stuttgart: Franz Steiner Verlag, 1991).

—— (ed.), *Analecta Paracelsica. Studien zum Nachleben Theophrast von Hohenheims im deutschen Kulturgebiet der frühen Neuzeit* (Heidelberger Studien zur Naturkunde der frühen Neuzeit, 4) (Stuttgart: Franz Steiner Verlag, 1994).

Temkin, Owsei, *The Falling Sickness. A History of Epilepsy from the Greeks to the Beginnings of Modern Neurology* (Baltimore, MD: Johns Hopkins University Press, 1971).

Tentler, Thomas N., *Sin and Confession on the Eve of the Reformation* (Princeton, NJ: Princeton University Press, 1977).

Todt, Sabine, *Kleruskritik, Frömmigkeit und Kommunikation in Worms im Mittelalter und in der Reformationszeit* (Stuttgart: Franz Steiner Verlag, 2005).

Töpfer, Bernhard, *Das kommende Reich des Friedens: Zur Entwicklung chiliastischer Zukunftshoffnungen im Hochmittelalter* (Berlin: Akademie-Verlag, 1964).

Tyson, Gerald P. and Sylvia S. Wagonheim (eds), *Print and Culture in the Renaissance. Essays on the Advent of Printing in Europe* (Newark, DE, etc.: University of Delaware Press, etc., 1986).

Ukena, Peter (ed.), *Ulrich von Hutten, Deutsche Schriften* (Munich: Winkler Verlag, 1970).

Vetter, Ferdinand (ed.), *Die Predigten Taulers* (Deutsche Texte des Mittelalters, 11), (Berlin: Weidmann, 1910).

Vögeli, Alfred (ed.), *Jörg Vögeli. Schriften zur Reformation in Konstanz 1519–1538*, 3 vols (Tübingen: Osianderische Buchhandlung, 1972–73).

Vogler, Günter, *Thomas Müntzer* (Berlin: Dietz Verlag, 1989).

Wagner, Andreas, 'Das Falsche der Religionen bei Sebastian Franck. Zur gesells-
chaftlichen Bedeutung des Spiritualismus der radikalen Reformation', doctoral
dissertation, Freien Universität Berlin, 2007.
Webster, Charles, 'Conrad Gessner and the Infidelity of Paracelsus', in Sarah Hutton
and John Henry (eds), *New Perspectives on Renaissance Thought: Essays ... in
Memory of Charles B. Schmitt* (London: Duckworth, 1990), 13–23.
—— *From Paracelsus to Newton. Magic and the Making of Modern Science* (Cambridge:
Cambridge University Press, 1982).
—— 'Paracelsus and Demons: Science as a Synthesis of Popular Belief', in Zambelli,
Scienze Credenze Occulte Livelli di Cultura, 3–20.
—— 'A Portrait of Paracelsus', in K. Bayertz and R. Porter (eds), *From Physico-
Theology to Bio-Technology: Essays in the Social and Cultural History of Biosciences: A
Festschrift for Mikulás Teich* (Clio Medica, 48) (Amsterdam: Rodopi, 1998), 54–75.
—— 'Paracelsus: Medicine as Popular Protest', in O.P. Grell and A. Cunningham (eds),
Medicine and the Reformation (London: Routledge, 1993), 57–77.
Weeks, Andrew, *Paracelsus. Speculative Theory and the Crisis of the Early Reformation*
(New York: State University of New York Press, 1997).
Weigelt, Horst, *Sebastian Franck und die lutherische Reformation* (Gütersloh: Gütersloher
Verlagshaus Gerd Mohn, 1972).
—— *Spiritualistische Tradition im Protestantismus. Die Geschichte des Schwenckfeldertums
in Schlesien* (Berlin, etc.: De Gruyter, 1973).
Weiß, Bardo, *Die deutschen Mystikerinnen und ihr Gottesbild*, 3 vols (Paderborn:
Ferdinand Schöningh, 2004).
Williams, George H., *The Radical Reformation* (London: Weidenfeld & Nicolson,
1962).
Williams, Gerhild Scholz and Charles D. Gunnoe Jr. (eds), *Paracelsian Moments.
Medicine and Astrology in Early Modern Europe* (Kirksville, MO: Truman State
University Press, 2002).
Windhorst, Christof, *Täuferisches Taufverständnis. Balthasar Hubmaiers Lehre zwischen
traditioneller und reformatorischer Theologie* (Studies in Medieval and Reformation
Thought, 16) (Leiden: Brill, 1976).
Wiswedel, Wilhelm, 'Die alten Täufergemeinden und ihr missionarisches Wirken',
Archiv für Reformationsgeschichte, 40 (1943), 183–200; 41 (1948), 115–32.
Wollgast, Siegfried, *Der deutsche Pantheismus im 16. Jahrhundert* (Berlin: VEB
Deutscher Verlag der Wissenschaften, 1972).
Wuttke, Dieter, 'Humanismus als integrative Kraft. Die Philosophia des deutschen
"Erzhumanisten" Conrad Celtis. Eine ikonologische Studie zu programmatischer
Graphik Dürers und Burgkmairs', *Artibus et Historiae*, 6 (1985), 65–99.
Wyser, Paul, 'Taulers Terminologie von Seelengrund', in Ruh, *Altdeutsche und altnieder-
ländische Mystik*, 324–52.
Zambelli, Paola (ed.), *Scienze credenze occulte livelli di cultura* (Florence: Olschki, 1982).
—— (ed.), *'Astrologi hallucinati'. Stars and the End of the World in Luther's Time* (Berlin:
De Gruyter, 1986).
Zorzin, Alejandro, *Karlstadt als Flugschriftenautor* (Göttingen: Vandenhoeck &
Ruprecht, 1990).
Zschoch, Hellmut, *Reformatorische Existenz und konfessionelle Identität. Urbanus Rhegius
als evangelischer Theologe in den Jahren 1520 bis 1530* (Tübingen: J.C.B. Mohr (Paul
Siebeck), 1995).

INDEX

peripatetic existence, 10–19, 36, 51–2, 58, 73–4, 172–6, 184, 254; portrait by AH, 18, 21, 273, 276; posthumous reputation, 1–2, 34–6, 62–5, 170, 244, 258; professional antagonists, 10–24, 36, 58, 247, 255, 259; prudence, 3, 11–12, 16, 27, 32–3, 97, 121, 175, 199, 225–6, 229; therapeutic practices, 52, 10–18, 29, 55–6, 247, 256, 261. See also Medical/ natural philosophical reformism of; Radical reformism of

Writings: and aspirations 7, 27, 34–6, 42–3, 50–8, 102–5, 176–7, 247–8, 251; astrological and prophetic, 15, 35, 62, 225–43; biblical commentaries, 35, 71, 76, 266; editors and editions, 1, 17–19, 34–7, 44, 62–4, 72–3, 204, 244–5, 248, 264, 290–1, 297, 298; Marian essays, 70–2, 200–1, 291; medical and scientific, 24–6, 50–8; religious, ethical and social, 27, 35, 50–1, 70–2, 176; *vita beata* sequence, 97.

Works cited in text: *Archidoxis*, 139; *Astronomia Magna*, 17–18, 62, 65, 67, 243; *Auslegung des cometen*, 35, 258, 260; *Auslegung der papstbilder*, 260, 288; *Bertheonea*, 104–5, 107–9; *De caduco matrices*, 103; *De causis morborum invisibilium*, 110, 165, 185–6; Commandments, commentary, 32–3, 258; *Elf tractat*, 140–1; *Erklärung der ganzen astronomie*, 67; *Von der franzö sischen krankheit*, 41, 260; *De genealogia Christi*, 30, 32, 139; *De gradibus, compositionibus*, 36; *Grosse Wundarznei*, 1, 15–16, 36, 227–8, 288; *Herbarius*, 49–50, 139, 141; *Intimatio*, 13, 35, 258; *De invocatione beatae Mariae*, 67; *Kärntner Schriften*, 17–18, 65; *Labyrinthus errantium medicorum*, 60–2, 110, 126–7; *Liber principiorum*, 111; *De martyrio Christi*, 32; Matthew commentaries, 70, 76, 92, 121, 265; *De natura rerum*, 240, 299; *Von den natürlichen dingen*, 141–2; *Opus paramirum*, 16, 41–2, 139, 165; *Paragranum*, 25–6, 105–8; *Practica gemach auff Europen*, 67, 225–6,

297; *Prognostikation* (1536), 70, 228, 234, 236–7, 260, 294–5, 297; *Prologus in vitam beatam*, 56, 92, 236; Psalms commentary, 71, 206–7; *De sacramento corporis Christi*, 41; *De secretis secretorum theologiae*, 240; *Septem punctis*, 18, 32, 71–92, 174–6, 179, 186–9, 200; *Sieben defensiones*, 60–1; *Volumen paramirum*, 113, 140; *Vorredt über die vier Evangelisten*, 32
Paracelsianism, 34–6, 132, 255
Patience, 31–2 53, 96–7, 129, 183, 218, 223, 231, 234
Patriarchs of Israel, 116–17, 122, 124–5, 159, 167, 242–3, 275
Patristic authorities, 79, 94, 201, 289
Peasantry, 11, 23, 51–2, 105–7, 174, 178, 181, 220–3, 231, 262, 272
Penance, sacrament of, 77, 87–90
Pentecost, 222–3
Petrarca-Meister, 260, 263, 280
Petrarch, 44, 260
Peypus, Friedrich, 225, 264
Pharisees, Sadducees, Scribes, Levites, 87, 91, 103–4, 106, 118, 124, 126, 189, 193, 198, 207, 218, 224
Philipp I, Markgraf von Baden, 11–12
Pico della Mirandola, Giovanni, 47, 66, 99, 110, 112, 132, 147–8, 158–9, 235, 250, 278, 280, 282, 296
Pietro d'Argellata, 114
Pilgrim ideal, 28–9, 92, 109, 179–80, 182–3, 198, 217, 237, 239, 251, 257, 287
Pilgrimage, relics, 12, 78–9, 86, 160–2
Plague, 152, 161–5, 213, 281, 287
Plato, 113, 116, 194, 270
Plentitude, 144–5, 165
Pliny (Gaius Plinius Secundus), 42, 148
Poetry, 25, 44, 97, 116–17, 121
Poison, in disease theory, 138–40, 147, 149–50, 152, 156, 160, 163–4, 281
Poor, the, poverty, 6, 21, 28, 84–7, 90, 92, 96–7, 103, 117–18, 124–5, 172, 180, 182–3, 189, 198, 200, 218, 230–3, 237, 239, 245–6, 255, 269, 284, 287
Posturing, prostration, scouging, 77–8, 267–8
Potentia dei absoluta/ordinata, 213, 229, 294